Medical Terminology *Express*

A Short-Course Approach by Body System

Barbara A. Gylys *(GĬL-ĭs)*, BS, MEd, CMA-A (AAMA)
Professor Emerita
College of Health and Human Service
Coordinator of Medical Assisting Technology
University of Toledo
Toledo, Ohio

Regina M. Masters, BSN, RN, CMA (AAMA), MEd
Director of Medical Education
Olympic Consulting Group, Ltd., Toledo, Ohio
Psychiatric Nursing Services, Flower Hospital
Sylvania, Ohio

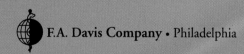

F.A. Davis Company • Philadelphia

F. A. Davis Company
1915 Arch Street
Philadelphia, PA 19103
www.fadavis.com

Printed in the United States of America

Last digit indicates print number: 10 9 8 7 6 5 4 3 2 1

Acquisitions Editor: Quincy McDonald
Manager of Content Development: George W. Lang
Developmental Editor: Brenna H. Mayer
Art and Design Manager: Carolyn O'Brien

As new scientific information becomes available through basic and clinical research, recommended treatments and drug therapies undergo changes. The author(s) and publisher have done everything possible to make this book accurate, up to date, and in accord with accepted standards at the time of publication. The author(s), editors, and publisher are not responsible for errors or omissions or for consequences from application of the book, and make no warranty, expressed or implied, in regard to the contents of the book. Any practice described in this book should be applied by the reader in accordance with professional standards of care used in regard to the unique circumstances that may apply in each situation. The reader is advised always to check product information (package inserts) for changes and new information regarding dose and contraindications before administering any drug. Caution is especially urged when using new or infrequently ordered drugs.

Library of Congress Cataloging-in-Publication Data

Gylys, Barbara A.
   Medical terminology express : a short-course approach by body system/Barbara A. Gylys, Regina M. Masters.
     p. ; cm.
   ISBN 978-0-8036-2388-0
1. Medicine--Terminology--Textbooks. I. Masters, Regina M., 1959 II. Title.
   [DNLM: 1. Terminology as Topic-Problems and Exercises. W15]
R123.G934 2011
610.1'4--dc2010

                                                      2010031790

This Book is Dedicated with Love

to my best friend, colleague, and husband, Julius A. Gylys
and
to my children, Regina Maria and Julius A., II
and
to Andrew Masters, Julia Masters, Caitlin Masters,
Michelle Bishop-Gylys, Anthony Bishop-Gylys, and Matthew Bishop-Gylys

−Barbara Gylys

to my mother, best friend, mentor, and co-author, Barbara A. Gylys
and
to my father, Julius A. Gylys
and
to my husband, Bruce Masters, and my children Andrew, Julia, and Caitlin,
all of whom have given me continuous encouragement and support

−Regina Masters

Acknowledgments

We wish to acknowledge the valuable contributions of F.A. Davis's editorial and production team who were responsible for this project:

- Quincy McDonald, Senior Acquisitions Editor, calmly guided the manuscript through the developmental and production phases of the process and helped ensure its excellence.
- Andy McPhee, Senior Acquisitions Editor, provided the overall design and layout. In addition, he was instrumental in assisting the authors in designing a wide variety of state-of-the-art pedagogical tools within the text and other supplemental materials.
- George W. Lang, Manager of Content Development, oversaw the entire production phase of the book and Activity Pack.
- Brenna H. Mayer, Developmental Editor, systematically and meticulously read the manuscript, helping it along at every stage. Her patience, creativity, and untiring assistance and support during this project are greatly appreciated, and the authors are grateful for all of her help.
- Margaret Biblis, Publisher, once again provided her support and efforts to this project.

We also acknowledge and thank our exceptionally dedicated publishing partners who helped guide and shape this large project:

- Stephanie A. Rukowicz, Departmental Assistant
- Robert Butler, Production Manager
- Yvonne N. Gillam, Developmental Editor
- Kate Margeson, Illustrations Coordinator
- Frank Musick, Developmental Editor, Electronic Publishing
- Carolyn O'Brien, Art and Design Manager
- David Orzechowski, Managing Editor
- Kirk Pedrick, Electronic Product Development Manager, Electronic Publishing
- Elizabeth Y. Stepchin, Developmental Associate.

We also we extend our sincerest gratitude to Neil Kelly, Director of Sales, and his staff of sales representatives, whose continued efforts will undoubtedly contribute to the success of this textbook.

Preface

Medical Terminology Express has evolved due to the growing demand for a straightforward, easy-to-understand short-course textbook. The book is written in an engaging, nontechnical language that relates to students of all backgrounds and levels of education and is designed as an uncomplicated passageway to learning the language of medicine. No natural science background is needed to absorb the information in the textbook. Keeping in mind that the needs of students from various educational environments differ, this text and its ancillary products are designed for use in colleges, universities, career schools, online courses, and other educational environments that offer a medical terminology course.

Although *Medical Terminology Express* has a unique approach that differs from any other medical terminology books we have authored, it still includes the same fundamental concepts of learning medical terminology, primarily by applying the principles of medical word building. The textbook and its complementary ancillary products are designed as competency-based instruments. They enable students to evaluate their understanding of medical terminology based on guidelines required by the major allied health accrediting agencies. The word-building and competency-based approaches are always evident in the educational materials we have published. Because this system of learning medical terminology has been so effective in numerous teaching environments and widely well received by educators and students, we continue to utilize the word-building and competency-based approaches in the textbooks and ancillary products we author. We have personally witnessed the success of these educational configurations during our many years of teaching medical terminology.

Various types of learning reinforcements are found throughout the *Medical Terminology Express* textbook and supplemental teaching aids available to students and instructors. The Activity Pack, Instructor's Resources, and DavisPlus website contain activities to supplement material covered in the textbook. All of them include testing tools to reinforce anatomy and physiology content. For those who require anatomy and physiology coverage, two anatomy and physiology activities, Anatomy Focus and Tag the Elements, are included for the 12 body-system chapters in the *Term-Plus* software packaged with some versions of the book. Nevertheless, the textbook emphasizes the understanding of the meaning of basic medical terms and demonstrates how the terms are used in the health care environment. The ability to communicate in the language of medicine provides students with additional confidence to become effective members of the health care team.

Textbook Overview

Each chapter begins with a set of objectives that outline the goals the student should be able to achieve upon completion of that chapter. By completing the reinforcing activities throughout the chapter, the student should be able to achieve the objectives in a structured manner.

Chapters 1 and 2. The first chapter is an **introduction to medical word building** followed by Chapter 2, which presents an **orientation to the body as a whole**. Knowledge of the descriptive terms introduced in Chapter 2 is an essential part of medical terminology and provides a basic foundation for a better understanding of the body-system chapters that follow. Most importantly, the descriptive terms are included in the language of medicine used by health care providers in the clinical environment.

Chapters 3 to 13. These chapters **introduce medical terminology related to a specific body system.** Each body-system chapter is arranged in the following sequence:

- The **Vocabulary Preview** includes terms, pronunciations, and meanings of medical words especially relevant to that chapter's body system so the student can easily understand the material presented in the chapter.
- The preview is followed by a description of the **Medical Specialty** or specialties related to the body system or systems covered in the chapter.
- The body system **Quick Study** presents a summary of the organs and functions of the specific body system covered in the chapter.
- The **Medical Word Building** tables introduce combining forms, suffixes, and prefixes related to the body system covered in the chapter. Each section on combining forms also includes an anatomical illustration of that system with combining forms listed for important structures. These tables also include learning activities that reinforce the word elements introduced.
- The **Additional Medical Vocabulary** section contains terms related to common signs, symptoms, diseases, and diagnoses; diagnostic, medical, and surgical procedures; and pharmacological agents used to treat diseases of the relevant body system. This section also presents dynamic illustrations that visually reinforce the disease or the medical or diagnostic procedure discussed.
- The **Closer Look** section presents extra information and reinforces key pathologies and medical procedures with dynamic illustrations related to the terminology covered in the given chapter.
- The **Chart Notes** section include chart note related to a medical specialty associated with the relevant body system to reinforce terminology covered in the chapter. The chart note is followed by an analysis exercise with an answer key to verify competency.
- At the end of key sections, an icon guides the student to **Multimedia Resources** that will enhance the study of these medical words. These powerful enhancements are packed with activities to ease the student's task of becoming proficient in the language of medicine. Three multimedia reinforcements are available:
  - the **Audio CD** packaged with this textbook, which offers *Listen and Learn* activities so the student can hear as well as read the medical terms reviewed in the chapter
  - the **DavisPlus** website *(http://davisplus.fadavis.com/gylys-express)*, which offers additional activities to accelerate retention.
  - *TermPlus* interactive software program (packaged with some versions), which enables students to monitor their progress in their study of medical terminology as well as record and send test scores via e-mail to their instructors.
- **Review exercises** are included throughout the text after each relevant section to provide instant review of the material learned. These exercises include **Medical Terminology Word Building, Additional Medical Vocabulary Recall,** and **Pronunciation and Spelling.** The **Demonstrate What You Know** review concludes each body-system chapter and provides a self-study check to determine retention level of material presented in the chapter. Each review section includes competency verifications with answer keys to help the student meet course requirements.

• Lastly, to improve your retention level of the chapter, a multimedia icon guides you to the DavisPlus site linked to the given chapter for additional reinforcement activities.

Appendices

Several appendices supplement the material in the chapters with additional information that aids in the learning process or provides information essential to meeting course requirements. Appendices include:

- **Appendix A: Glossary of Medical Word Elements,** a summary of word elements presented in the textbook as well as additional word elements the student may encounter in medical reports or discussions in the field of medicine
- **Appendix B: Answer Key,** which contains all of the answers for the activities in the textbook
- **Appendix C: Abbreviations and Symbols,** a summary of all the abbreviations with meanings presented in the textbook and additional abbreviations and symbols used in health care environments
- **Appendix D: Drug Classifications,** which provides a quick reference of common drug categories, including prescription and over-the-counter drugs used to treat signs, symptoms, and diseases of each body system
- **Appendix E: Medical Specialties,** a summary of medical specialties along with brief descriptions
- **Appendix F: Index of Diagnostic, Medical, and Surgical Procedures,** which provides a list of the diagnostic, medical, and surgical procedures covered in the textbook along with page numbers
- **Appendix G: Oncological Terms,** which provides a summary of oncology terms covered in the textbook along with page numbers.

Comprehensive Teaching and Learning Package

Medical Terminology Express: A Short-Course Approach by Body System is packaged with a selection of ancillary materials to benefit instructors and students. The rich array of teaching aids are available free of charge to instructors who adopt the textbook and students who purchase the textbook. The teaching aids contain considerable information and activities to reinforce, supplement, and enhance course content. The comprehensive teaching and learning package ensures students a program of excellence in a medical terminology curriculum. The ancillary products also help instructors plan course work and provide a rich array of presentations to reinforce the learning process. These teaching aids include the Instructor's Resources; DavisPlus, a web-based resource; an Audio CD, and *TermPlus,* an interactive CD-ROM available with some packages.

Instructor's Resources

The Instructor's Resources are a hearty collection of supplemental teaching aids for instructors to plan course work and enhance their presentations. It is also designed to help students learn the language of medicine commonly used in clinical environments. Instructors can easily implement the teaching tools in various educational settings, including the traditional classroom, distance learning, or independent studies. When instructors integrate the ancillary products into course content, they will help provide a sound foundation for students to develop an extensive medical vocabulary. In addition, its use guarantees a full program of excellence for students of all aptitudes, no matter what educational background they have. Access to the Instructor's Resources on DavisPlus will be provided to adopting instructors once they have filled out a short registration at the text's website at http://davisplus.fadavis.com/gylys-express. The Instructor's Resources include:

- **Activity Pack**
- **PowerPoint presentations,** including Lecture Notes with interactive exercises, and Name that Part, a body systems review
- **Image bank** with easily retrievable images of anatomical structures, pathological conditions, and diagnostic and therapeutic procedures
- **ExamView Pro computerized test bank,** a powerful, user-friendly test-generation program.

Activity Pack: Your Instructional Resource Kit

The Activity Pack is a resource full of instructional support for using the textbook and ancillary products. It is available in PDF format on the Instructor's Resources. In addition, instructors who wish to custom tailor the material can request the Activity Pack in a Microsoft Word document. The *Medical Terminology Express* Activity Pack includes:

- **Course Outlines.** Suggested course outlines help you determine a comfortable pace and plan the best method of covering the material presented in the textbook. It contains course outlines for a 10-week and a 15-week course. It also includes course outlines for textbooks packaged with *TermPlus* software.
- **Student- and Instructor-Directed Activities.** These activities offer a variety of activities for each body-system chapter. Activities can serve as course requirements or supplemental material. In addition, the instructor can assign them as individual or collaborative projects. For group projects, Peer Evaluation Forms are provided.
- **Anatomy questions.** Anatomical structures from each body-system chapter are provided to review or use as test questions. An answer key is also included.
- **Able to Label.** This testing device labels and reinforces the combining forms associated with the structures in each body-system chapter.
- **Supplemental Chart Notes and Analysis.** These exercises are provided for each body-system chapter. The notes are related to the medical specialty that reinforces terminology covered in the chapter.
- **Clinical Connection Activities.** These activities integrate clinical scenarios in each chapter as a solid reinforcement of content. Instructors can feel free to select activities they deem suitable for their course and decide whether the students should complete the activity independently, with peers, or as a group project.
- **Oral and Written Research Projects.** The research projects provide an opportunity for students to hone their research skills. The Community and Internet Resources section offers an updated list of technical journals, community organizations, and Internet sources that students can use to complete the oral and written projects. This section also contains a peer evaluation template for the oral and written research projects. These projects will add variety and interest to the course while reinforcing the learning process.
- **Pronunciation, Spelling, and Transcription Activity Template.** This template is designed to help evaluate student competency in pronunciation, spelling, and meaning of medical terms. It can also serve as an introduction to transcription skills.

- **Crossword Puzzles.** These fun, educational activities reinforce material covered in each body-system chapter. Instructors can use them for an individual or group activity, an extra credit opportunity, or just for fun. An answer key is included for each puzzle.
- **Anatomy Coloring Activities.** These activities are included for each body-system chapter to reinforce the positions of the main organs that compose a particular body system.
- **Chart Note Terminology Answer Keys.** This section contains the answers to the Terminology tables in the Chart Notes sections of the textbook. It provides instructional support in using the textbook and assists instructors in correcting the terminology assignments.

PowerPoint Presentations

Two PowerPoint presentations are included with this edition:

- **Name that Part** is a unique interactive PowerPoint presentation that allows you to guide students in identifying specific structures of a body system.
- **Lecture Notes with Interactive Exercises** include full-color illustrations from the textbook, followed by questions and answers relevant to the topic being discussed. This method helps reinforce the functions of each body system, the clinical application of medical terms, and the medical word-building system. Instructors can zoom in to enlarge images and test students' knowledge as they lead discussion of the content. In addition, links to other resources such as the Image Bank and Animations are summarized in notes so instructors are able to swap or add an illustration as well as present a reinforcing animation or assign it for students to view on the Student Resource section of the DavisPlus website. All Lecture Notes presentations related to a given chapter share a uniform structure:
  - *main structures and functions* of the body system with an interactive exercise
  - some of the *primary signs, symptoms, and diseases* of the body system with an interactive clinically related exercise
  - *common diagnostic procedures* used to evaluate pathological conditions of the various structures of the body system with an interactive word-building exercise
  - *common medical and surgical procedures* used to treat pathological conditions of the various structures of the given body system with an interactive clinically related exercise.
  - *common medications* prescribed for treatment of disorders of the body system discussed and includes an interactive clinically related exercise

Image Bank

Included in this edition is an Adobe Flash–based image bank that contains all illustrations from the textbook. It is fully searchable and allows users to zoom in and out and display a JPG image of an illustration that can be copied into a Microsoft Word document or PowerPoint presentation.

ExamView Pro Electronic Test Bank

This edition offers a powerful test-generating program called *ExamView Pro*. This program enables the instructor to create custom or randomly generated tests in a printable format from a test bank of more than 625 test items. The test bank includes multiple-choice, true-false, and matching questions. Because of the flexibility of the ExamView Pro test-generating program, instructors can edit questions in the test bank to meet their specific educational needs. Therefore, if instructors wish to restate, embellish, or streamline questions or change distractors, they can do so with little effort. They can also add questions to the test bank.

DavisPlus Website

The DavisPlus website, found at *http://davisplus.fadavis.com/gylys-express* is a companion study site for *Medical Terminology Express.* It provides activities to accelerate learning and reinforce information presented in each chapter. Special icons found within the chapters tells students when it is most advantageous to integrate the activities on the DavisPlus website into their studies. All online exercises provide instructions for completing the various activities. The multimedia activities available on DavisPlus include student and instructor resources.

Student Resources

- **Chart Notes Activities** for Chapters 3 to 13 allow students to click highlighted terms in the chart note, hear the pronunciation of key terms, and see the correct spelling of those terms.
- **Audio Exercises** are a replication of the audio CD key terms from the Medical Word Building tables. These exercises include spelling, pronunciation, and meaning of key terms and are downloadable to an iPod or MP3 player.
- Nearly 20 **Animations,** such as an exploration of the pathology of gastroesophageal reflux disease (GERD) and the various stages of pregnancy and delivery, are designed to help students better understand complex processes and procedures.
- **Interactive Exercises** include:
  - **flash-card activities** for preview and practice to reinforce word elements presented in the chapter
  - **word search games** that present a variety of medical terms to reinforce word recognition and spelling in a fun activity.

Instructor Resources

- **Lecture Notes PowerPoint presentation** with interactive exercises related to each body system
- **ExamView Pro Electronic Test Bank** with over 625 multiple-choice, short-answer, and vocabulary test items
- **Name that Part PowerPoint presentation**
- **Image Bank**
- **Activity Pack**

Audio CD

One audio CD is included free of charge in each textbook. The audio CD contains *Listen and Learn* exercises designed to strengthen the student's skill in spelling, pronouncing, and defining selected medical terms. They include pronunciation and spelling exercises for Chapters 2 through 13.

Medical secretarial and medical transcription students can also use the CD to learn beginning transcription skills by typing each word as it is pronounced. After typing the words, they can correct spelling by referring to the textbook or a medical dictionary. Finally, to evaluate student competency, a *Pronunciation, Spelling, and Transcription Activity Template* is provided in the Activity Pack on page 83.

TermPlus

TermPlus v3.0 is a powerful, interactive CD-ROM program offered with some texts, depending on which version has been selected. *TermPlus* is a competency-based, self-paced, multimedia program that includes graphics, audio, and a dictionary culled from *Taber's Cyclopedic Medical Dictionary,* 21st edition. Help menus provide navigational support. The software comes with numerous interactive learning activities, including:

- Anatomy Focus
- Tag the Elements (drag-and-drop)
- Spotlight the Elements
- Concentration
- Build Medical Words
- Programmed Learning
- Medical Vocabulary
- Chart Notes
- Spelling
- Crossword Puzzles
- Word Scramble
- Terminology Teaser

All activities can be graded and the results printed or e-mailed to an instructor. This feature makes the CD-ROM especially valuable as a distance-learning tool because it provides evidence of student drill and practice in various learning activities.

We are confident that students will enjoy *Medical Terminology Express* and that they will find learning the language of medicine to be an exciting, rewarding process that will help them succeed in the field of medicine. We welcome instructors and students to send comments and suggestions to F. A. Davis Company, 1915 Arch Street, Philadelphia, PA 19103. This feedback will help us better meet your educational needs in the second edition.

Barbara Gylys
Regina Masters

Reviewers

We greatly appreciate and extend a special thanks to the clinical reviewers and students who read and edited the manuscript and provided suggestions for the first edition of *Medical Terminology Express*. Their feedback undoubtedly helped improve the excellence of the final text and ancillary products.

We thank **Sandy Andreev,** BA, George Washington University, Washington, D.C., for her devotion to excellence which is evident in her meticulous review of the textbook, electronic test bank, and Activity Pack. Her forthright criticisms and helpful suggestions added immeasurably to the quality of the final text.

We are also grateful to **Andrew Masters,** BS, Miami University, Oxford, Ohio, and a graduate student at University of Toledo, Ohio, who worked through the final copy of the textbook and its ancillary products, including TermPlus software and provided invaluable feedback to the authors.

Clinical Reviewers

We express our appreciation to the following reviewers who, through their professionalism and skill, made this text possible and whose talents are reflected in the results.

Dianna Drury, BS, MT(ASCP)
Coordinator of Allied Health Curriculum
Health and Legal Department
El Centro College, Dallas, Texas

Jeanette Goodwin, BSN, CMA
Chair, Medical Assisting Program
Health Occupations Department
Southeast Community College, Lincoln, Nebraska

Jeanne S. Kelleher, MS RT(R)
Chairperson, Medical Imaging Department
Hudson Valley Community College, Troy,
* New York*

Tammy McClish, MEd, CMA, RT(R)(M)(QM)
Faculty
Allied Health Department
University of Akron, Akron, Ohio

Patricia S. Ottavio, PT, MPH
Assistant Dean
PTA Program
Northern Virginia Community College,
* Annandale, Virginia*

Lois Ricci, RNC, GNP, EdD
Education Coordinator
Center for Health in Aging
Department of Medicine
Emory University, Atlanta, Georgia

Janis Schiefelbein, RN, BC, MS, PhD
Associate Professor
Nursing
Pittsburg State University, Pittsburg, Kansas

Marilyn Turner, RN, CMA
Director, Medical Assisting Program
Ogeechee Technical College, Statesboro, Georgia

Kari Williams, BS, DC
Director
Medical Office Technology Program
Boulder County Campus
Front Range Community College, Boulder,
* Colorado*

Chapter Reviewers

The authors also acknowledge the assistance of the following individuals who reviewed the first stages of the manuscript.

Barbara J. Banning, MEd, OTR/L
Occupational Therapy Assistant Program
* Director*
Allied Health and Nursing
Augusta Technical College, Augusta, Georgia

Alice Clegg, MHEd
Lecturer/Advisor
Nursing and Allied Health
Dixie State College of Utah, St. George

Abigail C. Gilgeous Gordon, PT, DPT
Assistant Professor
Physical Therapy
Howard University, Washington, D.C.

Beverly K. Hogan, RN, MSN, APRN, BC
Doctoral Student
Medical Sociology
University of Alabama, Birmingham

Amy L Johns, BA, MM
Coordinator of Instructional Technology; Adjunct
* Instructor*
Moberly Area Community College, Moberly,
* Missouri*

Abigail Mitchell RN, MSN, RN, MSN, DHEd
Professor
Medical Assisting
Niagara County Community College, Sanborn,
* New York*
Graduate Nursing
D'Youville College, Buffalo, New York

Amy Richcreek, MSN, RN
Clinical Coordinator, Clinical Instructor
Nursing
Owens Community College, Toledo, Ohio

I. Christine Sproles, RN, CMT, BSN, MS
College Instructor
Business/Medical Office
Pensacola Christian College, Pensacola, Florida

Annmary E. Thomas, MEd, NREMT-P
Instructor
Allied Health
Community College of Philadelphia,
* Philadelphia, Pennsylvania*

Contents at a Glance

Contents

Appendices

Introduction to Medical Terminology

Objectives

Upon completion of this chapter, you will be able to:

- Identify and define the four elements used to build medical words.
- Apply the basic rules to define and build medical terms.
- Define and provide examples of surgical, diagnostic, pathological, and related suffixes.
- Apply rules learned in this chapter to write singular and plural forms of medical words.
- Practice pronouncing the medical terms presented in this chapter.
- Demonstrate your knowledge by successfully completing the activities in this chapter.

The language of medicine is a specialized vocabulary used by health care practitioners. Many current medical word elements originated as early as the 4th century B.C., when Hippocrates practiced medicine. With technological and scientific advancements in medicine, new terms have evolved to reflect these innovations. For example, radiographic terms, such as magnetic resonance imaging (MRI) and ultrasound (US), are now used to describe current diagnostic procedures.

Medical Word Elements

A medical word consists of some or all of the following elements:

- word root
- combining form
- suffix
- prefix.

How these elements are combined and whether all or some of them are present in a medical term determines the meaning of a word. To understand the meaning of medical words, it is important to learn how to divide them into their basic elements. The purpose of this chapter is to cover the basic principles of medical word building and how to pronounce the terms correctly. Thus, pronunciations are provided with all terms. In addition, pronunciation guidelines are located on the inside front cover of this book so you can refer to it throughout the chapters to help pronounce terms correctly.

Word Roots

A **word root** is the foundation of a medical term and contains its primary meaning. All medical terms have at least one word root. Examine the terms *tonsillitis*, *tonsillectomy*, *colitis*, and *colectomy* listed below to determine their basic elements (roots and suffixes) and meanings. You will note that the meaning of the word changes whenever you change one of the word elements. (In the examples that follow, word roots are in boldface and suffixes are in blue.)

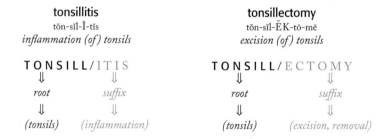

tonsillitis
tŏn-sĭl-Ī-tĭs
inflammation (of) tonsils

tonsillectomy
tŏn-sĭl-ĔK-tō-mē
excision (of) tonsils

TONSILL/ITIS
⇓   ⇓
root   *suffix*
⇓   ⇓
(tonsils)   *(inflammation)*

TONSILL/ECTOMY
⇓   ⇓
root   *suffix*
⇓   ⇓
(tonsils)   *(excision, removal)*

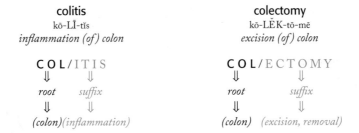

	colitis			colectomy	
	kō-LĬ-tĭs			kō-LĔK-tō-mē	
	inflammation (of) colon			*excision (of) colon*	

C O L / I T I S ⇓ ⇓ *root* *suffix* ⇓ ⇓ *(colon)(inflammation)*

C O L / E C T O M Y ⇓ ⇓ *root* *suffix* ⇓ ⇓ *(colon)* *(excision, removal)*

> **Word Analysis** The roots *tonsill* and *col* indicate body parts, the tonsils and colon, respectively. The suffix *-itis* means *inflammation;* the suffix *-ectomy* means *excision, removal.* By adding a different suffix to the root, the meaning of the word changes, as shown in the above examples.

Combining Forms

A **combining form** is created when a word root is combined with a vowel. The vowel, known as a *combining vowel*, is usually an *o*, but sometimes it is an *i* or *e*. The combining vowel has no meaning of its own but enables two word elements to be connected. Like the word root, the combining form is the basic foundation to which other word elements are added to build a complete medical word. In this text, a combining form will be listed as *word root/vowel* (such as *arthr/o, gastr/o, nephr/o, neur/o,* and *oste/o*), as illustrated in the examples below. The difficulty of pronouncing certain combinations of word roots requires insertion of a vowel. Like the word root, the combining form usually indicates a body part.

Examples of Combining Forms

Word Root	+	Combining Vowel	=	Combining Form	Meaning
arthr	+	o	=	arthr/o	joint
gastr	+	o	=	gastr/o	stomach
nephr	+	o	=	nephr/o	kidney
neur	+	o	=	neur/o	nerve
oste	+	o	=	oste/o	bone

Linking Suffixes

A combining form links with a suffix that begins with a consonant. Examples of suffixes that begin with a consonant are *-centesis* and *-pathy.* This linking is illustrated on the next page in the terms *arthr/o/centesis* and *gastr/o/pathy.*

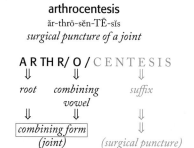

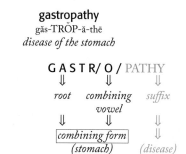

A word root links with a suffix that begins with a vowel. Examples of suffixes that begin with a vowel are *-itis* and *-ectomy*. This linking is illustrated below in the terms *arthr/itis* and *gastr/ectomy*.

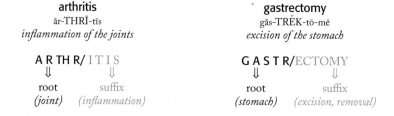

| Word Analysis | The roots *gastr* and *arthr* indicate body parts. The suffix *-itis* means *inflammation*; *-centesis* means *puncture*; *-pathy* means *disease*; and *-ectomy* means *excision, removal*. |

Suffixes

A **suffix** is a word element placed at the end of a word that changes the meaning of the word. In the terms *mast/ectomy* and *mast/itis*, the suffixes are *-ectomy* (excision, removal) and *-itis* (inflammation). Changing the suffix changes the meaning of the word. In medical terminology, a suffix usually describes a pathology (disease or abnormality), symptom, surgical or diagnostic procedure, or part of speech.

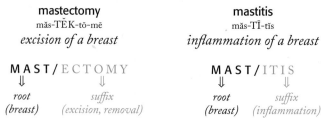

When studying medical terminology, try to learn the combining form rather than the root because the combining form makes most words easier to pronounce. In the example of arthrocentesis, the root without a connecting vowel would be written **arthrcentesis** (ăr-thr-sĕn-TĒ-sĭs). Spelled this way, the term is difficult to pronounce. By adding the vowel after the root, the word **arthrocentesis** (ăr-thrō-sĕn-TĒ-sĭs) is much easier to pronounce.

Word Analysis The root *mast* indicates the body part, the breast. The suffix *-ectomy* means *excision, removal;* the suffix *-itis* means *inflammation.* Adding different suffixes to the root *mast* changes the meaning of the word.

Prefixes

A **prefix** is a word element attached to the beginning of a word or word root. However, not all medical terms have a prefix. Adding or changing a prefix changes the meaning of the word. The prefix usually indicates a number, time, position, direction, or negation. Prefixes do not require adding a connecting vowel. Many prefixes in medical terms are the same as those used in the English language. Consider the following terms.

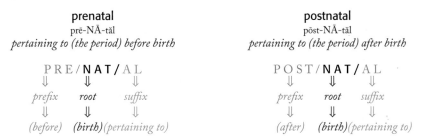

prenatal
prē-NĀ-tăl
pertaining to (the period) before birth

postnatal
pōst-NĀ-tăl
pertaining to (the period) after birth

PRE / **NAT** / AL
prefix   root   suffix
(before) (birth) (pertaining to)

POST / **NAT** / AL
prefix   root   suffix
(after)   (birth) (pertaining to)

Prefixes *pre-* and *post-* indicate a state of time. Both prefixes are attached directly to the word root that follows. In the above examples, *pre-* and *post-* are attached to the root *nat.* In this text, whenever a prefix stands alone, it will be followed by a hyphen, as in *pre-* and *post-.* Whenever a suffix stands alone, it will be preceded by a hyphen, as in *-al.*

Word Analysis The root *nat* means *birth;* the suffix *-al* means *pertaining to.*

Review Activity 1-1
Matching Word Elements

Match the numbered list items with their definitions in the right-hand column.

1. _____ *pre-* means
2. _____ basic components of words
3. _____ combining form
4. _____ combining vowel(s)
5. _____ *post-* means
6. _____ suffix *-itis*
7. _____ *gastr* means

a. foundation of a word, such as *cardi* and *arthr*
b. end of a word
c. beginning of a word
d. word root, suffix, combining form, and prefix
e. stomach
f. inflammation
g. arthr/o

8. _____ location of prefixes   h. "o" and "i"

9. _____ location of suffixes   i. after

10. _____ word root   j. before

Competency Verification: Check your answers in Appendix B, Answer Key, page 349. If you are not satisfied with your level of comprehension, review the terms in the table and retake the review.

Correct Answers: _____ × 10 = _____ % Score

Review Activity 1-2
Understanding Medical Word Elements

Fill in the following blanks to complete the sentences correctly.

1. The four elements used to form medical words are _____

   _____

2. A root is the main part or foundation of a word. In the words *arthritis, arthroma,* and *arthroscope,* the root is _____

Identify the following statements as true or false by circling *True* or *False* for each statement. If false, rewrite the statement correctly on the line provided.

3. A combining vowel is usually an *e*.   True False

   _____

4. A word root links a suffix that begins with a consonant.   True False

   _____

5. A combining vowel links multiple roots to each other.   True False

   _____

6. A combining form links a suffix that begins with a consonant.   True False

   _____

7. Whenever a prefix stands alone, it will be preceded by a hyphen.   True False

   _____

8. In the term *intramuscular, intra-* is the prefix.   True False

   _____

Underline the word root in each of following combining forms.

9. splen/o (spleen)

10. hyster/o (uterus)

11. enter/o (intestine)

12. neur/o (nerve)

13. ot/o (ear)

14. dermat/o (skin)

15. hydr/o (water)

 Competency Verification: Check your answers in Appendix B, Answer Key, page 349. If you are not satisfied with your level of comprehension, review the terms in the table and retake the review.

Correct Answers _____ × 6.67 = _____ **% Score**

Review Activity 1-3
Identifying Word Roots and Combining Forms

Underline the word roots in the following terms.

Medical Word	Meaning
1. nephritis	inflammation of the kidneys
2. arthrodesis	fixation of a joint
3. dermatitis	inflammation of the skin
4. arthrocentesis	surgical puncture of a joint
5. gastrectomy	excision of the stomach

Underline the following elements that are combining forms.

6. nephr	kidney
7. hepat/o	liver
8. arthr	joint
9. oste/o/arthr	bone, joint
10. cholangi/o	bile vessel

 Competency Verification: Check your answers in Appendix B, Answer Key, page 349. If you are not satisfied with your level of comprehension, review the terms in the table and retake the review.

Correct Answers _____ × 10 = _____ **% Score**

Defining and Building Medical Words

Defining and building medical words are crucial skills in mastering medical terminology. Following the basic guidelines will help develop these skills.

Defining Medical Words

Here are three steps for defining medical words using the term *oste/o/arthr/itis* (ŏs-tē-ō-ăr-THRĪ-tĭs) as an example.

1. Define the **suffix**, or last part of the word. In this case, *-itis*, which means *inflammation*.
2. Define the first part of the word (**word root** or **combining form**, or **prefix**). In this case, the combining form *oste/o* means *bone*.
3. Define the middle parts of the word (**word root** or **combining form**). In this case, *arthr* means *joint*. Table 1-1 further illustrates this process.

Table 1-1	**Defining Osteoarthritis**	
This table illustrates the three steps of defining a medical word using the example osteoarthritis.		
Combining Form	**Middle**	**Suffix**
oste/o	arthr	-itis
bone	joint	inflammation
(rule 2)	(rule 3)	(rule 1)

Building Medical Words

There are three rules for building medical words.

Rule #1

A word root links a suffix that begins with a vowel.

Word Root	+	Suffix	=	Medical Word	Meaning
append appendix	+	**-ectomy** excision, removal	=	**append/ectomy** ăp-ĕn-DĔK-tō-mē	excision of the appendix
gastr stomach	+	**-itis** inflammation	=	**gastr/itis** găs-TRĪ-tĭs	inflammation of the stomach

Rule #2

A combining form (root + *o*) links a suffix that begins with a consonant.

Combining Form	+	Suffix	=	Medical Word	Meaning
colon/o colon	+	**-scope** instrument for examining	=	**colon/o/scope** kō-LŎN-ō-skōp	instrument for examining the colon

Rule #3

A combining vowel links a root to another root to form a compound word. This rule holds true even if the next root begins with a vowel, as in *gastroenteritis*. Keep in mind that the rules for linking multiple roots to each other are slightly different from the rules for linking roots and combining forms to suffixes. Below are several examples.

Combining Form	+	Word Root	+	Suffix	=	Medical Word	Meaning
gastr/o stomach	+	**enter** intestine (usually small intestine)	+	**-itis** inflammation	=	**gastr/o/ enter/itis** găs-trō-ĕn-tĕr-Ī-tĭs	inflammation of stomach and intestine (usually small intestine)
		col colon	+	**-itis** inflammation	=	**gastr/o/col/ itis** găs-trō-kō-LĪ-tĭs	inflammation of stomach and colon

Combining Form	+	Word Root	+	Suffix	=	Medical Word	Meaning
oste/o (bone)	+	**chondr** cartilage	+	**-itis** inflammation	=	**osteochon-dritis** ŏs-tē-ō-kŏn-DRĪ-tĭs	inflammation of bone and cartilage
		arthr joint	+	**-itis** inflammation	=	**osteoarthritis** ŏs-tē-ō-ăr-THRĪ-tĭs	inflammation of bone and joint

Review Activity 1-4
Defining Medical Words

Use the following table to complete the statements below. The first one is completed for you.

Combining Forms	Suffixes and Prefixes	Meaning
append/o		*appendix*
arthr/o		*joint*
col/o		*colon*
enter/o		*intestine (usually small)*
gastr/o		*stomach*
mast/o		*breast*
oste/o		*bone*
	–centesis	*surgical puncture*
	–itis	*inflammation*
	–pathy	*disease*
	–scope	*instrument to view or examine*
	pre–	*before*
	post–	*after*

1. Mast/ectomy is an excision of a <u>*breast*</u>_____.

2. Tonsill/itis is an _____ of the tonsils.

3. A colon/o/scope is an instrument to examine the _____.

4. Oste/o/malacia is a softening of a _____ (singular).

5. Post/nat/al means pertaining to (the period) _____ birth.

6. Arthr/o/centesis is a surgical puncture of a _____.

7. Arthr/o/pathy is a _____ of the joints.

8. A prefix that means *before* is _____.

9. The combining form for *stomach* is _____.

10. The suffix for *disease* is _____.

11. The combining form for *breast* is _____.

12. The suffix that means *instrument to examine* is _____.

13. The combining form *append/o* refers to the _____.

14. Gastro/enter/itis is an inflammation of the stomach and the _____.

15. The suffix for *surgical puncture* is _____.

✓ **Competency Verification:** Check your answers in Appendix B, Answer Key, page 349. If you are not satisfied with your level of comprehension, review the terms in the table and retake the review.

Correct Answers _____ × 10 = _____ % Score

Review Activity 1-5
Defining and Building Medical Words

The three steps for defining medical words are:

1. Define the last part of the word, or **suffix.**

2. Define the first part of the word, or **prefix, word root,** or **combining form.**

3. Define the **middle of the word.**

First pronounce the term aloud. Then apply the above three steps to define the terms in the following table. If you are not certain of a definition, refer to Appendix A of this textbook which provides an alphabetical list of word elements and their definitions. The first one is completed for you.

Term	Definition
1. col/itis kō-LĪ-tĭs	*inflammation (of) colon*
2. gastr/o/scope GĂS-trō-skōp	
3. hepat/itis hĕp-ă-TĪ-tĭs	
4. pre/nat/al prē-NĀ-tăl	
5. tonsill/ectomy tŏn-sĭl-ĔK-tō-mē	
6. tonsill/itis tŏn-sĭl-Ī-tĭs	

Refer to the section "Building Medical Words" on page X to complete this activity. Write the number for the rule that applies to each listed term as well as a short summary of the rule. Use the abbreviations *WR* to designate a word root and *CF* to designate *combining form*. The first one is completed for you.

Term	Rule	Summary of the Rule
7. append/ectomy ăp-ĕn-DĔK-tō-mē	*1*	*A WR links a suffix that begins with a vowel.*
8. arthr/o/centesis ăr-thrō-sĕn-TĒ-sĭs		
9. col/ectomy kō-LĔK-tō-mē		
10. colon/o/scope kō-LŎN-ō-skōp		
11. gastr/itis găs-TRĪ-tĭs		
12. gastr/o/enter/o/col/itis găs-trō-ĕn-tĕr-ō-kŏl-Ī-tĭs		
13. arthr/o/pathy ăr-THRŎP-ă-thē		
14. oste/o/arthr/itis ŏs-tē-ō-ăr-THRĪ-tĭs		
15. oste/o/chondr/itis ŏs-tē-ō-kŏn-DRĪ-tĭs		

 Competency Verification: Check your answers in Appendix B, Answer Key, page 350. If you are not satisfied with your level of comprehension, review the terms in the table and retake the review.

Correct Answers _____ × 6.67 = _____ **% Score**

Pronunciation Guidelines

Although pronunciation of medical words usually follows the same rules that govern pronunciation of English words, some medical words may be difficult to pronounce when first encountered. Therefore, selected terms in this book include phonetic pronunciation. Diacritical marks and capitalization are used to aid pronunciation of terms throughout the text and to help understand pronunciation marks used in most dictionaries.

Pronunciation guidelines are located on the inside front cover of this book and at the end of selected tables. Use them whenever help is needed with pronunciation of medical words.

Review Activity 1-6

Understanding Pronunciations

Review the pronunciation guidelines (located inside the front cover of this book) and then underline the correct answer in each of the following statements.

1. The diacritical mark ‾ is called a (breve, macron).

2. The diacritical mark ˇ is called a (breve, macron).

3. The ‾ indicates the (short, long) sound of vowels.

4. The ˇ indicates the (short, long) sound of vowels.

5. The combination *ch* is sometimes pronounced like *(k, chiy)*. Examples are *ch*olesterol, *ch*olemia.

6. When *pn* is at the beginning of a word, it is pronounced only with the sound of *(p, n)*. Examples are *pn*eumonia, *pn*eumotoxin.

7. When *pn* is in middle of a word, the *p* *(is, is not)* pronounced. Examples are ortho*pn*ea, hyper*pn*ea.

8. When *i* is at the end of a word, it is pronounced like *(eye, ee)*. Examples are bronch*i*, fung*i*, nucle*i*.

9. For *ae* and *oe*, only the (first, second) vowel is pronounced. Examples are burs*ae*, pleur*ae*.

10. When *e* and *es* form the final letter or letters of a word, they are commonly pronounced as (combined, separate) syllables. Examples are syncop*e*, systol*e*, nar*es*.

 Competency Verification: Check your answers in Appendix B, Answer Key, page 351. If you are not satisfied with your level of comprehension, review the rules and retake the review.

Correct Answers _____ **× 10 =** _____ **% Score**

Review Activity 1-7

Plural Suffixes

When a word changes from a singular to a plural form, the suffix of the word is the part that changes. For example, the medical report may list one diagnos*is* or several diagnos*es*. The rules for forming plurals starting from the singular forms of the words are given in the inside back cover of this book. When in doubt about singular and plural word formations, refer to these rules or use a medical dictionary. Review the rules and use them to complete this activity. The first word is completed for you.

Singular	Plural	Rule
1. sarcoma săr-KŌ-mă	*sarcomata*	*Retain the* ma *and add* ta.
2. thrombus THRŎM-bŭs		

(Continued)

Singular	Plural	Rule
3. appendix ă-PĔN-dĭks		
4. diverticulum dī-vĕr-TĬK-ū-lŭm		
5. ovary Ō-vă-rē		
6. diagnosis dī-ăg-NŌ-sĭs		
7. lumen LŪ-mĕn		
8. vertebra VĔR-tĕ-bră		
9. thorax THŌ-răks		
10. spermatozoon spĕr-măt-ō-ZŌ-ŏn		

 Competency Verification: Check your answers in Appendix B, Answer Key, page 351. If you are not satisfied with your level of comprehension, review the rules for changing a singular word into its plural form (on inside back cover of this book) and retake the review.

Correct Answers _____ × **10 =** _____ **% Score**

Review Activity 1-8
Common Suffixes

In previous material, you were introduced to the principles of medical word building. You learned that a combining form is a word root + vowel and that the combining form is the main part or foundation of a medical term. Examples of combining forms are *gastr/o* (stomach), *dermat/o* (skin), and *nephr/o* (kidney). You also learned that a suffix is an element located at the end of a word and a prefix is an element located at the beginning of a word. This section presents common suffixes and prefixes used to construct medical terms. Some of these elements have already been introduced, but are now reinforced in the appropriate categorized tables below. Similar tables are included for each chapter in the book. Thus, the common elements in this section of the chapter will be reinforced throughout the textbook in numerous medical terms.

Surgical Suffixes

Common suffixes associated with surgical procedures, their meanings, and an example of a related term are listed in the table below. First, study the suffix as well as its meaning and practice pronouncing the term aloud. Then use the information provided to complete the meaning of each term. You may also refer to *Appendix A: Glossary of Medical Word Elements* to complete this exercise. To build a working vocabulary of medical terms and understand how those terms are used in the health care industry, it is important that you complete all of these exercises. The first one completed for you.

Suffix	Term	Meaning
-centesis surgical puncture	arthr/o/**centesis** ăr-thrō-sĕn-TĒ-sĭs *arthr/o:* joint	*Surgical puncture of a joint*
-clasis to break; surgical fracture	oste/o/**clasis** ŏs-tē–ŎK-lă-sĭs *oste/o:* bone	
-desis binding, fixation (of a bone or joint)	arth r/o/**desis** ăr-thrō-DĒ-sĭs *arthr/o:* joint	
-ectomy excision, removal	append/**ectomy** ăp-ĕn-DĔK-tō-mē *append:* appendix	
-lysis separation; destruction; loosening	thromb/o/**lysis** thrŏm-BŎL-ĭ-sĭs *thromb/o:* blood clot	
-pexy fixation (of an organ)	mast/o/**pexy** MĂS-tō-pĕks-ē *mast/o:* breast	
-plasty surgical repair	rhin/o/**plasty** RĪ-nō-plăs-tē *rhin/o:* nose	
-rrhaphy suture	my/o/**rrhaphy** mī-OR-ă-fē *my/o:* muscle	
-stomy forming an opening (mouth)	trache/o/**stomy** trā-kē-ŎS-tō-mē *trache/o:* trachea (windpipe)	
-tome instrument to cut	oste/o/**tome** ŎS-tē-ō-tōm *oste/o:* bone	

(Continued)

Suffix	Term	Meaning
-tomy incision	trache/o/**tomy** trā-kē–ŎT-ō–mē *trache/o:* trachea (windpipe)	
-tripsy crushing	lith/o/**tripsy** LĬTH-ō-trĭp-sē *lith/o:* stone, calculus	

Pronunciation Help	Long Sound Short Sound	ā in rāte ă in ălone	ē in rēbirth ĕ in ĕver	ī in īsle ĭ in ĭt	ō in ōver ŏ in nŏt	ū in ūnite ŭ in cŭt

 Competency Verification: Check your answers in Appendix B, Answer Key, page 351. If you are not satisfied with your level of comprehension, review the terms in the table and retake the review.

Diagnostic Suffixes

Common suffixes associated with diagnostic procedures, their meanings, and an example of a related term are listed in the table below. First, study the suffix as well as its meaning and practice pronouncing the term aloud. Then use the information provided to complete the meaning of each term. You may also refer to *Appendix A: Glossary of Medical Word Elements* to complete this exercise. To build a working vocabulary of medical terms and understand how those terms are used in the health care field, it is important that you complete all of these exercises. The first one is completed for you.

Suffix	Term	Meaning
-gram record, writing	electr/o/cardi/o/**gram** ē-lĕk-trō-KĂR-dē-ō-grăm *electr/o:* electricity *cardi/o:* heart	*Record of electrical activity of the heart*
-graph instrument for recording	cardi/o/**graph** KĂR-dē-ō-grăf *cardi/o:* heart	
-graphy process of recording	angi/o/**graphy** ăn-jē-ŎG-ră-fē *angi/o:* vessel (usually blood or lymph)	
-meter instrument for measuring	pelv/i/**meter*** pĕl-VĬM-ĕ-tĕr *pelv/i:* pelvis	

Suffix	Term	Meaning
-metry act of measuring	pelv/i/**metry*** pĕl-VĬM-ĕ-trē *pelv/i:* pelvis	
-scope instrument for examining	endo/**scope** ĔN-dō-skōp *endo-:* in, within	
-scopy visual examination	endo/**scopy** ĕn-DŎS-kō-pē *endo-:* in, within	

Pronunciation Help	Long Sound	ā in rāte	ē in rēbirth	ī in īsle	ō in ōver	ū in ūnite
	Short Sound	ă in ălone	ĕ in ĕver	ĭ in ĭt	ŏ in nŏt	ŭ in cŭt

*The i in pelv/i/meter *and* pelv/i/metry *are exceptions to the rule of using the connecting vowel o.*

 Competency Verification: Check your answers in Appendix B, Answer Key, page 352. If you are not satisfied with your level of comprehension, review the terms in the table and retake the review.

Pathological Suffixes

Common suffixes associated with pathologic (disease) conditions, their meanings, and an example of a related term are listed in the table below. First, study the suffix as well as its meaning and practice pronouncing the term aloud. Then use the information provided to complete the meaning of each term. You may also refer to *Appendix A: Glossary of Medical Word Elements* to complete this exercise. To build a working vocabulary of medical terms and understand how those terms are used in the health care industry, it is important that you complete all of these exercises. The first one is completed for you.

Suffix	Term	Meaning
-algia, -dynia pain	neur/**algia** nū-RĂL-jē-ă *neur:* nerve	*Pain in a nerve*
	ot/o/**dynia** ō-tō-DĬN-ē-ă *ot/o:* ear	
-cele hernia, swelling	hepat/o/**cele** hĕ-PĂT-ō-sēl *hepat/o:* liver	

(Continued)

Suffix	Term	Meaning
-ectasis dilation, expansion	bronchi/**ectasis** brŏng-kē-ĔK-tă-sĭs *bronchi:* bronchus (plural, bronchi)	
-edema swelling	lymph/**edema** lĭmf-ĕ-DĒ-mă *lymph:* lymph	
-emesis vomiting	hyper/**emesis** hī-pĕr-ĔM-ĕ-sĭs *hyper-:* excessive, above normal	
-emia blood condition	an/**emia** ă-NĒ-mē-ă *an-:* without, not	
-iasis abnormal condition (produced by something specific)	chol/e/lith/**iasis*** kō-lē-lĭ-THĪ-ă-sĭs *chol/e:* bile, gall *lith:* stone, calculus	
-itis inflammation	gastr/**itis** găs-TRĪ-tĭs *gastr:* stomach	
-lith stone, calculus	chol/e/**lith*** KŌ-lē-lĭth *chol/e:* bile, gall	
-malacia softening	chondr/o/**malacia** kŏn-drō-mă-LĀ-shē-ă *chondr/o:* cartilage	
-megaly enlargement	cardi/o/**megaly** kăr-dē-ō-MĔG-ă-lē *cardi/o:* heart	
-oma tumor	neur/**oma** nū-RŌ-mă *neur:* nerve	
-osis abnormal condition; increase (used primarily with blood cells)	cyan/**osis** sī-ă-NŌ-sĭs *cyan:* blue	

The e in chol/e/lithiasis and chol/e/lith are exceptions to the rule of using the connecting vowel o.

Suffix	Term	Meaning
-pathy disease	my/o/**pathy** mī-ŎP-ă-thē *my/o:* muscle	
-penia decrease, deficiency	erythr/o/**penia** ĕ-rĭth-rō-PĒ-nē-ă *erythr/o:* red	
-phobia fear	hem/o/**phobia** hē-mō-FŌ-bē-ă *hem/o:* blood	
-plegia paralysis	hemi/**plegia** hĕm-ē-PLĒ-jē-ă *hemi-:* one half	
-rrhage, -rrhagia bursting (of)	hem/o/**rrhage** HĔM-ĕ-rĭj *hem/o:* blood	
	men/o/**rrhagia** mĕn-ō-RĀ-jē-ă *men/o:* menses, menstruation	
-rrhea discharge, flow	dia/**rrhea** dī-ă-RĒ-ă *dia-:* through, across	
-rrhexis rupture	arteri/o/**rrhexis** ăr-tē-rē-ō-RĔK-sĭs *arteri/o:* artery	
-stenosis narrowing, stricture	arteri/o/**stenosis** ăr-tē-rē-ō-stĕ-NŌ-sĭs *arteri/o:* artery	
-toxic poison	hepat/o/**toxic** HĔP-ă-tō-tŏk-sĭk *hepat/o:* liver	
-trophy nourishment, development	dys/**trophy** DĬS-trō-fē *dys-:* bad; painful; difficult	

Pronunciation Help	Long Sound	ā in rāte	ē in rēbirth	ī in īsle	ō in ōver	ū in ūnite
	Short Sound	ă in ălone	ĕ in ĕver	ĭ in ĭt	ŏ in nŏt	ŭ in cŭt

Competency Verification: Check your answers in Appendix B, Answer Key, page 352. If you are not satisfied with your level of comprehension, review the terms in the table and retake the review.

Review Activity 1-9
Common Prefixes

Common prefixes, their meanings, and an example of a related term are listed in this table. First, study the prefix as well as its meaning and practice pronouncing the term aloud. Then use the information in the table below to complete the meaning of the terms. You may also refer to *Appendix A: Glossary of Medical Word Elements* to complete this exercise. To understand the meaning of medical terms, it is important to actively engage in activities of this type. Complete all of the exercises and you will master medical terminology. The first one is completed for you.

Prefix	Term	Meaning
a-*, an-** without, not	**a**/mast/ia ă-MĂS-tē-ă *mast:* breast *-ia:* condition	*Without a breast*
	an/esthesia ăn-ĕs-THĒ-zē-ă *-esthesia:* feeling	
circum-, peri- around	**circum**/duction sĕr-kŭm-DŬK-shŭn *-duction:* act of leading, bringing, conducting	
	peri/odont/al pĕr-ē-ō-DŎN-tăl *odont:* teeth *-al:* pertaining to	
dia-, trans- through, across	**dia**/therm/y DĪ-ă-thĕr-mē *therm:* heat *-y:* condition, process	
	trans/vagin/al trăns-VĂJ-ĭn-ăl *vagin:* vagina *-al:* pertaining to	

*The prefix a- is usually used before a consonant. **The prefix an- is usually used before a vowel.

Prefix	Term	Meaning
dipl-, diplo- double	**dipl**/opia dĭp-LŌ-pē-ă *-opia:* vision	
	diplo/bacteri/al dĭp-lō-băk-TĔR-ē-ăl *bacteri:* bacteria *-al:* pertaining to	
dys- bad, painful, difficult	**dys**/phonia dĭs-FŌ-nē-ă *-phonia:* voice	
endo-, intra- in, within	**endo**/crine ĔN-dō-krĭn *-crine:* secrete	
	intra/muscul/ar ĭn-tră-MŬS-kū-lăr *muscul:* muscle *-ar:* pertaining to	
homo-, homeo- same	**homo**/graft HŌ-mō-grăft *-graft:* transplantation	
	homeo/plasia hō-mē-ō-PLĀ-zē-ă *-plasia:* formation, growth	
hypo- under, below, deficient	**hypo**/derm/ic hī-pō-DĔR-mĭk *derm:* skin *-ic:* pertaining to	
macro- large	**macro**/cyte MĂK-rō-sīt *-cyte:* cell	
micro- small	**micro**/scope MĪ-krō-skōp *-scope:* instrument for examining	

(Continued)

Prefix	Term	Meaning
mono-, uni- one	**mono**/therapy MŎN-ō-thĕr-ă-pē *-therapy:* treatment	
	uni/nucle/ar ū-nĭ-NŪ-klē-ăr *nucle:* nucleus *-ar:* pertaining to	
post- after, behind	**post**/nat/al pōst-NĀ-tăl *nat:* birth *-al:* pertaining to	
pre-, pro- before, in front of	**pre**/nat/al prē-NĀ-tăl *nat:* birth *-al:* pertaining to	
	pro/gnosis prŏg-NŌ-sĭs *-gnosis:* knowing	
primi- first	**primi**/gravida prī-mĭ-GRĂV-ĭ-dă *-gravida:* pregnant woman	
retro- backward, behind	**retro**/version rĕt-rō-VĔR-zhŭn *-version:* turning	
super- upper, above	**super**/ior soo-PĒ-rē-or *-ior:* pertaining to	

Pronunciation Help	Long Sound	ā in rāte	ē in rēbirth	ī in īsle	ō in ōver	ū in ūnite
	Short Sound	ă in ălone	ĕ in ĕver	ĭ in ĭt	ŏ in nŏt	ŭ in cŭt

 Competency Verification: Check your answers in Appendix B, Answer Key, page 353. If you are not satisfied with your level of comprehension, review the terms in the table and retake the review.

 Multimedia Review. Enhance your study and reinforcement of word elements with the power of *DavisPlus*. Visit *http://davisplus.fadavis.com/gylys-express* for this chapter's flash-card activity. We recommend you complete the flash-card activity before continuing to the next chapter.

Body Structure

Objectives

Upon completion of this chapter, you will be able to:

- List the levels of organization of the human body.
- Understand the meanings and usage of terms related to direction, planes, quadrants, and regions of the body.
- Describe the standard positions of body placement that are used to perform patient examinations, x-rays, and medical and surgical procedures.
- Identify combining forms, suffixes, and prefixes associated with body structure.
- Recognize, pronounce, build, and spell medical terms and abbreviations associated with body structure.
- Demonstrate your knowledge of this chapter by successfully completing the activities in this chapter.

Vocabulary Preview

Terms	Meanings
anterior ăn-TĒR-ē-or *anter:* anterior, front *–ior:* pertaining to	Toward the front of the body, organ, or structure
anteroposterior ăn-těr-ō-pŏs-TĒR-ē-or	Pertaining to the front and back of the body or passing from the front to the back of the body
inferior ĭn-FĒ-rē-or *infer:* lower, below *–ior:* pertaining to	Pertaining to below, lower, or toward the tail
scan skăn	Process of using a moving device or a sweeping beam of radiation to produce images of an internal area, organ, or tissue of the body

Pronunciation Help	Long Sound	ā in rāte	ē in rēbirth	ī in īsle	ō in ōver	ū in ūnite
	Short Sound	ă in ălone	ě in ěver	ĭ in ĭt	ŏ in nŏt	ŭ in cŭt

Overview

This chapter provides an orientation to the body as a whole. Descriptive terms are used to describe the structural organization of the body. Included are terms that specify direction, position, and location of various organs in relationship to each other. Knowledge of the descriptive terms are an essential part of medical terminology and provide a basic foundation for a better understanding of the body system chapters that follow. Most importantly, they are included in the language of medicine used by health care providers in the clinical environment.

Levels of Organization

The human body consists of several structural and functional levels of organization. Each higher level increases in complexity because it incorporates the structures and functions of the previous level(s). Eventually, all levels contribute to the structure and function of the entire organism. (See Figure 2-1.) The levels of organization from the least to the most complex are the:

- **cellular level,** molecules combine to form cells, the basic structural and functional units of the body
- **tissue level,** groups of cells that work together to perform a specialized function
- **organ level,** structures that are composed of two or more different types of tissue; they have specific functions and usually have recognizable shapes
- **system level,** related organs with a common function; also called *organ-system level*
- **organism level,** collection of body systems that makes up the most complex level: a living human being. All parts of the human body functioning together constitute the total organism.

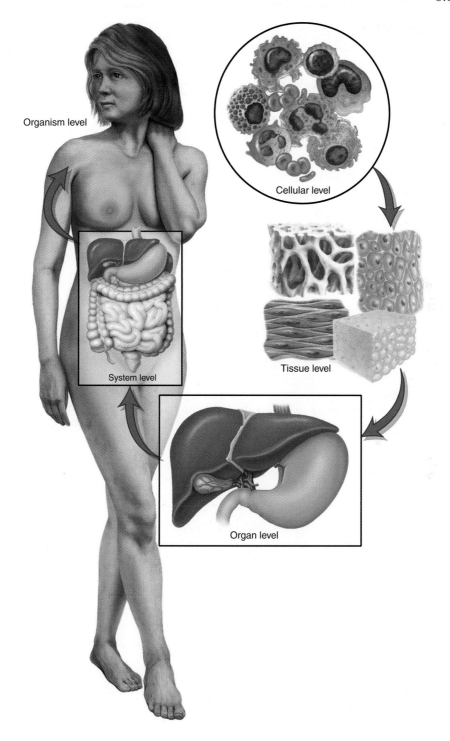

Organism level

Cellular level

Tissue level

System level

Organ level

Figure 2–1. Levels of organization of the human body. The body system illustrated is the digestive system.

Anatomical Position

Health care providers use directional terms to accurately identify location of diseases in the body. The terms also indicate the position of the body when performing diagnostic, surgical, and therapeutic procedures. That's why health care providers must visualize the body in a standard position. Without a standard position, directional terms are meaningless. In the field of medicine, the standard reference position of the body is known as the *anatomical position.* In anatomical position, the person stands erect, the eyes look straight ahead, the arms are at the sides of the body with the palms of the hand turned forward, the feet are parallel to one another and flat on the floor. (See Figure 2-2.)

Directional Terms

Directional terms describe the relationship of one body part to another in reference to the anatomical position. For example, if a person is in anatomical position, the toes are **anterior** to the

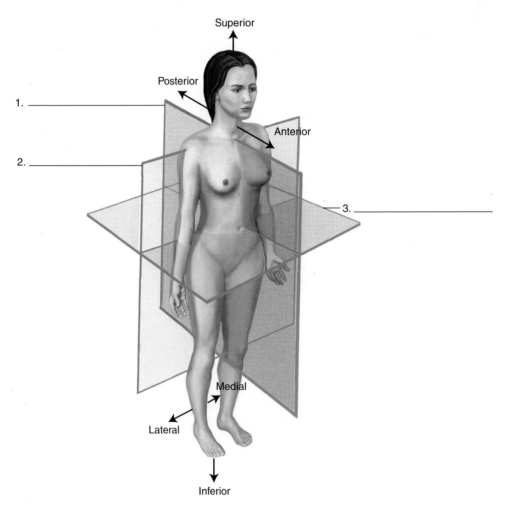

Figure 2–2. Anatomical position, directional terms, and body planes.

ankle, and the legs are **inferior** to the trunk. Locate the directional terms *anterior* and *inferior* in Figure 2-2. Physicians commonly use such terms in medical reports and to communicate with other health care providers and patients. For example, to explain the location, or position, of the liver to a patient who knows where the heart is, you can say that the heart is *superior* to, or *above*, the liver. You can also say the esophagus (throat) is *posterior* to, or *behind*, the trachea (windpipe).

Review Table 2-1 for a comprehensive summary of directional terms along with their definitions. These terms are used to describe the locations of organs in relationship to one another throughout

Table 2-1	Directional Terms	
Term	**Definition**	**Example**
Adduction	Movement toward the midline of the body	The arm moves from shoulder height to the side of the body.
Abduction	Movement away from the midline of the body	The arm moves from the side of the body to shoulder height.
Superior (cephalic, cranial)	Above or higher; toward the head	The chest is superior to the abdomen. The heart is superior to the stomach.
Inferior (caudal)	Below or lower; toward the tail	The intestines are inferior to the stomach. The legs are inferior to the trunk.
Anterior (ventral)	Front of the body; toward the front	The navel is on the anterior side of the body. The toes are anterior to the ankle.
Posterior (dorsal)	Back of the body; toward the back	The spinal column is on the posterior side of the body. The heel is posterior to the toes.
Medial	Pertaining to the middle; toward the midline	The mouth is medial to the cheeks.
Lateral	Pertaining to the side; toward the side	The eyes are lateral to the nose.
External	Outside, exterior to	The ribs are external to the lungs.
Internal	Within, interior to	The brain is internal to the skull.
Superficial	Toward or on the surface	A scrape from a fall is a superficial wound.
Deep	Away from the surface	A bullet wound can penetrate deep into the abdomen.
Proximal	Near the point of attachment to the trunk or a structure	The ankle is proximal to the foot.
Distal	Farther from the point of attachment to the trunk or a structure	The toes are distal to the ankle.
Parietal	Pertaining to the outer wall of a cavity	The parietal pleura lines the chest cavity.
Visceral	Pertaining to the organs within a cavity	The visceral pleura covers the lungs.

the body. In the table, opposing terms are presented consecutively to aid memorization. A graphic illustration of some of these terms is also depicted in Figure 2-2.

Body Planes

A **plane** is an imaginary flat surface that separates two portions of the body or an organ. Reference of body planes helps you understand the anatomical relationship of one body part to another.

Body planes are also used to describe the location of x-ray images. For example, an **anteroposterior** chest x-ray is taken in the frontal (coronal) plane. Prior to the development of computed tomography (CT) scanning, which displays an image along a transverse plane, conventional x-ray images were on a vertical plane. Thus, the dimensions of body irregularities were difficult, if not impossible, to ascertain.

Label the three body planes in Figure 2-2 as you read the following material.

1. **Median plane** — vertical plane that passes through the midline of the body and divides the body or organ into equal right and left sides; also called *midsagittal plane.*
2. **Frontal plane** — plane that divides the body into **anterior** (front) and **posterior** (back) portions; also called *coronal plane.*
3. **Horizontal plane** — plane that separates the body into **superior** (upper) and **inferior** (lower) portions; also called *transverse plane.*

Quadrants and Regions

The abdominopelvic region is divided into quadrants and regions, each of which has specific uses in communicating between health care providers.

Abdominopelvic Quadrants

Four quadrants identify the placement of internal organs in the abdominopelvic cavity. Generally, quadrants are used to report the findings of a clinical examination or an exploratory surgery. For example, a physician may describe a patient's abdominal pain in the left upper quadrant (LUQ). This quadrant indicates different clinical possibilities than if the pain was in the right lower quadrant (RLQ). Quadrants are also used to describe the location of surgical procedures, incision sites, or tumors. Use these abbreviations and locations to label the quadrants in Figure 2-3A.

1. Right upper quadrant (RUQ) — contains the right lobe of the liver, the gallbladder, part of the pancreas, and part of the small and large intestine
2. Right lower quadrant (RLQ) — contains part of the small and large intestine, the appendix, the right ovary, the right fallopian tube, and the right ureter
3. Left upper quadrant (LUQ) — contains the left lobe of the liver, the stomach, the spleen, part of the pancreas, and part of the small and large intestine
4. Left lower quadrant (LLQ) — contains part of the small and large intestine, the left ovary, the left fallopian tube, and the left ureter.

Abdominopelvic Regions

The abdominopelvic cavity can be divided into nine regions. While quadrants are normally used to describe and diagnose conditions, region designations are used mainly to indicate the location of

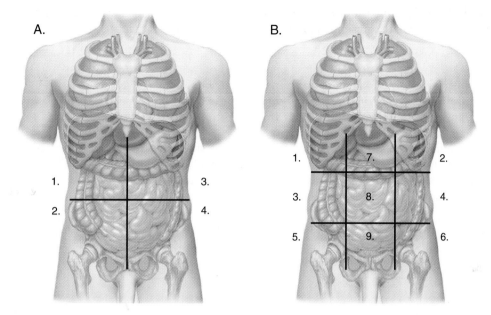

Figure 2–3. Regions and quadrants. (A) Four quadrants of the abdomen. (B) Nine regions of the abdomen.

internal organs. For example, the liver is located in the epigastric and right hypochondriac regions. Identify the nine regions in Figure 2-3B as you read the following information.

1. Right hypochondriac — upper right region located under the cartilage of the ribs
2. Left hypochondriac — upper left region located under the cartilage of the ribs
3. Right lumbar — middle right region located near the waist
4. Left Lumbar — middle left region located near the waist
5. Right iliac — lower right region located near the groin (also called *right inguinal region*)
6. Left iliac — lower left region located near the groin (also called *left inguinal region*)
7. Epigastric — middle region located above the stomach
8. Umbilical — middle region located in the area of the umbilicus, or navel
9. Hypogastric — lower middle region located below the stomach and umbilical region

Positioning for Examinations and Treatments

To provide a comfortable environment for patients during an examination, surgery, or therapeutic treatment, it is customary to expose only the body part that is being examined or treated. Draping sheets are used to cover the body while the patient lies on the examining table and also prior to surgery.

Various body positions are employed during medical examinations, x-rays, surgeries, and therapeutic treatments. The position used depends on the procedure or treatment as well as the sex of the patient. Seven basic patient positions used for medical examinations, therapeutic treatments, and surgeries are illustrated in Figure 2-4 and discussed below. These terms are found in different types of medical reports, including the physical examination, radiographic report, and operative report:

1. **Knee-chest position.** Patient is assisted into a kneeling position with the buttocks elevated. The head and chest are on the table, and the arms are extended above the head and flexed at the elbow. This position facilitates examination of the rectum.
2. **Lithotomy position.** Patient is assisted into a **supine** (lying on the back) position. The legs are sharply flexed at the knees, and the feet are placed in stirrups. This position is used for vaginal examination and the Papanicolaou (Pap) test.
3. **Dorsal recumbent position.** Patient is assisted into a supine position. The legs are sharply flexed at the knees, and the feet are placed on the table. This position is used to examine the vagina and rectum in the female and the rectum in the male.
4. **Sims position.** Patient is assisted into a side-lying position on the left side. The left arm is placed behind the body and the right arm is moved forward and flexed at the elbow. Both legs are flexed at the knee, but the right leg is sharply flexed and positioned next to the left leg, which is slightly flexed. This position is used to examine the vagina and rectum in the female and the rectum in the male. Sims position is also used to administer an enema.

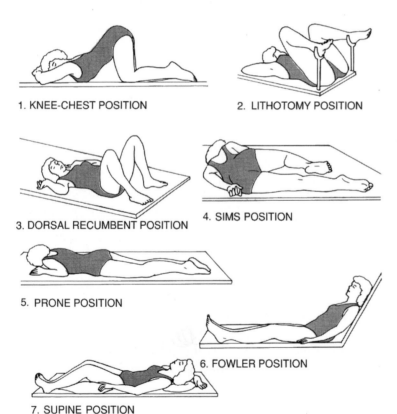

Figure 2–4. Basic patient positioning for medical examination.

5. **Prone position.** Patient is assisted to lie flat on the abdomen with the head turned slightly to the side. The arms are extended above the head or alongside the body. Prone position is used to examine the back, spine, and lower extremities.

6. **Fowler position.** Patient is assisted into a semi-sitting position. The head of the examination table is tilted to produce a 45- to 60-degree angle with patient's knees bent or not bent. An angle of 45 degrees or more is considered *high Fowler position;* an angle of approximately 30 degrees is considered *semi-Fowler position.* This position promotes lung expansion. It is used if the patient has difficulty breathing.

7. **Supine position.** Patient is assisted to lie flat on their back with arms at the sides. This position is used to examine the chest, heart, abdomen, and extremities. It is also used to examine the head and neck as well as in certain neurologic reflex testing.

Two other commonly used positions are the erect standing position and Trendelenburg position. The **erect standing position,** also referred to as the *anatomical position,* is illustrated in Figure 2-2. In anatomical position, and depending on the type of examination, the patient may be instructed to bend over, walk, or move specific body parts in a particular manner. The physician observes these movements to determine the patient's level of coordination, strength, flexibility, balance, and range of motion. In the **Trendelenburg position,** the patient is lying flat on his or her back and the entire examination table is tilted with the head of the table down. This position is used for therapeutic treatments, such as postural drainage in patients who have thick respiratory secretions.

 Competency Verification: Check your labeling of Figure 2-2, and Figure 2-3A in Appendix B, Answer Key, page 355.

Medical Word Building

Building medical words using word elements related to body structure will enhance your understanding of those terms and reinforce your ability to use terms correctly.

Combining Forms

Begin your study of body structure terminology by reviewing their associated combining forms (CFs) as outlined in the tables below. This introductory study of CFs provides an understanding of the construction and meanings of medical terms related to body regions, body structures, as well as the use of directional terms. You may also refer to *Appendix A: Glossary of Medical Word Elements* to complete this exercise.

Combining Form	Meaning	Medical Word	Meaning
Body Regions			
abdomin/o	abdomen	**abdomin/**al (ăb-DŎM-ĭ-năl) *-al:* pertaining to	*pertaining to the abdomen*
caud/o	tail	**caud/**ad (KAW-dăd) *-ad:* toward	

(Continued)

Combining Form	Meaning	Medical Word	Meaning
Body Regions			
cephal/o	head	**cephal/**ad (SĔF-ă-lăd) *-ad:* toward	
cervic/o	neck; cervix uteri (neck of uterus)	**cervic/**al (SĔR-vĭ-kăl) *-al:* pertaining to	
crani/o	cranium (skull)	**crani/**al (KRĀ-nē-ăl) *-al:* pertaining to	
gastr/o	stomach	**gastr/**ic (GĂS-trĭk) *-ic:* pertaining to	
ili/o	ilium (lateral, flaring portion of the hip bone)	**ili/**ac (ĬL-ē-ăk) *-ac: pertaining to*	
inguin/o	groin	**inguin/**al (ĬNG-gwĭ-năl) *-al:* pertaining to	
lumb/o	loins (lower back)	**lumb/**ar (LŬM-băr) *-ar:* pertaining to	
pelv/i* **pelv/o**	pelvis	**pelv/i/**meter (pĕl-VĬM-ĕ-tĕr) *-meter:* instrument for measuring **pelv/**ic (PĔL-vĭc) *-ic:* pertaining to	
spin/o	spine	**spin/**al (SPĪ-năl) *-al:* pertaining to	
thorac/o	chest	**thorac/**ic (thō-RĂS-ĭk) *-ic:* pertaining to	
umbilic/o	umbilicus, navel	**umbilic/**al (ŭm-BĬL-ĭ-kăl) *-al:* pertaining to	
Directional Terms			
anter/o	anterior, front	**anter/**ior (ăn-TĔR-ē-ōr) *-ior:* pertaining to	
dist/o	far, farthest	**dist/**al (DĬS-tăl) *-al:* pertaining to	

*The i in pelv/i/meter *is an exception to the rule of using the connecting vowel o.*

Combining Form	Meaning	Medical Word	Meaning
Directional Terms			
dors/o	back (of the body)	**dors/al** (DOR-săl) *-al:* pertaining to	
infer/o	lower, below	**infer/ior** (ĭn-FĒ-rē-or) *-ior:* pertaining to	
later/o	side, to one side	**later/al** (LĂT-ĕr-ăl) *-al:* pertaining to	
medi/o	middle	**medi/al** (MĒ-dē-ăl) *-al:* pertaining to	
poster/o	back (of the body), behind, posterior	**poster/ior** (pŏs-TĒR-ē-or) *-ior:* pertaining to	
proxim/o	near, nearest	**proxim/al** (PRŎK-sĭm-ăl) *-al:* pertaining to	
super/o**	upper, above	**super/ior** (soo-PĒ-rē-or) *-ior:* pertaining to	
ventr/o	belly, belly side	**ventr/al** (VĔN-trăl) *-al:* pertaining to	
Other Combining Forms Related to Body Structure			
cyt/o	cell	**cyt/o/meter** (sī-TŎM-ĕ-tĕr) *-meter:* instrument for measuring	
hist/o	tissue	**hist/o/lysis** (hĭs-TŎL-ĭ-sĭs) *-lysis:* separation; destruction; loosening	
nucle/o	nucleus	**nucle/ar** (NŪ-klē-ăr) *-ar:* pertaining to	
radi/o	radiation, x-ray; radius (lower arm bone on the thumb side)	**radi/o/graphy** (rā-dē-ŎG-ră-fē) *-graphy:* process of recording	

**The CF super/o can also be used as prefix.

Suffixes and Prefixes

In the table below, suffixes and prefixes are listed alphabetically and other word parts are defined as needed. Review the medical word and study the elements that make up the term. Then complete the meaning of the medical words in the right-hand column. You may also refer to *Appendix A: Glossary of Medical Word Elements* to complete this exercise.

Word Element	Meaning	Medical Words	Meaning
Suffixes			
-ad	toward	medi/**ad** (MĒ-dē-ăd) *medi/o:* middle	
-al	pertaining to	coron/**al** (kŏ -RŌN-ăl) *coron:* heart	
-algia, **-dynia**	pain	cost/**algia** (kŏs-TĂL-jē-ă) *cost:* ribs thorac/o/**dynia** (thō-răk-ō-DĬN-ē-ă) *thorac/o:* chest	
-gen, **-genesis**	forming, producing, origin	path/o/**gen** (PĂTH-ō-jĕn) *path/o:* disease carcin/o/**genesis** (kăr-sĭ-nō-JĚN-ĕ-sĭs) *carcin/o:* cancer	
-logist	specialist in the study of	hist/o/**logist** (hĭs-TŎL-ō-jĭst) *hist/o:* tissue	
-logy	study of	eti/o/**logy** (ē-tē-ŎL-ō-jē) *eti/o:* cause	
-lysis	separation; destruction; loosening	cyt/o/**lysis** (sī-TŎL-ĭ-sĭs) *cyt/o:* cell	
-meter	instrument used to measure	therm/o/**meter** (thĕr-MŎM-ĕ-tĕr) *therm/o:* heat	

Word Element	Meaning	Medical Words	Meaning
Suffixes			
-plasia	formation, growth	hyper/**plasia** (hī-pĕr-PLĀ-zē-ă) *hyper-:* excessive, above normal	
-toxic	poison	hepat/o/**toxic** (HĔP-ă-tō-tŏk-sĭk) *hepat/o:* liver	
Prefixes			
bi-	two	**bi**/later/al (bī-LĂT-ĕr-ăl) *later:* side, to one side *-al:* pertaining to	
epi-	above, on	**epi**/gastr/ic (ĕp-ĭ-GĂS-trĭk) *gastr:* stomach *-ic:* pertaining to	
infra-	below, under	**infra**/cost/al (ĭn-fră-KŎS-tăl) *cost:* ribs *-al:* pertaining to	
trans-	across, through	**trans**/vagin/al (trăns-VĂJ-ĭn-ăl) *vagin:* vagina *-al:* pertaining to	

 Competency Verification: Check your answers in Appendix B, Answer Key, page 355. If you are not satisfied with your level of comprehension, review the terms in the table and retake the review.

 Listen and Learn, the audio CD-ROM included in this book, will help you master pronunciation of selected medical words. Use it to practice pronunciations of the medical terms in the above "Word Building" tables and for instructions to complete the *Listen and Learn* exercise.

 Flash-Card Activity. Enhance your study and reinforcement of this chapter's word elements with the power of *DavisPlus* flash-card activity. Do so by visiting *http://davisplus.fadavis.com/ gylys-express*. We recommend you complete the flash-card activity before continuing with the next section.

Medical Terminology Word Building

In this section, combine the word parts you have learned to construct medical terms related to body structures. The first one is an example completed for you.

Use *caud/o* (tail) to build words that mean:

1. toward the tail *caudad* _____

2. pertaining to the tail _____

Use *thorac/o* (chest) to build words that mean:

3. surgical puncture of the chest _____

4. pertaining to the chest _____

5. surgical repair of the chest _____

Use *gastr/o* (stomach) to build words that mean:

6. pertaining to the stomach _____

7. surgical repair of the stomach _____

Use *pelv/i* (pelvis) to build words that mean:

8. pertaining to the pelvis _____

9. instrument to measure the pelvis _____

Use *abdomin/o* (abdomen) to build words that mean:

10. pertaining to the abdomen _____

11. surgical repair of the abdomen _____

Use *crani/o* (cranium [skull]) to build words that mean:

12. pertaining to the cranium (skull) _____

13. surgical repair of the cranium (skull) _____

Use *medi/o* (middle) to build words that mean:

14. pertaining to the middle _____

15. toward the middle _____

Use *cyt/o* (cell) to build words that mean:

16. study of cells _____

17. specialist in the study of cells _____

18. destruction, dissolution, or separation of a cell _____

Use *hist/o* (tissue) to build words that mean:

19. study of tissues _____

20. specialist in the study of tissues _____

 Competency Verification: Check your answers in Appendix B, Answer Key, page 357. Review material that you did not answer correctly.

Correct Answers _____ **× 5 =** _____ **%**

Additional Medical Vocabulary

The following table lists additional terms related to the body as a whole. Recognizing and learning these terms will help you understand the connection between common signs, symptoms, and diseases and their diagnoses. It also provides the rationale behind methods of medical and surgical treatments selected for a particular disorder.

Signs, Symptoms, and Diseases

adhesion ăd-HĒ-zhŭn	Band of scar tissue binding anatomical surfaces that are normally separate from each other
inflammation ĭn-flă-MĀ-shun	Protective response of body tissues to irritation, infection, or allergy
sepsis SĚP-sĭs	Body's inflammatory response to infection in which there is fever, elevated heart and respiratory rate, and low blood pressure

Diagnostic Procedures

endoscopy ĕn-DŎS-kō-pē *endo-:* in, within *-scopy:* visual examination	Visual examination of the interior of organs and cavities with a specialized lighted instrument called an *endoscope* (See Figure 2-5.)

fluoroscopy
floo-or-ŎS-kō-pē
fluor/o: luminous,
    fluorescence
-scopy: visual
    examination
	Radiographic procedure that uses a fluorescent screen instead of a photographic plate to produce a visual image from x-rays that pass through the patient, resulting in continuous imaging of the motion of internal structures and immediate serial images

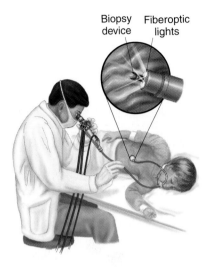

Biopsy device   Fiberoptic lights

Figure 2–5. Endoscopy.

magnetic resonance imaging (MRI) măg-NĔT-ĭc RĔZ-ĕn-ăns ĬM-ĭj-ĭng	Radiographic technique that uses electromagnetic energy to produce multiplanar cross-sectional images of the body (See Figure 2-6E.)
nuclear scan NŪ-klē-ăr	Diagnostic technique that produces an image of an organ or area by recording the concentration of a radiopharmaceutical substance called a *tracer;* usually introduced into the body by ingestion, inhalation, or injection (See Figure 2-6C.)
radiography rā-dē-ŎG-ră-fē *radi/o:* radiation, x-ray; radius (lower arm bone on the thumb side) *-graphy:* process of recording	Production of captured shadow images on photographic film through the action of ionizing radiation passing through the body from an external source (See Figure 2-6A.)

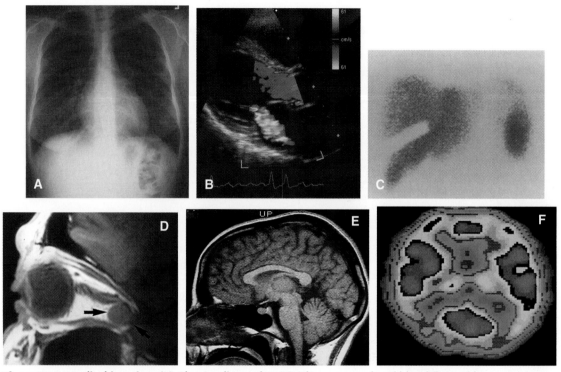

Figure 2–6. Medical imaging. (A) Chest radiography, (B) Ultrasonography of blood flow with color indicating direction, (C) Nuclear scan of liver and spleen, (D) CT scan of eye (lateral view), (E) MRI scan of head, (F) PET scan of brain.

radiopharmaceutical rā-dē-ō-fărm-ă-SŪ-tĭ-kăl *radi/o:* radiation, x-ray; radius (lower arm bone on thumb side) *pharmaceutic:* drug, medicine *-al:* pertaining to	Drug that contains a radioactive substance, which travels to an area or a specific organ that will be scanned

tomography
tō-MŎG-ră-fē
   tom/o: to cut
   -graphy: process of
      recording
	Radiographic technique that produces a film representing a detailed cross-section of tissue structure at a predetermined depth

computed tomography (CT) scan
kŏm-PŪ-tĕd
tō-MŎG-ră-fē
   tom/o: to cut
   -graphy: process of
      recording
	Narrow beam of x-rays with a contrast medium (provides more detail) or without a contrast medium that targets a specific organ or body area to produce multiple cross-sectional images for detecting such pathological conditions as tumors or metastases (See Figure 2-6D.)

positron emission tomography (PET) scan
PŎZ-ĭ-trŏn
ē-MĬSH-ŭn
tō-MŎG-ră-fē
   tom/o: to cut
   -graphy: process of
      recording
	Nuclear imaging study that combines CT with radiopharmaceuticals to produce a cross-sectional image of radioactive dispersements in a section of the body to reveal the areas where the radiopharmaceutical is being metabolized and where there is a deficiency in metabolism; useful in evaluating Alzheimer disease and epilepsy (See Figure 2-6F.)

single-photon emission computed tomography (SPECT) scan
SĬNG-gŭl FŌ-tŏn
ē-MĬ -shŭn
cŏm-PŪ-tĕd
tō-MŎG-ră-fē
   tom/o: to cut
   -graphy: process of
      recording
	Nuclear imaging study that scans organs after injection of a radioactive tracer and employs a specialized gamma camera that detects emitted radiation to produce a three-dimensional image from a composite of numerous views; used to show how blood flows to an organ and helps determine how well it is functioning

ultrasonography (US)
ŭl-tră-sŏn-ŎG-ră-fē
   -ultra: excess, beyond
   son/o: sound
   -graphy: process of
      recording
	Imaging technique that uses high-frequency sound waves (ultrasound) that bounce off body tissues and are recorded to produce an image of an internal organ or tissue (See Figure 2-6B.)

Pronunciation Help	Long Sound	ā in rāte	ē in rēbirth	ī in īsle	ō in ōver	ū in ūnite
	Short Sound	ă in ălone	ĕ in ĕver	ĭ in ĭt	ŏ in nŏt	ŭ in cŭt

Additional Medical Vocabulary Recall

Match the medical term(s) below with the definitions in the numbered list.

adhesion	inflammation	radiopharmaceutical
CT scan	MRI	sepsis
endoscope	nuclear scan	SPECT
endoscopy	PET	tomography
fluoroscopy	radiography	US

1. _____ uses a narrow beam of x-rays generate multiple views of a specific organ or body area in cross-sectional images.

2. _____ directs x-rays through the body to a fluorescent screen to view organs in motion, such as the digestive tract and heart.

3. _____ employs high-frequency sound waves to produce images of internal structures of the body.

4. _____ employs magnetic energy to produce cross-sectional images.

5. _____ is a type of nuclear scan that uses radiopharmaceuticals to reveal areas where the radiopharmaceutical is metabolized.

6. _____ is a specialized lighted instrument used to view interior of organs and cavities.

7. _____ is the body's protective response to irritation, infection, or allergy.

8. _____ is similar to PET, but employs a specialized gamma camera that detects emitted radiation to produce a three-dimensional image.

9. _____ produces a film representing a detailed cross-section of tissue structure at a predetermined depth; three types include CT, PET, and SPECT.

10. _____ is a drug that contains a radioactive substance that travels to an area or a specific organ to be scanned.

11. _____ is a procedure to enable visualization of the interior of organs and cavities with a lighted instrument.

12. _____ is an imaging technique that relies on the use of a tracer to diagnose a disease.

13. _____ is a band of scar tissue that binds anatomical surfaces that normally are separate from each other.

14. _____ is production of shadow images on photographic film.

15. _____ is the body's inflammatory response to infection, in which there is fever, elevated heart rate and respiratory rate, and low blood pressure.

Competency Verification: Check your answers in Appendix B, Answer Key, on page 357. Review material that you did not answer correctly.

Correct Answers _____ × **6.67** = _____ %

Pronunciation and Spelling

Use the following list to practice correct pronunciation and spelling of medical terms. First practice the pronunciation aloud. Then write the correct spelling of the term. The first word is completed for you.

Pronunciation	Spelling
1. bī-LĂT-ĕr-ăl	*bilateral*
2. ăd-HĒ-zhŭn	
3. SĔR-vĭ-kăl	
4. KRĀ-nē-ăl	
5. DĬS-tăl	
6. ĕn-DŎS-kō-pē	
7. floo-or-ŎS-kō-pē	
8. ĭn-flă-MĀ-shun	
9. LŬM-băr	
10. rā-dē-ō-fărm-ă-SŪ-tĭ-kăl	
11. rā-dē-ŎG-ră-fē	
12. SĔP-sĭs	
13. sĭg-MOY-dō-skōp	
14. SPĔK-ū-lŭm	
15. tō-MŎG-ră-fē	

Competency Verification: Check your answers in Appendix B, Answer Key, on page 357. Review material that you did not answer correctly.

Correct Answers: _____ × **6.67** = _____ %

Abbreviations

This section introduces abbreviations associated with body structure and radiology.

Abbreviation	Meaning	Abbreviation	Meaning
Body Structure and Related			
ant	anterior	LUQ	left upper quadrant
AP	anteroposterior	PA	posteroanterior
Bx, bx	biopsy	RLQ	right lower quadrant
CXR	chest x-ray; chest radiograph	RUQ	right upper quadrant
LAT, lat	lateral	Sx	symptom
LLQ	left lower quadrant	Tx	treatment
Radiology			
CT	computed tomography	PET	positron emission tomography
CXR	chest x-ray, chest radiograph	US	ultrasound; ultrasonography
MRI	magnetic resonance imaging	SPECT	single photon emission computed tomography

Demonstrate What You Know!

To evaluate your understanding of body regions and directional terms, match each term in Column A with its meaning in Column B.

Column A

1. umbilical _____

2. iliac _____

3. cervical _____

4. cephalad _____

5. cranial _____

6. epigastric _____

7. thoracic _____

8. inguinal _____

9. anterior _____

10. proximal _____

11. lateral _____

12. posterior _____

13. caudad _____

14. ventral _____

15. distal _____

Column B

a. pertaining to the skull

b. pertaining to the groin

c. pertaining to the chest

d. toward the front (of the body)

e. nearest the point of attachment

f. pertaining to the belly side or front of the body

g. farthest from the point of attachment

h. toward the head

i. middle region located near the navel

j. pertaining to the neck

k. pertaining to the side

l. toward the tail

m. middle region located above the stomach

n. pertaining to the ilium

o. pertaining to the back (of body), behind

 Competency Verification: Check your answers in Appendix B, Answer Key, page 357. Review material that you did not answer correctly.

 Multimedia Review. If you are not satisfied with your retention level of the body structure chapter, go to *http://davisplus.fadavis.com/gylys-express* to complete the website activities linked to this chapter. It is your choice whether or not you want to take advantage of these reinforcement exercises before continuing with the next chapter.

Integumentary System

MULTIMEDIA STUDY TOOLS.
To enrich your medical terminology skills, look for this multimedia icon throughout the text. It will help alert you to when it is best to use the various multimedia resources available with this textbook to enhance your studies.

Objectives

Upon completion of this chapter, you will be able to:

- Describe types of medical treatment provided by dermatologists.
- List three primary functions of the skin.
- Identify the two layers and the three accessory organs of the skin.
- Identify three underlying structures of the skin.
- Identify combining forms, suffixes, and prefixes associated with the integumentary system.
- Recognize, pronounce, build, and spell medical terms, and abbreviations associated with the integumentary system.
- Demonstrate your knowledge by successfully completing the activities in this chapter.

Vocabulary Preview

Term	Meaning
avascular ă-VĂS-kū-lăr *a:* without, not *vascul:* vessel (usually blood or lymph *-ar:* pertaining to	Pertaining to a type of tissue that does not have blood vessels
cutaneous kū-TĀ-nē-ŭs *cutane:* skin *-ous:* pertaining to	Pertaining to the skin
dermis DĔR-mĭs *derm:* skin *-is:* noun ending	Deeper layer of skin composed of nerves, blood vessels, hair follicles, and sebaceous (oil) and sudoriferous (sweat) glands
epidermis ĕp-ĭ-DĔR-mĭs *epi-:* above, upon *derm:* skin *-is:* noun ending	Outer protective layer of skin that covers the body and does not have a blood or nerve supply
lesion LĒ-zhŭn	Wound, injury, or pathological change in body tissue
sebaceous sē-BĀ-shŭs	Pertaining to sebum, an oily fatty substance secreted by the sebaceous glands
subcutaneous sŭb-kū-TĀ-nē-ŭs *sub:* under, below *cutane:* skin *-ous:* pertaining to	Pertaining to under the skin
sudoriferous soo-dor-ĬF-ĕr-ŭs	Pertaining to or producing sweat
systemic sĭs-TĔM-ĭk	Pertaining to a system or the whole body rather than a localized area
therapeutic thĕr-ă-PŪ-tĭk *therapeut:* treatment *-ic:* pertaining to	Pertaining to treating, remediating, or curing a disorder or disease

Term	Meaning
vascular VĂS-kū-lăr *vascul:* vessel (usually blood or lymph *-ar:* pertaining to	Pertaining to or containing blood vessels

Pronunciation Help	Long Sound	ā in rāte	ē in rēbirth	ī in īsle	ō in ōver	ū in ūnite
	Short Sound	ă in ălone	ĕ in ĕver	ĭ in ĭt	ŏ in nŏt	ŭ in cŭt

Dermatology

The integumentary system is associated with the medical specialty of **dermatology**. Physicians who specialize in treating integumentary disorders are called *dermatologists*. These specialists focus on diseases of the skin and the relationship of a **cutaneous lesion** to a **systemic** disease.

Various surgical and **therapeutic** procedures are used to treat integumentary disorders, including skin transplantations, ultraviolet light therapy, and various medications. The dermatologist's practice includes treatment of skin disorders caused by internal diseases of the body. Examples are pressure ulcers that result from poor circulation and skin lesions that result from diabetes or syphilis. The dermatologist's scope of practice also includes management of skin cancers, moles, and other skin tumors. The dermatologist also uses various techniques to enhance and correct cosmetic skin defects and prescribes measures to maintain healthy skin.

Integumentary System Quick Study

The term **integumentary**, also known as *skin*, is derived from the Latin word *integumentum*, which means a *covering*. The skin is the largest organ of the body, consisting of several kinds of tissues that are structurally arranged to function together. Its elaborate system of distinct tissues includes glands that produce several types of secretions, nerves that transmit impulses, and blood vessels that help regulate body temperature. The skin itself skin contains two layers:

1. The **epidermis,** the outer layer that protects the body from the environment, prevents the entry of harmful substances, and performs many vital functions. The epidermis is **avascular** because it is composed of epithelial tissue and does not contain blood vessels.
2. The **dermis,** the skin's inner layer, is rich with blood vessels, nerve endings, **sebaceous** (oil) and **sudoriferous** (sweat) glands, and hair follicles. The **subcutaneous** tissue, which lies just beneath the dermis, binds the dermis to underlying structures. The main functions of the subcutaneous tissue are to protect the tissues and organs underneath it and to prevent heat loss.

Anatomical structures known as the accessory organs of the skin are also located within the dermis. They include, nails, sweat glands, and sebaceous glands. (See *Integumentary System*, page 48.)

 An extensive anatomy and physiology review is included in *TermPlus*, the powerful, interactive CD-ROM program.

Medical Word Building

Building medical words using word elements related to the integumentary system will enhance your understanding of those terms and reinforce your ability to use terms correctly.

Combining Forms

Begin your study of integumentary terminology by reviewing the organs and their associated combining forms (CFs) and other word elements, which are illustrated in the figure *Integumentary System* below.

Integumentary System

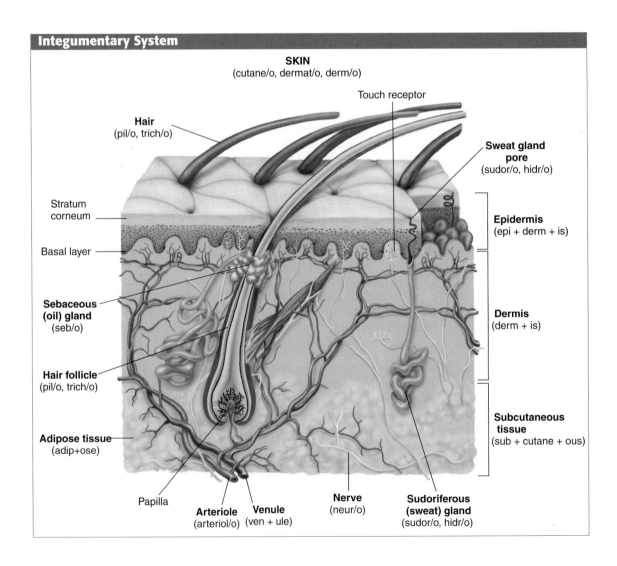

SKIN
(cutane/o, dermat/o, derm/o)

Touch receptor

Hair
(pil/o, trich/o)

Sweat gland pore
(sudor/o, hidr/o)

Stratum corneum

Epidermis
(epi + derm + is)

Basal layer

Sebaceous (oil) gland
(seb/o)

Dermis
(derm + is)

Hair follicle
(pil/o, trich/o)

Subcutaneous tissue
(sub + cutane + ous)

Adipose tissue
(adip+ose)

Papilla

Arteriole
(arteriol/o)

Venule
(ven + ule)

Nerve
(neur/o)

Sudoriferous (sweat) gland
(sudor/o, hidr/o)

In the table below, CFs are listed alphabetically and other word parts are defined as needed. Review the medical word and study the elements that make up the term. Then complete the meaning of the medical words in the right-hand column. The first one is completed for you. You may also refer to *Appendix A: Glossary of Medical Word Elements* to complete this exercise.

Combining Form	Meaning	Medical Word	Meaning
adip/o	fat	**adip/o**/cele (ĂD-ĭ-pō-sēl) *-cele:* hernia, swelling	*hernia containing fat or fatty tissue*
lip/o		**lip/o**/cyte (LĬP-ō-sīt) *-cyte:* cell	
steat/o		**steat**/oma (stē-ă-TŌ-mă) *-oma:* tumor	
cutane/o	skin	sub/**cutane**/ous (sŭb-kū-TĀ-nē-ŭs) *sub-:* under, below *-ous:* pertaining to	
dermat/o		**dermat/o**/logist (dĕr-mă-TŎL-ō-jĭst) *-logist:* specialist in the study of	
derm/o		hypo/**derm**/ic (hī-pō-DĔR-mĭk) *hypo-:* under, below, deficient *-ic:* pertaining to	
cyan/o	blue	**cyan**/osis (sī-ă-NŌ-sĭs) *-osis:* abnormal condition; increase (used primarily with blood cells)	
erythem/o	red	**erythem**/a (ĕr-ĭ-THĒ-mă) *-a:* noun ending	
erythemat/o		**erythemat**/ous (ĕr-ĭ-THĔM-ă-tŭs) *-ous:* pertaining to	
erythr/o		**erythr/o**/cyte (ĕ-RĬTH-rō-sīt) *-cyte:* cell	

(Continued)

Combining Form	Meaning	Medical Word	Meaning
hidr/o*	sweat	**hidr**/osis (hī-DRŌ-sĭs) *–osis:* abnormal condition; increase (used primarily with blood cells)	
sudor/o		**sudor**/esis (sū-dō-RĒ-sĭs) *–esis:* condition	
ichthy/o	dry, scaly	**ichthy**/osis (ĭk-thē-Ō-sĭs) *–osis:* abnormal condition; increase (used primarily with blood cells)	
kerat/o	horny tissue; hard; cornea	**kerat**/osis (kĕr-ă-TŌ-sĭs) *–osis:* abnormal condition; increase (used primarily with blood cells)	
melan/o	black	**melan**/oma (mĕl-ă-NŌ-mă) *–oma:* tumor	
myc/o	fungus (plural, *fungi)*	dermat/o/**myc**/osis (dĕr-mă-tō-mī-KŌ-sĭs) *dermat/o:* skin *–osis:* abnormal condition; increase (used primarily with blood cells)	
onych/o	nail	**onych**/o/malacia (ŏn-ĭ-kō-mă-LĀ-shē-ă) *–malacia:* softening	
pil/o	hair	**pil**/o/nid/al (pī-lō-NĪ-dăl) *nid:* nest *–al:* pertaining to	
trich/o		**trich**/o/pathy (trĭk-ŎP-ă-thē) *–pathy:* disease	

*Do not mistake hidr/o (sweat) for hydr/o (water).

Combining Form	Meaning	Medical Word	Meaning
scler/o	hardening; sclera (white of eye)	scler/o/derma (sklĕr-ō-DĔR-mă) *-derma:* skin	
seb/o	sebum, sebaceous	seb/o/rrhea (sĕb-or-Ē-ă) *-rrhea:* discharge, flow	
squam/o	scale	squam/ous (SKWĀ-mŭs) *-ous:* pertaining to	
therm/o	heat	therm/al (THĔR-măl) *-al:* pertaining to	
xer/o	dry	xer/o/derma (zē-rō-DĔR-mă) *-derma:* skin	

Suffixes and Prefixes

In the table below, suffixes and prefixes are listed alphabetically and other word parts are defined as needed. Review the medical word and study the elements that make up the term. Then complete the meaning of the medical words in the right-hand column. You may also refer to *Appendix A: Glossary of Medical Word Elements* to complete this exercise.

Word Element	Meaning	Medical Word	Meaning
Suffixes			
-cyte	cell	leuk/o/**cyte** (LOO-kō-sīt) *leuk/o:* white	
-derma	skin	py/o/**derma** (pī-ō-DĔR-mă)	
-oma	tumor	carcin/**oma** (KĂR-sĭ-NŌ-mă) *carcin:* cancer Get a closer look at carcinomas on page 63 and page 64.	
-phoresis	carrying, transmission	dia/**phoresis** (dī-ă-fō-RĒ-sĭs) *dia-:* through, across	

(Continued)

Word Element	Meaning	Medical Word	Meaning
Suffixes			
-plasty	surgical repair	dermat/o/**plasty** (DĚR-mă-tō-plăs-tē) *dermat/o:* skin	
-therapy	treatment	cry/o/**therapy** (krī-ō-THĔR-ă-pē) *cry/o:* cold	
Prefixes			
an-	without, not	**an**/hidr/osis (ăn-hī-DRŌ-sĭs) *hidr:* sweat *-osis:* abnormal condition; increase (used primarily with blood cells)	
epi-	above, upon	**epi**/derm/oid (ĕp-ĭ-DĚR-moyd) *derm:* skin *-oid:* resembling	
homo-	same	**homo**/graft (HŌ-mō-grăft) *-graft:* transplantation	
hyper-	excessive, above normal	**hyper**/hidr/osis (hī-pĕr-hī-DRŌ-sĭs) *hidr:* sweat *-osis:* abnormal condition; increase (used primarily with blood cells)	

 Competency Verification: Check your answers in Appendix B, Answer Key, page 358. If you are not satisfied with your level of comprehension, review the terms in the table and retake the review.

 Listen and Learn, the audio CD-ROM included in this book, will help you master pronunciation of selected medical words. Use it to practice pronunciations of the medical terms in the above "Word Building" tables and for instructions to complete the *Listen and Learn* exercise.

 Flash-Card Activity. Enhance your study and reinforcement of this chapter's word elements with the power of the DavisPlus flash-card activity. Do so by visiting *http://davisplus.fadavis.com/gylys-express.* We recommend you complete the flash-card activity before continuing with the next section.

Medical Terminology Word Building

In this section, combine the word parts you have learned to construct medical terms related to the integumentary system.

Use *adip/o* or *lip/o* (fat) to build medical words that mean:

1. tumor consisting of fat _____

2. cell consisting of fat _____

Use *ichthy/o* (dry, scaly) to build a word that means:

3. abnormal condition of dry, scaly (skin) _____

Use *onych/o* (nail) to build medical words that mean:

4. tumor of the nail _____

5. disease of nails _____

6. softening of nails _____

Use *trich/o* (hair) to build medical words that mean:

7. disease of the hair _____

8. abnormal condition of the hair _____

Use *xer/o* (dry) to build medical words that mean:

9. skin that is dry _____

10. abnormal condition of dryness _____

Use the suffix *-cyte* (cell) to build medical words that mean:

11. red cell _____

12. white cell _____

13. black cell _____

Use prefixes *an-* (without, not) or *hyper-* (excessive, above normal) to build medical words that mean:

14. abnormal condition without sweat _____

15. abnormal condition of excessive sweat _____

Competency Verification: Check your answers in Appendix B, Answer Key, on page 359. Review material that you did not answer correctly.

Correct Answers _____ × **6.67 =** _____ **%**

Additional Medical Vocabulary

The following tables list additional terms related to the integumentary system. Recognizing and learning these terms will help you understand the connection between common signs, symptoms, diseases, and their diagnoses. Included are medical and surgical procedures as well as pharmacological agents used to treat diseases.

Signs, Symptoms, and Diseases

abrasion ă -BRĀ-zhŭn	Scraping or rubbing away of a surface, such as skin, by friction
abscess ĂB-sĕs	Localized collection of pus at the site of an infection (characteristically a staphylococcal infection)
furuncle FŪ-rŭng-kl	Abscess that originates in a hair follicle; also called *boil*
carbuncle KĂR-bŭng-kl	Cluster of furuncles in the subcutaneous tissue (See Figure 3-1.)
acne ĂK-nē	Inflammatory disease of sebaceous follicles of the skin, marked by comedos (blackheads), papules, and pustules (small skin lesion filled with purulent material)
alopecia ăl-ō-PĒ-shē-ă	Absence or loss of hair, especially of the head; also known as *baldness*

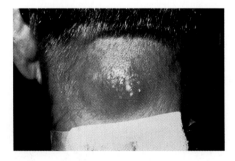

Figure 3–1. Dome-shaped abscess that has formed a furuncle in hair follicles of the neck. (From Goldsmith, LA, Lazarus, GS, and Tharp, MD: *Adult and Pediatric Dermatology: A Color Guide to Diagnosis and Treatment.* FA Davis, Philadelphia, 1997, p 364, with permission.)

burn	Tissue injury caused by contact with a thermal, chemical, electrical, or radioactive agent
first-degree (superficial)	Mild burn affecting the epidermis and characterized by redness and pain with no blistering or scar formation
second-degree (partial thickness)	Burn affecting the epidermis and part of the dermis and characterized by redness, blistering or larger bullae, and pain with little or no scarring (See Figure 3-2.)
third-degree (full thickness)	Severe burn characterized by destruction of the epidermis and dermis with damage to the subcutaneous layer, leaving the skin charred black or dry white in appearance with insensitivity to touch

carcinoma kăr-sĭ-NŌ-mă	Uncontrolled growth of abnormal cells in the body; also called *malignant cells*
melanoma mĕl-ă-NŌ-mă	Malignant tumor that originates in melanocytes and is considered the most dangerous type of skin cancer, which, if not treated early, becomes difficult to cure and can be fatal

 Get a closer look at carcinomas, page 63 and page 64.

comedo KŎM-ē-dō	Discolored, dried sebum plugging an excretory duct of the skin; also called *blackhead*

cyst SĬST	Closed sac or pouch in or under the skin with a definite wall that contains fluid, semifluid, or solid material
pilonidal pī-lō-NĪ-dăl	Growth of hair in a dermoid cyst or in a sinus opening on the skin
sebaceous sē-BĀ-shŭs	Cyst filled with sebum (fatty material) from a sebaceous gland

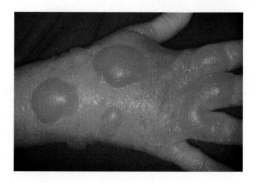

Figure 3–2. Second-degree (partial thickness burn). (From Goldsmith, LA, Lazarus, GS, and Tharp, MD: *Adult and Pediatric Dermatology: A Color Guide to Diagnosis and Treatment.* FA Davis, Philadelphia, 1997, p 318, with permission.)

eczema ĔK-zĕ-mă	Redness of skin caused by swelling of the capillaries (See Figure 3-3.)
gangrene GĂNG-grēn	Death of tissue, usually resulting from loss of blood supply

hemorrhage
HĔM-ĕ-rĭj
   hem/o: blood
   -rrhage: bursting forth (of)
	External or internal loss of a large amount of blood in a short period

contusion kŏn-TOO-zhŭn	Hemorrhage of any size under the skin in which the skin is not broken; also known as a *bruise*
ecchymosis ĕk-ĭ-MŌ-sĭs	Skin discoloration consisting of a large, irregularly formed hemorrhagic area with colors changing from blue-black to greenish brown or yellow; commonly called a *bruise* (See Figure 3-4.)
petechia pē-TĒ-kē-ă	Minute, pinpoint hemorrhagic spot of the skin that is a smaller version of an ecchymosis

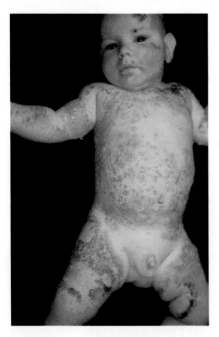

Figure 3–3. Scattered eczema of the trunk of an infant. (From Goldsmith, LA, Lazarus, GS, and Tharp, MD: *Adult and Pediatric Dermatology: A Color Guide to Diagnosis and Treatment.* FA Davis, Philadelphia, 1997, p 243, with permission.)

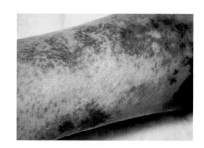

Figure 3–4. Ecchymosis. (From Harmening, DM: *Clinical Hematology and Fundamentals of Hemostasis,* ed 4. FA Davis, Philadelphia, 2001, p 489, with permission.)

hematoma hēm-ă-TŌ-mă *hemat:* blood *-oma:* tumor	Elevated, localized collection of blood trapped under the skin that usually results from trauma
hirsutism HŬR-sūt-ĭzm	Excessive growth of hair in unusual places, especially in women; may be due to hypersecretion of testosterone
ichthyosis ĭk-thē-Ō-sĭs *ichthy/o:* dry, scaly *-osis:* abnormal condition; increase (used primarily with blood cells)	Genetic skin disorder in which the skin is dry and scaly, resembling fish skin due to a defect in keratinization (See Figure 3-5.)
impetigo ĭm-pĕ-TĪ-gō	Bacterial skin infection characterized by isolated pustules that become crusted and rupture

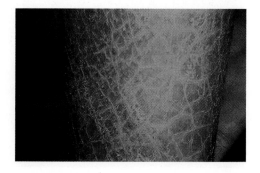

Figure 3–5. Ichthyosis. (From Goldsmith, LA, Lazarus, GS, and Tharp, MD: *Adult and Pediatric Dermatology: A Color Guide to Diagnosis and Treatment.* FA Davis, Philadelphia, 1997, p 129, with permission.)

keloid KĒ-lŏyd	Overgrowth of scar tissue at the site of a skin injury (especially a wound, surgical incision, or severe burn) due to excessive collagen formation during the healing process
psoriasis sō-RĪ-ă-sĭs	Chronic skin disease characterized by itchy red patches covered with silvery scales (See Figure 3-6.)
scabies SKĀ-bēz	Contagious skin disease transmitted by the itch mite
skin lesions LĒ-zhŭnz	Areas of pathologically altered tissue caused by disease, injury, or a wound due to external factors or internal disease
tinea TĬN-ē-ă	Fungal infection whose name commonly indicates the body part affected, such as tinea pedis (athlete's foot); also called *ringworm*
ulcer ŬL-sĕr	Lesion of the skin or mucous membranes marked by inflammation, necrosis, and sloughing of damaged tissues
pressure ulcer	Skin ulceration caused by prolonged pressure, usually in a person who is bedridden; also known as *decubitus ulcer* or *bedsore*

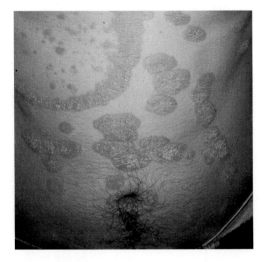

Figure 3–6. Psoriasis. (From Goldsmith, LA, Lazarus, GS, and Tharp, MD: *Adult and Pediatric Dermatology: A Color Guide to Diagnosis and Treatment.* FA Davis, Philadelphia, 1997, p 258, with permission.)

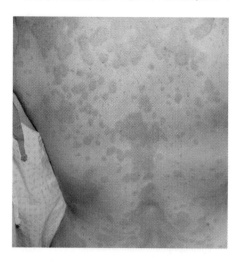

Figure 3–7. Urticaria. (From Goldsmith, LA, Lazarus, GS, and Tharp, MD: *Adult and Pediatric Dermatology: A Color Guide to Diagnosis and Treatment.* FA Davis, Philadelphia, 1997, p 209, with permission.)

urticaria ŭr-tĭ-KĂR-ē-ă	Allergic reaction of the skin characterized by eruption of pale red elevated patches that are intensely itchy; also called *wheals (hives)* (See Figure 3-7.)
verruca vĕr-ROO-kă	Rounded epidermal growth caused by a virus; also called *wart*
vesicle VĔS-ĭ-kl	Small blister-like elevation on the skin containing a clear fluid; large vesicles are called *bullae* (singular: bulla)
vitiligo vĭt-ĭl-Ī-gō	Localized loss of skin pigmentation characterized by milk-white patches; also called *leukoderma* (See Figure 3-8.)
wheal hwēl	Smooth, slightly elevated skin that is white in the center with a pale red periphery; also called *hives* if itchy

Diagnostic Procedures

biopsy (bx)
BĪ-ŏp-sē
   bi: life
   -opsy: view of
	Removal of a small piece of living tissue from an organ or other part of the body for microscopic examination to confirm or establish a diagnosis, estimate prognosis, or follow the course of a disease

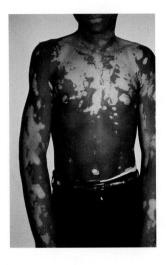

Figure 3–8. Vitiligo. (From Goldsmith, LA, Lazarus, GS, and Tharp, MD: *Adult and Pediatric Dermatology: A Color Guide to Diagnosis and Treatment.* FA Davis, Philadelphia, 1997, p 121, with permission.)

skin test	Any test in which a suspected allergen or sensitizer is applied to or injected into the skin to determine the patient's sensitivity to it (See Figure 3-9.)

Medical and Surgical Procedures

cryosurgery krī-ō-SĔR-jĕr-ē *cry/o:* cold	Use of subfreezing temperature, commonly with liquid nitrogen, to destroy abnormal tissue cells, such as unwanted, cancerous, or infected tissue

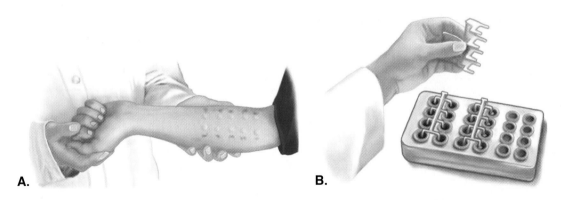

A.   **B.**

Figure 3–9. Skin tests. (A) Intradermal allergy test reactions. (B) Scratch (prick) skin test kit for allergy testing.

debridement dā-brēd-MŎN *or* dĭ-BRĒD-mĕnt	Removal of foreign material, damaged tissue, or cellular debris from a wound or burn to prevent infection and promote healing
fulguration fŭl-gū-RĀ-shŭn	Tissue destruction by means of high-frequency electric current; also called *electrodesiccation*
incision and drainage (I&D)	Incision of a lesion, such as an abscess, followed by the drainage of its contents
Mohs surgery mōz	Surgical procedure used primarily to treat skin neoplasms in which tumor tissue fixed in place is removed layer by layer for microscopic examination until the entire tumor is removed
skin graft	Surgical procedure to transplant healthy tissue by applying it to an injured site

allograft
   ĂL-ō-grăft
     allo: other, differing
       from normal
     -graft: transplantation
	Transplantation of healthy tissue from one person to another person; also called *homograft*

autograft
   AW-tō-grăft
     auto: self, own
     -graft: transplantation
	Transplantation of healthy tissue from one site to another site in the same individual

synthetic sĭn-THĔT-ĭk	Transplantation of artificial skin produced from collagen fibers arranged in a lattice pattern

xenograft
   ZĔN-ō-grăft
     xen/o: foreign, strange
     -graft: transplantation
	Transplantation (dermis only) from a foreign donor (usually a pig) and transferred to a human; also called *heterograft*

skin resurfacing	Procedure that repairs damaged skin, acne scars, fine or deep wrinkles, or tatoos or improves skin tone irregularities through the use of topical chemicals, abrasion, or laser
chemical peel	Use of chemicals to remove outer layers of skin to treat acne scarring and general keratoses as well as for cosmetic purposes to remove fine wrinkles on the face; also called *chemabrasion*
cutaneous laser kū-TĀ-nē-ŭs *cutane:* skin *-ous:* pertaining to	Any of several laser treatments employed for cosmetic and plastic surgery
dermabrasion DĔRM-ă-brā-zhŭn	Removal of acne scars, nevi, tattoos, or fine wrinkles on the skin through the use of sandpaper, wire brushes, or other abrasive materials on the epidermal layer

Pharmacology

antibiotics ăn-tĭ-bī-ŎT-ĭks	Kill bacteria that cause skin infections
antifungals ăn-tĭ-FŬNG-găls	Kill fungi that infect the skin
antipruritics ăn-tĭ-proo-RĬT-ĭks	Reduce severe itching
corticosteroids kor-tĭ-kō-STĔR-oyds	Anti-inflammatory agents that treat skin inflammation

Pronunciation Help	Long Sound Short Sound	ā in rāte ă in ălone	ē in rēbirth ĕ in ĕver	ī in īsle ĭ in ĭt	ō in ōver ŏ in nŏt	ū in ūnite ŭ in cŭt

Closer Look

Take a closer look at these integumentary disorders to enhance your understanding of the medical terminology associated with them.

Basal Cell Carcinoma

Basal cell carcinoma, the most common type of **nonmelanoma skin cancer,** is a cancerous tumor **(malignancy)** of the basal layer of the epidermis, or hair follicles. Basal cell carcinoma is commonly caused by overexposure to sunlight. Although basal cell carcinomas rarely invade distant structures of the body **(metastasize),** they tend to recur—especially those that are larger than 2 cm. However, this skin cancer can invade the tissue sufficiently to destroy an ear, nose, or eyelid. Basal cell carcinoma is most prevalent in blond, fair-skinned men and is the most common malignant tumor affecting white people. Although these tumors grow slowly, they commonly ulcerate as they increase in size and develop crusting that is firm to the touch. Depending on the location, size, and depth of the lesion, treatment includes surgical excision, **curettage and electrodessication, cryosurgery,** or **radiation therapy.** The illustration below shows a late stage of basal cell carcinoma (A) and common sites of basal cell carcinoma (B).

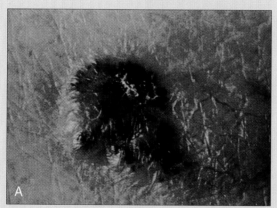
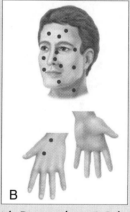

(From Goldsmith, LA, Lazarus, GS, and Tharp, MD: *Adult and Pediatric Dermatology: A Color Guide to Diagnosis and Treatment.* FA Davis, Philadelphia, 1997, p 144, with permission.)

(Continued)

Closer Look–cont'd

Squamous Cell Carcinoma

Squamous cell carcinoma (SCC) is the second most common form of nonmelanoma skin cancer after basal cell carcinoma. When caught and treated early, it rarely causes further problems. Untreated, SCC can grow large or metastasize, causing serious complications.

The incidence of skin cancers is rising every year; likely due to increased sun exposure. Most squamous cell carcinomas result from prolonged exposure to **ultraviolet (UV) radiation,** either from sunlight or from tanning beds or lamps. Avoiding UV light as much as possible is the best protection. Sunscreen is an important part of a sun-safety program, but by itself doesn't completely prevent squamous cell carcinoma or other types of skin cancer. The illustration below shows squamous cell carcinoma on the skin (A) and common sites on sun-exposed areas of the skin (B).

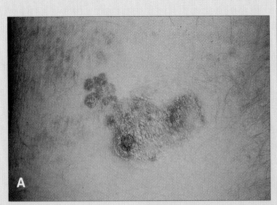
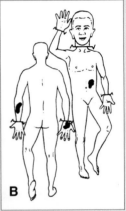

(From Goldsmith, LA, Lazarus, GS, and Tharp, MD: *Adult and Pediatric Dermatology: A Color Guide to Diagnosis and Treatment.* FA Davis Philadelphia, 1997, p 237, with permission.)

Additional Medical Vocabulary Recall

Match the medical term(s) below with the definitions in the numbered list.

alopecia	debridement	pressure ulcer
autograft	dermabrasion	scabies
biopsy	eczema	tinea
comedo	hirsutism	verruca
cryosurgery	metastasize	vitiligo

1. _____ is a rounded epidermal growth caused by a virus.

2. _____ is localized loss of skin pigmentation characterized by appearance of milk-white patches.

3. _____ is a fungal skin disease, commonly called ringworm, whose name indicates the body part affected.

4. _____ is ulceration caused by prolonged pressure; also called decubitus ulcer.

5. _____ is a general term for an itchy red rash that may become crusted, thickened, or scaly.

6. _____ is a type of skin graft taken from a different site of the same patient's body

7. _____ refers to excision of a small piece of living tissue from an organ or other part of the body for microscopic examination.

8. _____ refers to use of revolving wire brushes or sandpaper to remove superficial scars on the skin.

9. _____ is excessive growth of hair, in unusual places, especially in women.

10. _____ refers to use of liquid nitrogen to destroy or eliminate abnormal tissue cells.

11. _____ refers to removal of foreign material and dead or damaged tissue, especially in a wound.

12. _____ is a contagious skin disease transmitted by the itch mite.

13. _____ is absence or loss of hair, especially of the head; baldness.

14. _____ is a blackhead.

15. _____ means to spread or invade distant structures of the body.

 Competency Verification: Check your answers in Appendix B, Answer Key, on page 359. Review material that you did not answer correctly.

Correct Answers _____ × **6.67 =** _____ %

Pronunciation and Spelling

Use the following list to practice correct pronunciation and spelling of medical terms. Practice the pronunciation aloud and then write the correct spelling of the term. The first word is completed for you.

Pronunciation	Spelling
1. ă-BRĀ-zhŭn	*abrasion*
2. ĂB-sĕs	
3. ĂK-nē	
4. ăl-ō-PĒ-shē-ă	
5. BĪ-ŏp-sē	
6. krī-ō-THĔR-ă-pē	
7. dī-ă-fō-RĒ-sĭs	
8. ĕp-ĭ-DĔR-moyd	
9. ĕr-ĭ-THĔM-ă-tŭs	
10. FŪ-rŭng-kl	
11. KĒ-lŏyd	
12. hēm-ă-TŌ-mă	
13. HŬR-sūt-ĭzm	
14. LĒ-zhŭnz	
15. ŏn-ĭ-kō-mă-LĀ-shē-ă	
16. pē-TĒ-kē-ă	
17. SKĀ-bēz	
18. sō-RĪ-ă-sĭs	
19. sĕb-or-Ē-ă	
20. vĭt-ĭl-Ī-gō	

 Competency Verification: Check your answers in Appendix B, Answer Key, on page 359. Review material that you did not answer correctly.

Correct Answers: _____ × 5 = _____ %

Abbreviations

The table below introduces abbreviations associated with the integumentary system.

Abbreviation	Meaning	Abbreviation	Meaning
Bx, bx	biopsy	IMP	impression (synonymous with *diagnosis*)
CA	cancer; chronological age; cardiac arrest	PE	physical examination; pulmonary embolism; pressure-equalizing (tube)
Derm	dermatology	SCC	squamous cell carcinoma
FH	family history	subcu, Sub-Q, subQ	subcutaneous (injection)
I&D	incision and drainage; irrigation and debridement	UV	ultraviolet
IM	intramuscular	WBC	white blood count

Chart Notes

Chart notes comprise part of the medical record and are used in various types of health care facilities. The chart notes that follow were dictated by the patient's physician and reflect common clinical events using medical terminology to document the patient's care. By studying and completing the terminology and chart note analysis sections below you will learn and understand terms associated with the medical specialty of dermatology.

Terminology

The following terms are linked to chart notes in the specialty of dermatology. First, practice pronouncing each term aloud. Then, use a medical dictionary such as *Taber's Cyclopedic Medical Dictionary, Appendix A: Glossary of Medical Word Elements*, page 337, or other resources to define each term.

Term	Meaning
Bartholin gland BĂR-tō-lĭn	
colitis kō-LĪ-tĭs	

(Continued)

Term	Meaning
diabetes mellitus dī-ă-BĒ-tēz MĔ-lĭ-tŭs	
diaphoresis dī-ă-fō-RĒ-sĭs	
enteritis ĕn-tĕr-Ī-tĭs	
erythematous ĕr-ĭ-THĔM-ă-tŭs	
FH	
histiocytoma hĭs-tē-ō-sī-TŌ-mă	
macules MĂK-ūlz	
papules PĂP-ūlz	
pruritus proo-RĪ-tŭs	
psoriasis sō-RĪ-ă-sĭs	
sclerosed sklĕ-RŌST	
sinusitis sī-nŭs-Ī-tĭs	
syncope SĬN-kō-pē	
vulgaris vŭl-GĂ-rĭs	

Visit *http://DavisPlus.fadavis.com/gylys-express* for the terminology pronunciation exercise associated with this chart note.

Psoriasis

Read the chart note below aloud. Underline any term you have trouble pronouncing or cannot define. If needed, refer to the Terminology section above for correct pronunciations and meanings of terms.

This is a 32-year-old female who experienced intermittent psoriasis since her early teens in various stages of severity. Her condition has become more troublesome over the past year because of an increase of symptoms after being exposed to the sun. Her past history indicates she had chronic sinusitis of 3 years' duration. Her Bartholin gland was excised in 20xx. She has had pruritus of the scalp and abdominal regions. There is no FH of psoriasis. An uncle has had diabetes mellitus since age 43. Patient has occasional abdominal pains accompanied with diaphoresis and/or syncope. PE showed the patient has psoriatic involvement of the scalp, external ears, trunk, and, to a lesser degree, on the legs. There are many scattered erythematous (light ruby colored) thickened plaques covered by thick yellowish white scales. A few areas on the legs and arms show multiple, sclerosed, brown macules and papules.

Diagnoses:
1. Psoriasis vulgaris.
2. Multiple histiocytomas.
3. Abdominal pains, by history.
4. Rule out colitis, regional enteritis.

Chart Note Analysis

From the chart note above, select the medical word that means

1. discolored area on the skin that is not elevated: _____

2. condition that comes and goes: _____

3. fainting episode: _____

4. common or ordinary: _____

5. inflammation of the colon: _____

6. of long duration: _____

7. hardened: _____

8. inflammation of small intestine: _____

9. severe itching: _____

10. mucous gland at the vaginal opening: _____

11. skin disease characterized by itchy red patches covered with silvery scales: _____

12. redness of the skin due to capillary dilation: _____

13. inflammation of the sinus cavity: _____

14. elevated lesion containing pus,(as seen in acne and psoriasis) is known as: _____

15. synonymous with hyperhidrosis and sudoresis: _____

✓ **Competency Verification:** Check your answers in Appendix B, Answer Key, on page 359.
Review material that you did not answer correctly.

Correct Answers: _____ × **6.67 =** _____ %

Demonstrate What You Know!

To evaluate your understanding of how medical terms you have studied in this and previous chapters are used in a clinical environment, complete the numbered sentences by selecting an appropriate term from the list below.

antibiotic	ichthyosis	pyoderma
carcinoma	lipocyte	psoriasis
dermatologist	mycosis	sebaceous
dermis	onychomalacia	sudoriferous
epidermis	onychopathy	xenograft

1. Layer of skin containing blood vessels, oil and sweat glands, and hair follicles is the _____.

2. When a person sweats, the _____ glands are working.

3. If there is disease of the nail bed, the condition is charted _____.

4. The Dx for a patient with a fungal infection of the skin is _____.

5. A skin transplantation from a foreign donor to a human is a(n) _____.

6. Layer of skin that does not have blood or nerve supplies is the _____.

7. A physician who specializes in treating skin disorders is known as a _____.

8. _____ glands are oil-producing glands of the skin.

9. The Dx of a patient with a cancerous tumor is _____.

10. Hereditary skin disorder characterized by fine, small flaky, white scales is called _____.

11. A patient who exhibits softening of the nails has the condition called _____.

12. A(n) _____ kills bacteria that cause skin infections.

13. A fat-storing cell is called a(n) _____.

14. Chronic skin disease characterized by itchy red patches covered with silvery scales is _____.

15. The medical term for pus in the skin is _____.

Competency Verification: Check your answers in Appendix B, Answer Key, on page 360. Review material that you did not answer correctly.

Correct Answers: _____ × **6.67** = _____ %

Multimedia Review. If you are not satisfied with your retention level of the integumentary chapter, go to *http://davisplus.fadavis.com/gylys-express* to complete the website activities linked to this chapter. It is your choice whether or not you want to take advantage of these reinforcement exercises before continuing with the next chapter.

Respiratory System

MULTIMEDIA STUDY TOOLS.
To enrich your medical terminology skills, look for this multimedia icon throughout the text. It will help alert you to when it is best to use the various multimedia resources available with this textbook to enhance your studies.

Objectives

Upon completion of this chapter, you will be able to:

- Identify four types of medical treatment provided by pulmonary specialists.
- List three primary functions of the respiratory system.
- Identify the primary structures of the respiratory system.
- Briefly describe the pathway of inhaled and exhaled air through the respiratory tract.
- Identify combining forms, suffixes, and prefixes associated with the respiratory system.
- Recognize, pronounce, build, and spell medical terms and abbreviations associated with the respiratory system.
- Demonstrate your knowledge by successfully completing the activities in this chapter.

Vocabulary Preview

Term	Meaning
diagnosis dī-ăg-NŌ-sĭs *dia-:* through, across *gnos:* knowing *-is:* noun ending	Identification of a disease or condition by a scientific evaluation of physical signs, symptoms, history, laboratory test results, and procedures
pulmonary PŬL-mō-nĕ-rē *pulmon:* lung *-ary:* pertaining to	Pertaining to the lungs or the respiratory system
respiration rĕs-pĭr-Ā-shŭn	Molecular exchange of oxygen and carbon dioxide within the body's tissues; also called *breathing, pulmonary ventilation,* or *ventilation*
thoracic thō-RĂS-ĭk *thorac:* chest *-ic:* pertaining to	Pertaining to the thorax or thoracic cage (bony enclosure formed by the sternum, costal cartilages, ribs, and the bodies of the thoracic vertebrae)
vascular VĂS-kū-lăr *vascul:* vessel (usually blood or lymph) *-ar:* pertaining to	Pertaining to a blood vessel

Pronunciation Help	Long Sound	ā in rāte	ē in rēbirth	ī in īsle	ō in ōver	ū in ūnite
	Short Sound	ă in ălone	ĕ in ĕver	ĭ in ĭt	ŏ in nŏt	ŭ in cŭt

Pulmonology

The respiratory system is associated with the medical specialty of **pulmonology**, also known as ***pulmonary*** medicine. This branch of medicine focuses on treatment of diseases involving the structures of the lower respiratory tract, including the lungs, their airways, and the chest wall (**thoracic** cage).

Medical doctors who treat respiratory disorders are called *pulmonologists. Pulmonologists* treat such pulmonary disorders as asthma, **emphysema**, chronic **bronchitis**, occupational and industrial lung disease, and **pulmonary vascular** disease. Pulmonologists also care for patients who require specialized ventilator support and lung transplantation.

In general, pulmonologists diagnose and manage pulmonary disorders and acute and chronic respiratory failure. **Diagnosis** and management of pulmonary disorders may include administering pulmonary function tests, arterial blood gas analysis, chest x-rays, and chemical or microbiological tests.

Respiratory System Quick Study

The **respiratory system** consists of the nose, pharynx, larynx, trachea, bronchial tubes, lungs, and breathing muscles. All of these organs work together to perform the mechanical and, for the most part, unconscious mechanism of **respiration.** Respiration, or breathing, consists of external and internal processes:

- In **external respiration,** oxygen (O_2) is inhaled into the lungs and absorbed into the bloodstream. Carbon dioxide leaves the bloodstream and enters the lungs where it is expelled during exhalation.
- In **internal respiration,** oxygen and carbon dioxide (CO_2) are exchanged at the cellular level. Oxygen leaves the bloodstream and is delivered to the tissue cells, where it is used for energy. In exchange, carbon dioxide enters the bloodstream from the tissues and is transported back to the lungs for removal. (See *Respiratory System,* page 76.)

 An extensive anatomy and physiology review is included in *TermPlus,* the powerful, interactive CD-ROM program.

Medical Word Building

Building medical words using word elements related to the respiratory system will enhance your understanding of those terms and reinforce your ability to use terms correctly.

Combining Forms

Begin your study of respiratory terminology by reviewing the organs and their associated combining forms (CFs), which are illustrated in the figure *Respiratory System* on the next page.

Respiratory System

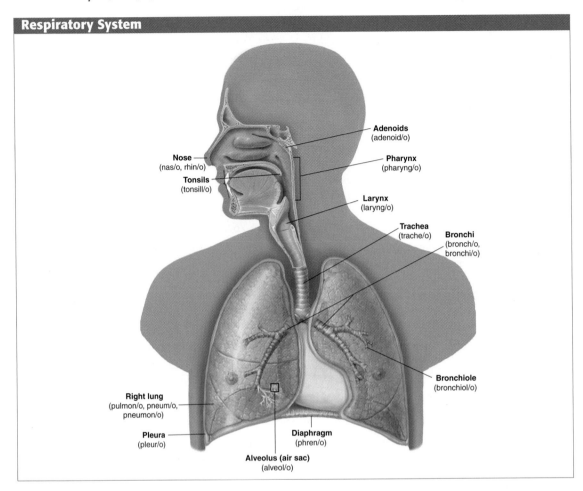

In the table below, CFs are listed alphabetically and other word parts are defined as needed. Review the medical word and study the elements that make up the term. Then complete the meaning of the medical words in the right-hand column. The first one is completed for you. You may also refer to *Appendix A: Glossary of Medical Word Elements* to complete this exercise.

Combining Form	Meaning	Medical Word	Meaning
Upper Respiratory Tract			
adenoid/o	adenoids	**adenoid**/ectomy (ăd-ĕ-noyd-ĔK-tō-mē) *-ectomy:* excision, removal	*excision of the adenoids*
laryng/o	larynx (voice box)	**laryng/o**/scope (lăr-ĬN-gō-skōp) *-scope:* instrument for examining	

Combining Form	Meaning	Medical Word	Meaning
Upper Respiratory Tract			
nas/o	nose	**nas**/al (NĂ-zl) *-al:* pertaining to	
rhin/o		**rhin/o**/rrhea (rī-nō-RĒ-ă) *-rrhea:* discharge, flow	
pharyng/o	pharynx (throat)	**pharyng/o**/spasm (far-ĬN-gō-spăzm) *-spasm:* involuntary contraction, twitching	
tonsill/o	tonsils	**tonsill**/ectomy (tŏn-sĭl-ĔK-tō-mē) *-ectomy:* excision, removal	
trache/o	trachea (windpipe)	**trache/o**/tomy (trā-kē-ŎT-ō-mē) *-tomy:* incision	
Lower Respiratory Tract			
alveo/o	alveolus; air sac	**alveo**/ar (ăl-VĒ-ō-lăr) *-ar:* pertaining to	
bronch/o	bronchus (plural, bronchi)	**bronch/o**/scopy (brŏng-KŎS-kō-pē) *-scopy:* visual examination Get a closer look at bronchoscopy on page 91.	
bronchi/o		**bronchi**/ectasis (brŏng-kē-ĔK-tă-sĭs) *-ectasis:* expansion, dilation	
bronchiol/o	bronchiole	**bronchiol**/itis (brŏng-kē-ō-LĪ-tĭs) *-itis:* inflammation	
phren/o	diaphragm	**phren**/algia (frĕ-NĂL-jē-ă) *-algia:* pain	

(Continued)

Combining Form	Meaning	Medical Word	Meaning
Lower Respiratory Tract			
pleur/o	pleura	**pleur/o**/dynia (ploo-rō-DĬN-ē-ă) *-dynia:* pain	

pneum/o	air; lung	**pneum**/o/melan/osis
		(nū-mō-měl-ăn-Ō-sĭs)
		melan: black
		  -osis: abnormal condi-
		    tion; increase
		    (used primarily
		    with blood cells	

pneumon/o		**pneumon**/ia (nū-MŌ-nē-ă) *-ia:* condition	
pulmon/o	lung	**pulmon/o**/logist (pŭl-mŏ-NŎL-ŏ-jĭst) *-logist:* specialist in the study of	
thorac/o	chest	**thorac/o**/pathy (thō-răk-ŎP-ă-thē) *-pathy:* disease	
Other Related Combining Forms			
aer/o	air	**aer/o**/phagia (ěr-ō-FĀ-jē-ă) *-phagia:* swallowing, eating	
cyan/o	blue	**cyan**/osis (sī-ă-NŌ-sĭs) *-osis:* abnormal condi- tion; increase (used primarily with blood cells)	
mastoid/o	mastoid process (houses air cells which direct sound waves into the inner ear)	**mastoid**/itis (măs-toyd-Ī-tĭs) *-itis:* inflammation	
muc/o	mucus	**muc**/oid (MŪ-koyd) *-oid:* resembling	

Combining Form	Meaning	Medical Word	Meaning
Other Related Combining Forms			
myc/o	fungus	**myc**/osis (mī-KŌ-sĭs) *-osis:* abnormal condition; increase (used primarily with blood cells)	
orth/o	straight	**orth/o/pnea** (or-THŎP-nē-ă) *-pnea:* breathing	
py/o	pus	**py/o/**thorax (pī-ō-THŌ-răks) *-thorax:* chest	

Suffixes and Prefixes

In the table below, suffixes and prefixes are listed alphabetically and other word parts are defined as needed. Review the medical word and study the elements that make up the term. Then complete the meaning of the medical words in the right-hand column. You may also refer to *Appendix A: Glossary of Medical Word Elements* to complete this exercise.

Word Element	Meaning	Medical Word	Meaning
Suffixes			
-oma	tumor	chondr/**oma** (kŏn-DRŌ-mă) *chondr/o:* cartilage	
-plasty	surgical repair	rhin/o/**plasty** (RĪ-nō-plăs-tē) *rhin/o:* nose	
-plegia	paralysis	laryng/o/**plegia** (lă-rĭn-gō-PLĒ-jē-ă) *laryng/o:* larynx (voice box)	
Prefixes			
a-	without, not	**a/**pnea (ăp-NĒ-ă) *-pnea:* breathing Get a closer look at apnea on page 92.	

(Continued)

Word Element	Meaning	Medical Word	Meaning
Prefixes			
brady-	slow	**brady**/pnea (brăd-ĭp-NĒ-ă) *-pnea:* breathing	
dys-	bad; painful; difficult	**dys**/pnea (dĭsp-NĒ-ă) *-pnea:* breathing	
eu-	good, normal	**eu**/pnea (ūp-NĒ-ă) *-pnea:* breathing	
tachy-	rapid	**tachy**/pnea (tăk-ĭp-NĒ-ă) *-pnea:* breathing	

 Competency Verification: Check your answers in Appendix B, Answer Key, page 360. If you are not satisfied with your level of comprehension, review the terms in the table and retake the review.

 Listen and Learn, the audio CD-ROM included in this book, will help you master pronunciation of selected medical words. Use it to practice pronunciations of the medical terms in the above "Word Building" tables and for instructions to complete the *Listen and Learn* exercise.

 Flash-Card Activity. Enhance your study and reinforcement of this chapter's word elements with the power of the DavisPlus flash-card activity. Do so by visiting *http://davisplus.fadavis.com/gylys-express.* We recommend you complete the flash-card activity before continuing with the next section.

Medical Terminology Word Building

In this section, combine the word parts you have learned to construct medical terms related to the respiratory system.

Use *rhin/o* (nose) to build words that mean:

1. surgical repair of the nose _____

2. watery discharge from the nose _____

Use *laryng/o* larynx (voice box) to build words that mean:

3. paralysis of the larynx _____

4. inflammation of the larynx _____

Use *bronch/o* or *bronchi/o* (bronchus) to build words that mean:

5. dilation or expansion of the bronchus _____

6. visual examination of the bronchus _____

Use *pleur/o* (pleura) to build words that mean:

7. pain in the pleura _____

8. inflammation of the pleura _____

Use *cyan/o* (blue) to build a word that means:

9. abnormal condition of blue (skin) _____

Use *-pnea* (breathing) to build words that mean:

10. difficult or painful breathing _____

11. slow breathing _____

12. rapid breathing _____

13. good or normal breathing_____

Use *-thorax* (chest) to build a word that means:

14. pus in the thorax _____

Use *-phagia* (swallowing) to build a word that means:

15. swallowing air_____

Competency Verification: Check your answers in Appendix B, Answer Key, on page 361. Review material that you did not answer correctly.

Correct Answers _____ × **6.67 =** _____ %

Additional Medical Vocabulary

The following tables list additional terms related to the respiratory system. Recognizing and learning these terms will help you understand the connection between common signs, symptoms, and diseases and their diagnoses. Included are medical and surgical procedures as well as pharmacological agents used to treat diseases.

Signs, Symptoms, and Diseases

abnormal breath sounds	Abnormal sounds heard during inhalation or expiration, with or without a stethoscope
crackles KRĂK-ălz	Fine crackling or bubbling sounds, commonly heard during inspiration when there is fluid in the alveoli; also called *rales*.
friction rub	Dry, grating sound heard with a stethoscope during auscultation (listening for sounds within the body)
rhonchi RŎNG-kī	Loud coarse or snoring sounds heard during inspiration or expiration; caused by obstructed airways
stridor STRĪ-dor	High-pitched, musical sound made on inspiration; caused by an obstruction in the trachea or larynx
wheezes HWĒZ-ĕz	Continuous high-pitched whistling sounds, usually during expiration; caused by narrowing of an airway
acidosis ăs-ĭ-DŌ-sĭs *acid:* acid *-osis:* abnormal condition; increase (used primarily with blood cells)	Excessive acidity of blood due to an accumulation of acids or an excessive loss of bicarbonate caused by abnormally high levels of carbon dioxide (CO_2) in the body
acute respiratory distress syndrome (ARDS) ă-KŪT RĔS-pĭ-ră-tō-rē dĭs-TRĔS SĬN-drōm	Life-threatening build-up of fluid in the air sacs (alveoli), caused by vomit into the lungs (aspiration), inhaling chemicals, pneumonia, septic shock, or trauma, that prevents enough oxygen from passing into the bloodstream; also called *adult respiratory distress syndrome (ARDS)*
anosmia ăn-ŎZ-mē-ă *an-:* without, not *-osmia:* smell	Absence or decrease in the sense of smell
anoxia ăn-ŎK-sē-ă *an:* without, not *-oxia:* oxygen	Total absence of O_2 in body tissues; caused by a lack of O_2 in inhaled air or by obstruction that prevents O_2 from reaching the lungs

asphyxia
ăs-FĬK-sē-ă
> *as-:* without, not
> *-phyxia:* pulse

Condition of insufficient intake of oxygen due to choking, toxic gases, electric shock, drugs, drowning, smoke, or trauma

asthma
ĂZ-mă

Inflammatory airway disorder that results in attacks of wheezing, shortness of breath that gets worse with exercise or activity, and coughing (with or without sputum)

 Get a closer look at COPD and asthma on page 93.

atelectasis
ăt-ĕ-LĔK-tă-sĭs
> *atel:* incomplete; imperfect
> *-ectasis:* dilation, expansion

Collapse of lung tissue, which prevents the respiratory exchange of oxygen and carbon dioxide and is caused by a variety of conditions including obstruction of foreign bodies, excessive secretions, or pressure on the lung from a tumor

bronchitis
brŏng-KĪ-tĭs
> *bronch:* bronchus (plural, bronchi)
> *-itis:* inflammation

Acute or chronic inflammation of mucous membranes of the bronchial airways caused by irritation, infection, or both

 Get a closer look at COPD and bronchitis on page 93.

coryza
kŏ-RĪ-ză

Acute inflammation of the nasal passages accompanied by profuse nasal discharge; also called a *cold*

croup
croop

Acute respiratory syndrome that occurs primarily in children and infants and is characterized by laryngeal obstruction and spasm, barking cough, and stridor

cystic fibrosis (CF) SĬS-tĭk fĭ-BRŌ-sĭs *cyst:* bladder *-ic:* pertaining to *fibr:* fiber, fibrous tissue *-osis:* abnormal condition; increase (used primarily with blood cells)	Genetic disease that is one of the most common types of chronic lung disease in children and young adults and causes thick, sticky mucus to build up in the lungs and digestive tract, possibly resulting in early death
emphysema ĕm-fĭ-SĒ-mă	Chronic obstructive pulmonary disease (COPD) that makes it difficult to breathe and is characterized by loss of elasticity of the lung tissue that causes the small airways to collapse during forced exhalation Get a closer look at COPD and emphysema on page 93.
epistaxis ĕp-ĭ-STĂK-sĭs *epi-:* above, upon *-staxis:* dripping, oozing (of blood)	Hemorrhage from the nose; also called *nosebleed*
hypercapnia hī-pĕr-KĂP-nē-ă *hyper-:* excessive, above normal *-capnia:* carbon dioxide (CO_2)	Greater than normal amounts of carbon dioxide in the blood
hypoxemia hī-pŏks-Ē-mē-ă *hyp-:* under, below, deficient *ox:* oxygen *-emia:* blood condition	Deficiency of oxygen in the blood; usually a sign of respiratory impairment

hypoxia hī-PŎKS-ē-ă *hyp-:* under, below, deficient *-oxia:* oxygen	Deficiency of oxygen in body tissues; usually a sign of respiratory impairment
influenza ĭn-floo-ĔN-ză	Acute, contagious respiratory infection characterized by sudden onset of fever, chills, headache, and muscle pain
otitis media (OM) ō-TĪ-tĭs MĒ-dē-ă *ot:* ear *-itis:* inflammation *med:* middle *-ia:* condition **exudative** ĔKS-ū-dă-tĭv	Inflammation of the middle ear, commonly the result of an upper respiratory infection (URI) with symptoms of otodynia; may be treated with myringotomy or tympanostomy tubes OM with the presence of fluid, such as pus or serum
pertussis pĕr-TŬS-ĭs	Acute infectious disease characterized by a "whoop"-sounding cough; also called *whooping cough*
pleurisy PLOO-rĭs-ē *pleur:* pleura *-isy:* state of; condition	Inflammation of the pleural membrane characterized by a stabbing pain that is intensified by deep breathing or coughing
pneumothorax nū-mō-THŌ-răks *pneum/o:* air, lung *-thorax:* chest	Collection of air or gas in the pleural cavity, causing the complete or partial collapse of a lung (See Figure 4-1.)
sudden infant death syndrome (SIDS)	Completely unexpected and unexplained death of an apparently well, or virtually well, infant; also called *crib death*

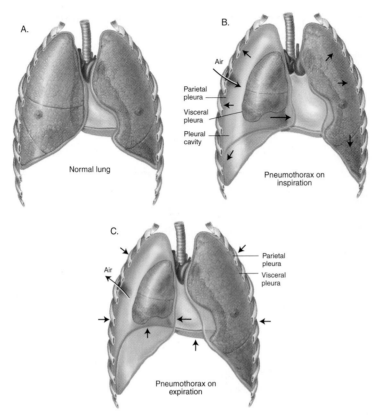

Figure 4–1. Pneumothorax. (A) Normal lung. (B) Pneumothorax on inspiration. (C) Pneumothorax on expiration.

Diagnostic Procedures

arterial blood gases (ABGs) ăr-TĒ-rē-ăl *arteri:* artery *-al:* pertaining to	Group of tests that measure the oxygen and carbon dioxide concentration in an arterial blood sample
Mantoux test măn-TŪ	Intradermal test to determine recent or past exposure to tuberculosis (TB)

pulmonary function tests (PFTs) PŬL-mō-ně-rē *pulmon:* lung 　*-ary:* pertaining to	Variety of tests used to determine the capacity of the lungs to exchange O_2 and CO_2 efficiently

Medical and Surgical Procedures

cardiopulmonary resuscitation (CPR) kăr-dē-ō-PŬL-mō-něr-ē rě-sŭs-ĭ-TĀ-shŭn *cardi/o:* heart *pulmon:* lung 　*-ary:* pertaining to	Basic emergency procedure for life support, consisting of artificial respiration and manual external cardiac massage
endotracheal intubation ĕn-dō-TRĀ-kē-ăl ĭn-tū-BĀ-shŭn *endo:* in, within *trache:* trachea 　　(windpipe) 　*-al:* pertaining to	Procedure in which an airway catheter is inserted through the mouth or nose into the trachea in patients who are unable to breathe on their own or to administer oxygen, medication, or anesthesia
postural drainage	Use of body positioning to assist in the removal of secretions from specific lobes of the lung, bronchi, or lung cavities
thoracocentesis thō-ră-cō-sĕn-TĒ-sĭs *thorac/o:* chest *-centesis:* surgical 　　puncture	Use of a needle to collect pleural fluid for laboratory analysis or remove excess pleural fluid or air from the pleural space; also called *thoracentesis* (See Figure 4-2.)

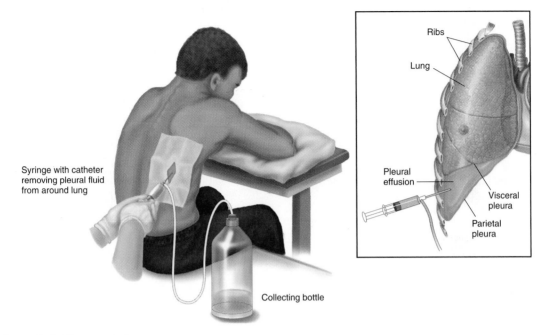

Figure 4–2. Thoracentesis.

tracheostomy trā-kē-ŎS-tō-mē *trache/o:* trachea (windpipe) *-stomy:* forming an opening (mouth)	Incision into the trachea (tracheotomy) and creation of a permanent opening through which a tracheostomy tube is inserted to keep the opening patent (accessible or wide open) (See Figure 4-3.)

Pharmacology

bronchodilators brŏng-kō-DĪ-lā-tŏrs	Dilate constricted airways by relaxing muscle spasms in the bronchial tubes through oral administration or inhaled via a metered-dose inhaler (MDI)
corticosteroids kor-tĭ-kō-STĔR-oyds	Suppress the inflammatory reaction that causes swelling and narrowing of the bronchi

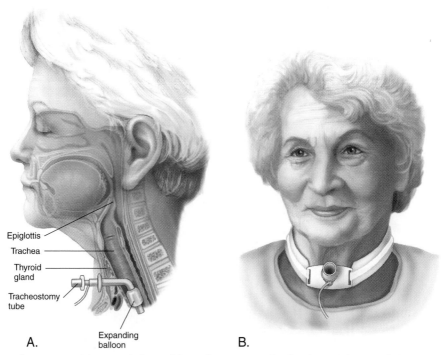

Epiglottis

Trachea

Thyroid gland

Tracheostomy tube

A.

Expanding balloon

B.

Figure 4–3. Tracheostomy. (A) Lateral view with tracheostomy tube in place. (B) Frontal view.

expectorants ĕk-SPĔK-tō-rănts	Improve the ability to cough up mucus from the respiratory tract
metered-dose inhaler (MDI)	Device that enables the patient to self-administer a specific amount of medication into the lungs through inhalation (See Figure 4-4.)
nebulized mist treatment (NMT) NĔB-ū-līzd	Method of administering medication directly into the lungs using a device (nebulizer) that produces a fine spray; also called *aerosol therapy* (See Figure 4-5.)

Pronunciation Help	Long Sound	ā in rāte	ē in rēbirth	ī in īsle	ō in ōver	ū in ūnite
	Short Sound	ă in ălone	ĕ in ĕver	ĭ in ĭt	ŏ in nŏt	ŭ in cŭt

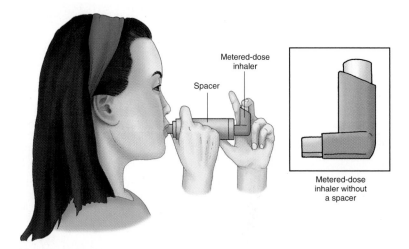

Figure 4–4. Metered-dose inhaler.

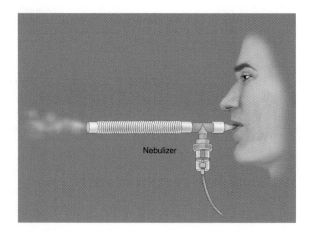

Figure 4–5. Nebulizer.

Closer Look

Take a closer look at these respiratory disorders to enhance your understanding of the medical terminology associated with them.

Bronchoscopy

Bronchoscopy, a type of endoscopic procedure, is the visual examination of the interior bronchi using a flexible fiberoptic instrument with a light **(bronchoscope).** It is inserted either through the nose **(transnasally)** or through the mouth. This procedure may be performed to remove obstructions, obtain a **biopsy specimen,** or observe directly for pathological changes. In children, this procedure may be used to remove foreign objects that have been inhaled. In adults, the procedure is most commonly used to take samples of suspicious lesions **(biopsy)** and for culturing specific areas in the lung. The cavity, organ, or canal being examined dictates the name of the endoscopic procedure, such as *cystoscopy, gastroscopy,* or *bronchoscopy.* The illustration below shows bronchoscopy of the left bronchus.

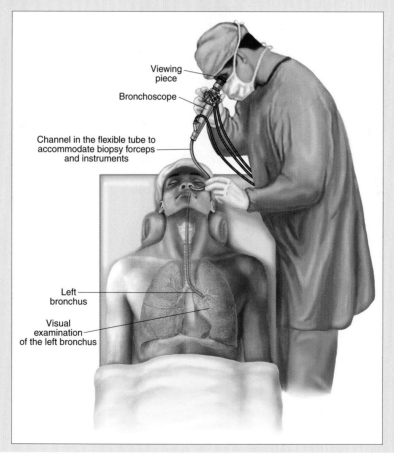

(Continued)

Closer Look—cont'd

Apnea

Apnea is a temporary cessation of breathing. *Sleep apnea* refers to a sudden cessation of breathing during sleep that can result in hypoxia and lead to cognitive impairment, **hypertension,** and **arrhythmias.** *Obstructive sleep apnea* (**OSA**) involves a physical obstruction in the upper airways. The condition is usually marked by recurrent sleep interruptions, choking and gasping spells on awakening, and drowsiness caused by loss of normal sleep. **Continuous positive airway pressure (CPAP)** is a gentle ventilator support used to keep the airways open. Uncorrected, the disorder commonly leads to central sleep apnea, pulmonary failure, and cardiac abnormalities. The illustration below shows the airway obstruction caused by enlarged tonsils that eventually leads to obstructive sleep apnea (A) and the CPAP machine used to treat sleep apnea (B).

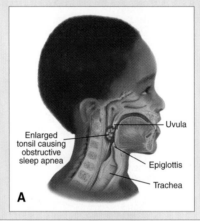

A

Enlarged tonsil causing obstructive sleep apnea

Uvula

Epiglottis

Trachea

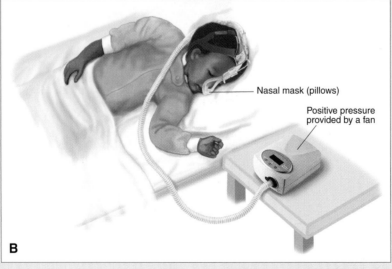

B

Nasal mask (pillows)

Positive pressure provided by a fan

Closer Look—cont'd

COPD

Chronic obstructive pulmonary disease (COPD), a group of respiratory disorders, is characterized by chronic, partial obstruction of the bronchi and lungs that makes it difficult to breathe. Three major disorders included in COPD are asthma, chronic bronchitis, and emphysema. In COPD, the airway passages become clogged with mucus. Although air reaches the alveoli in the lungs during inhalation, it may not be able to escape during exhalation. COPD tends to be progressive and irreversible. Smoking, prolonged exposure to polluted air, **respiratory infections**, and allergies are predisposing factors to the disease. Thus **bronchodilators** and **corticosteroids** are commonly prescribed to help alleviate the symptoms of COPD. The illustration below shows the inflamed airways and excessive mucus involved in chronic bronchitis (A), the distended bronchioles and alveoli associated with emphysema (B), and the narrowed bronchial tubes and swollen mucous membranes associated with asthma (C).

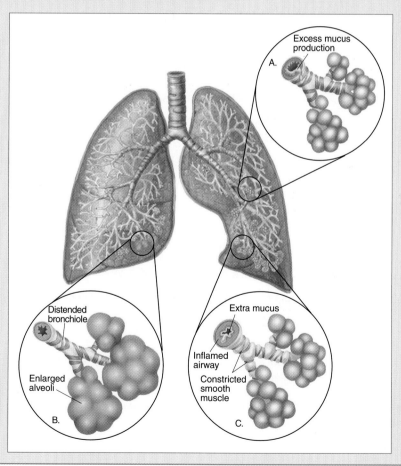

Additional Medical Vocabulary Recall

Match the medical term(s) below with the definitions in the numbered list.

ABGs	CF	Mantoux
anosmia	corticosteroids	PFT
asthma	croup	pleurisy
atelectasis	epistaxis	pneumothorax
bronchodilators	hypoxemia	stridor

1. _____ is an inflammation of the pleura.

2. _____ is an acute respiratory syndrome of childhood characterized by laryngeal obstruction and spasm, barking cough, and stridor.

3. _____ is a deficiency of oxygen in the blood.

4. _____ are hormonal agents that reduce edema and inflammation.

5. _____ is a disease that causes severe congestion within the lungs and digestive system due to production of thick mucus.

6. _____ is a high-pitched musical sound made on inspiration resulting from an obstruction of air passages.

7. _____ is a respiratory disorder marked by recurrent attacks of difficult or labored breathing accompanied by wheezing.

8. _____ are drugs that dilate the bronchioles and bronchi to increase airflow.

9. _____ refers to a collection of air or gas in the pleural cavity.

10. _____ involve analyzing oxygen and carbon dioxide concentrations in an arterial blood sample.

11. _____ is a hemorrhage from the nose; also called *nosebleed*.

12. _____ is an absence or decrease in the sense of smell.

13. _____ refers to any of several tests used to evaluate respiratory function.

14. _____ is an intradermal test to determine recent or past exposure to tuberculosis.

15. _____ is a collapse of lung tissue, preventing the respiratory exchange of oxygen and carbon dioxide.

Competency Verification: Check your answers in Appendix B, Answer Key, on page 361. Review material that you did not answer correctly.

Correct Answers _____ × **6.67 =** _____ %

Pronunciation and Spelling

Use the following list to practice correct pronunciation and spelling of medical terms. Practice the pronunciation aloud and then write the correct spelling of the term. The first word is completed for you.

Pronunciation	Spelling
1. ăs-ĭ-DŌ-sĭs	*acidosis*
2. ĕr-ō-FĂ-jē-ă	
3. ăn-ŎZ-mē-ă	
4. ăs-FĬK-sē-ă	
5. ĂZ-mă	
6. ăt-ĕ-LĔK-tă-sĭs	
7. brăd-ĭp-NĒ-ă	
8. brŏng-kē-ĔK-tă-sĭs	
9. brŏng-kō-DĪ-lā-tŏrz	
10. brŏng-KŎS-kō-pē	
11. ĕm-fĭ-SĒ-mă	
12. kor-tĭ-kō-STĒR-oydz	
13. kŏ-RĪ-ză	
14. KRĂK-ăl	
15. dĭsp-NĒ-ă	
16. hī-pŏks-Ē-mē-ă	
17. hī-PŎKS-ē-ă	
18. pĕr-TŬS-ĭs	
19. PLOO-rĭs-ē	
20. RŎNG-kī	

 Competency Verification: Check your answers in Appendix B, Answer Key, on page 362. Review material that you did not answer correctly.

Correct Answers: _____ × 5 = _____ %

Abbreviations

The table below introduces abbreviations associated with the respiratory system.

Abbreviation	Meaning	Abbreviation	Meaning
ABG	arterial blood gas(es)	NMT	nebulized mist treatment
ARDS	adult respiratory distress syndrome; acute respiratory distress syndrome	OM	otitis media
CF	cystic fibrosis	OP	outpatient; operative procedure
CO_2	carbon dioxide	O_2	oxygen
COPD	chronic obstructive pulmonary disease	OSA	obstructive sleep apnea
CPAP	continuous positive airway pressure	PFT	pulmonary function test
CPR	cardiopulmonary resuscitation	TB	tuberculosis
Dx	diagnosis	UPP	uvulopalatopharyngoplasty
IV	intravenous	URI	upper respiratory infection
MDI	metered-dose inhaler		

Chart Notes

Chart notes make up part of the medical record and are used in various types of health care facilities. The chart notes below were dictated by the patient's physician and reflect common clinical events using medical terminology to document the patient's care. By studying and completing the terminology and chart note analysis sections below you will learn and understand terms associated with the medical specialty of pulmonary medicine.

Terminology

The following terms are linked to chart notes in the medical specialty of pulmonology; also called *pulmonary medicine.* Practice pronouncing each term aloud and then use a medical dictionary such as *Taber's Cyclopedic Medical Dictionary, Appendix A: Glossary of Medical Word Elements,* page 337, or other resources to define each term.

Term	Meaning
anesthesia ăn-ĕs-THĒ-zē-ă	
biopsy BĪ-ŏp-sē	
carcinoma kăr-sĭ-NŌ-mă	
diagnosis dī-ăg-NŌ-sĭs	
expired	
fascia FĂSH-ē-ă	
hemorrhage HĔM-ĕ-rĭj	
lymph node lĭmf nōd	
meatus mē-Ā-tŭs	
metastatic mĕt-ă-STĂT-ĭk	
necropsy NĔK-rŏp-sē	
papillary PĂP-ĭ-lăr-ē	
pathologic păth-ō-LŎJ-ĭk	
pneumonia nū-MŌ-nē-ă	
polypectomy pŏl-ĭ-PĔK-tō-mē	
polypoid PŎL-ē-poyd	

(Continued)

Term	Meaning
pulmonary PŬL-mō-nĕ-rē	
snare snār	
submaxillary sŭb-MĂK-sĭ-lĕr-ē	

 Visit *http://davisplus.fadavis.com/gylys-express* for the terminology pronunciation exercise associated with this chart note.

Airway Obstruction

Read the chart note below aloud. Underline any term you have trouble pronouncing and or cannot define. If needed, refer to the Terminology section above for correct pronunciations and meanings of terms.

This 45-year-old-white male was seen 2 years ago because of upper airway obstruction due to large polyps in the right nasal cavity. On examination, a large polypoid mass filled most of the right nasal cavity. The mass originated in the middle meatus. With use of a nasal snare, polypectomy was performed to remove several sections. There was a slight hemorrhage. On the next day, a 4- × 3-cm oval soft mass was excised from beneath the left submaxillary region, with the patient under local anesthesia. The mass was just beneath the superficial fascia and appeared to be an enlarged lymph node unconnected with the nasal disease.

Pathologic diagnosis of the nasal growth was low grade papillary carcinoma. The diagnosis of the lymph node was metastatic carcinoma. A chest film was taken that indicated the presence of pulmonary densities attributed to unresolved pneumonia. Also, a needle biopsy of the enlarged liver nodes yielded no results.

The patient expired at home after discharge from the hospital and no necropsy was obtained.

Chart Note Analysis

From the chart note, select the medical word that means

1. resembling a polyp: _____

2. an opening: _____

3. removal of a small piece of tissue for microscopic examination: _____

4. pertaining to a carcinoma that has spread to a distant site: _____

5. excision of a polyp: _____

6. wire loop instrument used for excision of polyps: _____

7. abnormal bursting forth of blood: _____

8. administered substance that results in a loss of feeling sensation: _____

9. metric abbreviation that refers to a unit of length: _____

10. tumor that is cancerous: _____

Competency Verification: Check your answers in Appendix B, Answer Key, on page 362. Review material that you did not answer correctly.

Correct Answers: _____ × 10 = _____ %

Demonstrate What You Know!

To evaluate your understanding of how medical terms you have studied in this and previous chapters are used in a clinical environment, complete the numbered sentences by selecting an appropriate term from the list below.

alveoli	diaphragm	laryngoscope	pneumonia
apnea	emphysema	O_2	rhonchi
bronchioles	hypoxia	pharyngitis	tachypnea
CO_2	laryngectomy	phrenalgia	tracheotomy

1. An incision of the trachea to allow for oxygen exchange is called _____.

2. The exchange of oxygen and carbon dioxide takes place in the lungs in small sacs called _____.

3. A person with CA of the voice box may undergo the surgery called _____.

4. _____ is one of the major disorders included in COPD.

5. To view the voice box of a patient with nodules on the vocal cords, the physician uses a(n) _____.

6. A patient with streptococcal infection of the throat has a condition called_____.

7. Patients who suffer from asthma have spasms of the _____.

8. Temporary cessation of breathing is known as _____.

9. _____ is a snoring sound heard during inspiration or expiration that is caused by obstructed airways.

10. The chemical symbol for oxygen is _____.

11. Acute inflammation of the lungs, caused by a bacterium, is called _____.

12. A pain the diaphragm is charted with a Dx of _____.

13. _____ is a deficiency of oxygen in body tissues.

14. The muscle that separates the lungs from the abdominal cavity is called the _____.

15. A patient who is breathing rapidly is charted with a Dx of _____.

Competency Verification: Check your answers in Appendix B, Answer Key, on page 362. Review material that you did not answer correctly.

Correct Answers: _____ × 6.67 = _____ %

Multimedia Review. If you are not satisfied with your retention level of the respiratory chapter, go to *http://davisplus.fadavis.com/gylys-express* to complete the website activities linked to this chapter. It is your choice whether or not you want to take advantage of these reinforcement exercises before continuing with the next chapter.

Cardiovascular System

MULTIMEDIA STUDY TOOLS.
To enrich your medical terminology skills, look for this multimedia icon throughout the text. It will help alert you to when it is best to use the various multimedia resources available with this textbook to enhance your studies.

Objectives

Upon completion of this chapter, you will be able to:

- Describe types of medical treatment provided by cardiologists
- Name five structures of the cardiovascular system.
- Discuss the primary function of the cardiovascular system.
- Identify combining forms, suffixes, and prefixes associated with the cardiovascular and system.
- Recognize, pronounce, build, and spell medical terms and abbreviations associated with the cardiovascular system.
- Demonstrate your knowledge by successfully completing the activities in this chapter.

Vocabulary Preview

Term	Meaning
angioplasty ĂN-jē-ō-plăs-tē *angi/o:* essel (usually blood or lymph) *-plasty:* surgical repair	Surgical procedure that opens a blocked artery by inflating a small balloon within a catheter to widen and restore blood flow in the artery
arteries ĂR-tĕr-ēz	Large blood vessels that carry oxygenated blood away from the heart
capillaries KĂP-ĭ-lăr-ēz	Microscopic blood vessels joining arterioles and venules
congenital kŏn-JĔN-ĭ-tăl	Pertaining to presence of a disorder at the time of birth, which may result from genetic or environmental causes
metabolism mĕ-TĂB-ō-lĭzm	Sum of all physical and chemical changes that take place within an organism
myocardium mī-ō-KĂR-dē-ŭm *my/o:* muscle *cardi:* heart *-um:* structure, thing	Middle layer of the walls of heart that is composed of cardiac muscle
veins vānz	Vessels that return deoxygenated blood to the heart

Pronunciation Help	Long Sound	ā in rāte	ē in rēbirth	ī in īsle	ō in ōver	ū in ūnite
	Short Sound	ă in ălone	ĕ in ĕver	ĭ in ĭt	ŏ in nŏt	ŭ in cŭt

Cardiology

The medical specialty of **cardiology** focuses on medical, surgical, and therapeutic treatments of heart diseases. Generally, three types of cardiology specialists provide medical care: the **cardiologist,** the **pediatric cardiologist,** and the **cardiac surgeon.** The cardiologist specializes in treating adults, and the pediatric cardiologist specializes in treating infants, children, and adolescents. Surgeries performed by the cardiac surgeon include but are not limited to coronary artery bypass, **angioplasty,** pacemaker insertion, valve replacement or repair, heart transplantation, and repairs of **congenital** heart diseases.

Cardiovascular System Quick Study

The **cardiovascular (CV) system** is composed of the heart, which is essentially a muscular pump, and an extensive network of blood vessels. The main purpose of the CV system, also called the *circulatory system*, is to deliver oxygen, nutrients, and other essential substances to body cells and remove waste products of cellular **metabolism.** This process is carried out by a complex network of blood vessels that includes **arteries, capillaries,** and **veins**—all of which are connected to the heart. Circulation of blood through the heart and body depends on contraction of the heart, or the heartbeat. The heart also contracts and relaxes in a regular rhythm that is coordinated by a series of nodes and nerve tissues in the conduction system of the heart. A contraction is known as **systole,** and the resting period between contractions when the heart fills with blood is known as **diastole.** A healthy CV system is vital to a person's survival. A CV system that does not provide adequate circulation deprives tissues of oxygen and nutrients and fails to remove waste products. These problems result in irreversible cell changes that could be life-threatening. (See *Cardiovascular System*, page 104.)

 An extensive anatomy and physiology review is included in *TermPlus,* the powerful, interactive CD-ROM program.

Medical Word Building

Building medical words using word elements related to the cardiovascular system will enhance your understanding of those terms and reinforce your ability to use terms correctly.

Combining Forms

Begin your study of cardiovascular terminology by reviewing the organs and their associated combining forms (CFs), which are illustrated in the figure *Cardiovascular System* on the next page.

Cardiovascular System

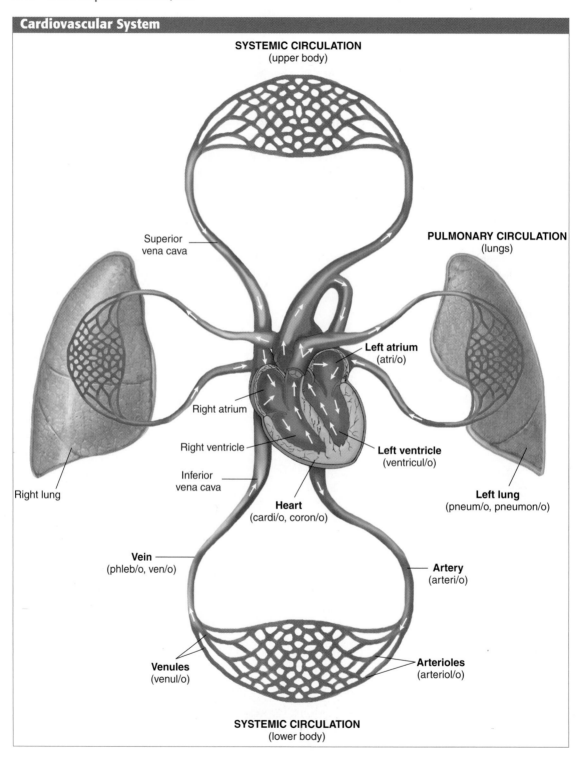

SYSTEMIC CIRCULATION
(upper body)

PULMONARY CIRCULATION
(lungs)

Superior
vena cava

Left atrium
(atri/o)

Right atrium

Right ventricle

Left ventricle
(ventricul/o)

Inferior
vena cava

Right lung

Left lung
(pneum/o, pneumon/o)

Heart
(cardi/o, coron/o)

Vein
(phleb/o, ven/o)

Artery
(arteri/o)

Venules
(venul/o)

Arterioles
(arteriol/o)

SYSTEMIC CIRCULATION
(lower body)

In the table below, CFs are listed alphabetically and other word parts are defined as needed. Review the medical word and study the elements that make up the term. Then complete the meaning of the medical words in the right-hand column. The first one is completed for you. You may also refer to *Appendix A: Glossary of Medical Word Elements* to complete this exercise.

Combining Form	Meaning	Medical Word	Meaning
Cardiovascular System			
aneurysm/o	widening, widened blood vessel	**aneurysm/o**/rrhaphy (ăn-ū-rĭz-MOR-ă-fē) *-rrhaphy:* suture	suture (of the sac) of an aneurysm
arteri/o	artery	**arteri/o**/scler/osis (ăr-tē-rē-ō-sklĕ-RŌ-sĭs) *scler:* hardening; sclera (white of eye) *-osis:* abnormal condition; increase (used primarily with blood cells) Get a closer look at coronary artery disease on page 119.	
ather/o	fatty plaque	**ather/**oma (ăth-ĕr-Ō-mă) *-oma:* tumor	
atri/o	atrium	**atri/**um (Ā-trē-ŭm) *-um:* structure, thing	
cardi/o	heart	**cardi/o**/megaly (kăr-dē-ō-MĔG-ă-lē) *-megaly:* enlargement	
coron/o		**coron/**ary (KOR-ō-nă-rē) *-ary:* pertaining to	
phleb/o	vein	**phleb/**itis (flĕb-Ī-tĭs) *-itis:* inflammation	
ven/o		**ven/**ous (VĒ-nŭs) *-ous:* pertaining to	
thromb/o	blood clot	**thromb/o**/lysis (thrŏm-BŎL-ĭ-sĭs) *-lysis:* separation; destruction; loosening	

(Continued)

Combining Form	Meaning	Medical Word	Meaning
Cardiovascular System			
varic/o	dilated vein	**varic**/ose (VĂR-ĭ-kōs) *-ose:* pertaining to sugar ◯ Get a closer look at varicose veins on page 120.	
vas/o	vessel; vas deferens; duct	**vas/o**/spasm (VĂS-ō-spăzm) *-spasm:* involuntary contraction, twitching	
vascul/o	vessel	**vascul**/ar (VĂS-kū-lăr) *-ar:* pertaining to	
ventricul/o	ventricle (of heart or brain)	inter/**ventricul**/ar (ĭn-tĕr-vĕn-TRĬK-ū-lăr) *inter-:* between *-ar:* pertaining to	

Suffixes and Prefixes

In the table below, suffixes and prefixes are listed alphabetically and other word parts are defined as needed. Review the medical word and study the elements that make up the term. Then complete the meaning of the medical words in the right-hand column. You may also refer to *Appendix A: Glossary of Medical Word Elements* to complete this exercise.

Word Element	Meaning	Medical Words	Meaning
Suffixes			
-cardia	heart condition	tachy/**cardia** (tăk-ē-KĂR-dē-ă) *tachy-:* rapid	
-gram	record, writing	electr/o/cardi/o/**gram** (ē-lĕk-trō-KĂR-dē-ō-grăm) *electr/o:* electricity *cardi/o:* heart	
-graph	instrument for recording	electr/o/cardi/o/**graph** (ē-lĕk-trō-KĂR-dē-ŏ-grăf) *electr/o:* electricity *cardi/o:* heart	

Word Element	Meaning	Medical Words	Meaning
Suffixes			
-graphy	process of recording	angi/o/**graphy** (ăn-jē-ŎG-ră-fē) *angi/o:* vessel (usually blood or lymph)	
-stenosis	narrowing, stricture	aort/o/**stenosis** (ā-or-tō-stĕn-Ō-sĭs) *aort/o:* aorta	
Prefixes			
brady-	slow	**brady/**cardi/ac (brăd-ē-KĂR-dē-ăk) *cardi:* heart -*ac:* pertaining to	
endo-	in, within	**endo/**cardi/um (ĕn-dō-KĂR-dē-ŭm) *cardi:* heart -*um:* structure, thing	
epi-	above, upon	**epi/**cardi/um (ĕp-ĭ-KĂR-dē-ŭm) *cardi:* heart -*um:* structure, thing	
peri-	around	**peri/**cardi/um (pĕr-ĭ-KĂR-dē-ŭm) *cardi:* heart -*um:* structure, thing	

 Competency Verification: Check your answers in Appendix B, Answer Key, page 362. If you are not satisfied with your level of comprehension, review the terms in the table and retake the review.

 Listen and Learn, the audio CD-ROM included in this book, will help you master pronunciation of selected medical words. Use it to practice pronunciations of the medical terms in the above "Word Building" tables and for instructions to complete the *Listen and Learn* exercise.

 Flash-Card Activity. Enhance your study and reinforcement of this chapter's word elements with the power of the DavisPlus flash-card activity. Do so by visiting *http://davisplus.fadavis.com/ gylys-express.* We recommend you complete the flash-card activity before continuing with the next section.

Medical Terminology Word Building

In this section, combine the word parts you have learned to construct medical terms related to the cardiovascular system.

Use *ather/o* (fatty plaque) to build words that mean:

1. tumor of fatty plaque _____

2. hardening of fatty plaque _____

Use *phleb/o* (vein) to build words that mean:

3. inflammation of a vein (wall) _____

4. abnormal condition of a blood clot in a vein _____

Use *ven/o* (vein) to build words that mean:

5. pertaining to a vein _____

6. spasm of a vein _____

Use *cardi/o* (heart) to build words that mean:

7. specialist in the study of the heart _____

8. instrument for recording the electrical activity of the heart _____

9. enlargement of the heart _____

Use *angi/o* (vessel) to build words that mean:

10. disease of blood vessels _____

11. tumor of a vessel _____

Use *-stenosis* (narrowing, stricture) to build words that mean:

12. narrowing of the aorta _____

13. stricture of an artery _____

Use *-cardia* (heart condition) to build words that mean:

14. rapid heart rate _____

15. slow heart rate _____

Competency Verification: Check your answers in Appendix B, Answer Key, on page 363. Review material that you did not answer correctly.

Correct Answers _____ × **6.67 =** _____ %

Additional Medical Vocabulary

The following tables list additional terms related to the cardiovascular system. Recognizing and learning these terms will help you understand the connection between common signs, symptoms, and diseases. Included are medical and surgical procedures as well as pharmacological agents used to treat diseases.

Signs, Symptoms, and Diseases

aneurysm ĂN-ū-rĭzm	Localized dilation of a blood vessel wall (usually an artery) due to a congenital defect or weakness in the vessel wall (See Figure 5-1.)
angina pectoris ăn-JĪ-nă PĔK-tō-rĭs	Mild to severe pain or pressure in the chest caused by ischemia; also called *angina*

arrhythmia
ă-RĬTH-mē-ă
    a-: without, not
rrhythm: rhythm
    -ia: condition
	Irregularity or loss of rhythm of the heartbeat; also called *dysrhythmia*

fibrillation fĭ-brĭl-Ā-shŭn	Irregular, random contraction of heart fibers that commonly occurs in the atria or ventricles of the heart and is usually described by the part that is contracting abnormally, such as atrial fibrillation or ventricular fibrillation

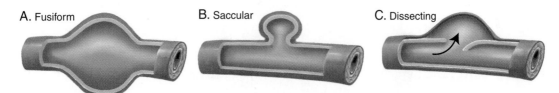

Figure 5–1. Aneurysms. (A) Fusiform aneurysm with dilation of entire circumference of the artery. (B) Saccular aneurysm with bulging on only one side of the artery wall. (C) Dissecting aneurysm with tear (dissection) in the wall of an artery because of bleeding into the weakened wall, which splits the wall (more common in the aorta).

arteriosclerosis

ăr-tē-rē-ō-sklĕ-RŌ-sĭs

arteri/o: artery
  scler: hardening, sclera
    (white of eye)
  -osis: abnormal con-
    dition; increase
    (used primarily
    with blood cells)

Thickening, hardening, and loss of elasticity of arterial walls; also called *hardening of the arteries*

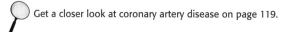 Get a closer look at coronary artery disease on page 119.

atherosclerosis

ăth-ĕ-rō-sklĕ-RŌ-sĭs

ather/o: fatty plaque
  scler: hardening, sclera
    (white of eye)
  -osis: abnormal condi-
    tion; increase
    (used primarily
    with blood cells)

Most common form of arteriosclerosis caused by accumulation of fatty substances within the arterial walls, resulting in partial and, eventually, total blockage (See Figure 5-2.)

bruit

brwē

Soft blowing sound heard on auscultation caused by turbulent blood flow

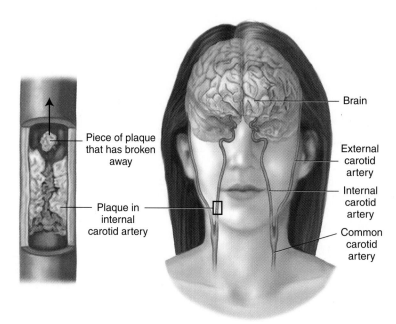

Figure 5–2. Atherosclerosis of the internal carotid artery.

embolus
ĔM-bō-lŭs
   embol: embolus (plug)
    –us: condition;
      structure
	Mass of undissolved matter (commonly a blood clot, fatty plaque, or air bubble) that travels through the bloodstream and becomes lodged in a blood vessel

heart block	Disease of the electrical system of the heart, which controls activity of heart muscle
first-degree	Atrioventricular (AV) block in which the atrial electrical impulses are delayed by a fraction of a second before being conducted to the ventricles
second-degree	AV block in which only some atrial electrical impulses are conducted to the ventricles
third-degree	AV block in which no electrical impulses reach the ventricles; also called *complete heart block (CHB)*
heart failure (HF)	Condition in which the heart cannot pump enough blood to meet the metabolic requirement of body tissues; formerly called *congestive heart failure (CHF)*

hypertension (HTN)
hī-pĕr-TĔN-shŭn
   hyper: excessive, above
     normal
   –tension: to stretch
	Consistently elevated blood pressure, causing damage to the blood vessels and, ultimately, the heart

ischemia
ĭs-KĒ-mē-ă
   isch: to hold back
   –emia: blood
	Inadequate supply of oxygenated blood to a body part due to an interruption of blood flow
	
	 Get a closer look at ischemia due to coronary artery disease on page 119.

mitral valve prolapse (MVP) MĪ-trăl vălv PRŌ-lăps	Structural abnormality in which the mitral (bicuspid) valve does not close completely, resulting in a backflow of blood into the left atrium with each contraction
murmur MĔR-mĕr	Abnormal sound heard on auscultation caused by defects in the valves or chambers of the heart

myocardial infarction (MI) mī-ō-KĂR-dē-ăl ĭn-FĂRK-shŭn *my/o:* muscle *cardi:* heart *-al:* pertaining to	Necrosis of a portion of cardiac muscle caused by partial or complete occlusion of one or more coronary arteries; also called *heart attack*
patent ductus arteriosus PĂT-ĕnt DŬK-tŭs ăr-tē-rē-Ō-sĭs	Failure of the ductus arteriosus (which connects the pulmonary artery to the aortic arch in a fetus) to close after birth, resulting in an abnormal opening between the pulmonary artery and the aorta
Raynaud disease rā-NŌ	Severe, sudden vasoconstriction and spasm in fingers and toes followed by cyanosis after exposure to cold temperature or emotional stress; also called *Raynaud phenomenon*
rheumatic heart disease rū-MĂT-ĭk	Streptococcal infection that causes damage to the heart valves and heart muscle, most commonly in children and young adults
stroke strōk	Damage to part of the brain due to interruption of its blood supply caused by bleeding within brain tissue or, more commonly, blockage of an artery; also called *cerebrovascular accident (CVA)*
thrombus THRŎM-bŭs *thromb:* blood clot *us:* condition; structure	A stationary blood clot formed within a blood vessel or within the heart, commonly causing vascular obstruction; also called *blood clot*
deep vein thrombosis (DVT) dēp vān thrŏm-BŌ-sĭs *thromb:* blood clot *-osis:* abnormal condition; increased (used primarily with blood cells)	Formation of a blood clot in a deep vein of the body, occurring most commonly in the iliac and femoral veins

transient ischemic attack (TIA) TRĂN-zhĕnt ĭs-KĒ-mĭk	Blood supply to part of the brain is briefly interrupted but does not cause permanent brain damage and may be a warning sign of a more serious and debilitating stroke in the future; also called *ministroke*

Diagnostic Procedures

cardiac catheterization KĂR-dē-ăk kăth-ĕ-tĕr-ĭ-ZĀ-shŭn *cardi:* heart *-ac:* pertaining to	Insertion of a small tube (catheter) through an incision into a large vein, usually of an arm (brachial approach) or leg (femoral approach), that is then threaded through a blood vessel until it reaches the heart (See Figure 5-3.)
cardiac enzyme studies KĂR-dē-ăk ĔN-zīm	Battery of blood tests performed to determine the presence of cardiac damage
echocardiography (ECHO) ĕk-ō-kăr-dē-ŎG-ră-fē *echo-:* repeated sound *cardi/o:* heart *-graphy:* process of recording	Ultrasound technique used to image the heart and evaluate how the heart's chambers and valves are working and to diagnose and detect pathological conditions

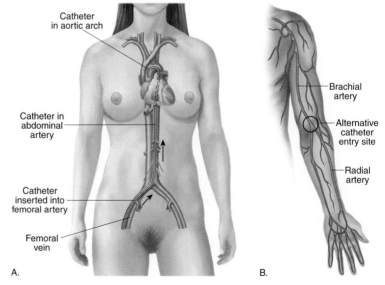

Catheter in aortic arch

Catheter in abdominal artery

Catheter inserted into femoral artery

Femoral vein

Brachial artery

Alternative catheter entry site

Radial artery

A.

B.

Figure 5–3. Cardiac catheterization. (A) Catheter insertion into a femoral vein or artery. (B) Catheter insertion into a brachial or radial artery.

electrocardiography (ECG) ē-lĕk-trō-kăr-dē-ŎG-ră-fē *electr/o:* electricity *cardi/o:* heart *-graphy:* process of recording	Creation and study of graphic recordings (electrocardiograms) produced by electric activity generated by the heart muscle; also called *cardiography*
Holter monitor HŎL-tĕr MŎN-ĭ-tor	Monitoring device worn by a patient that records prolonged electrocardiograph readings (usually 24 hours) on a portable tape recorder while the patient conducts normal daily activities (See Figure 5-4.)
stress test **nuclear**	Electrocardiography (ECG) taken under controlled exercise stress conditions (typically using a treadmill) while measuring oxygen consumption ECG that utilizes a radioisotope to evaluate coronary blood flow

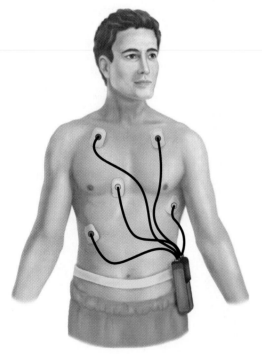

Figure 5–4. Holter monitor.

troponin I TRŌ-pō-nĭn	Blood test that measures protein released into the blood by damaged heart muscle (not skeletal muscle) and is a highly sensitive, specific indicator of recent myocardial infarction (MI)

Medical and Surgical Procedures

angioplasty ĂN-jē-ō-plăs-tē	Surgery that opens a blocked artery by inflating a small balloon within a catheter to widen and restore blood flow in the artery (See Figure 5-5.)
coronary artery bypass graft (CABG) KOR-ō-nă-rē ĂR-tĕr-ē *coron:* heart *-ary:* pertaining to	Angioplasty in which peripheral vein(s) are removed and each end of the vein is sutured onto the coronary artery to create new routes around narrowed and blocked arteries, allowing sufficient blood flow to deliver oxygen and nutrients to the heart muscle (See Figure 5-6.)
cardioversion căr-dē-ō-VĔR-zhŭn *cardi/o:* heart *-version:* turning	Restoration of normal heart rhythm by applying an electrical countershock to the chest using a device called a *defibrillator;* also called *defibrillation*

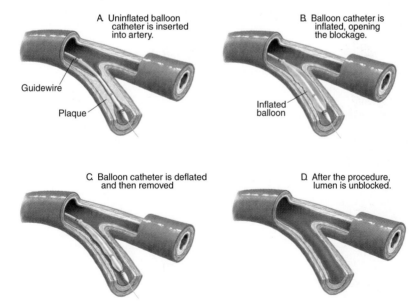

A. Uninflated balloon catheter is inserted into artery.

B. Balloon catheter is inflated, opening the blockage.

Guidewire

Plaque

Inflated balloon

C. Balloon catheter is deflated and then removed

D. After the procedure, lumen is unblocked.

Figure 5–5. Balloon angioplasty.

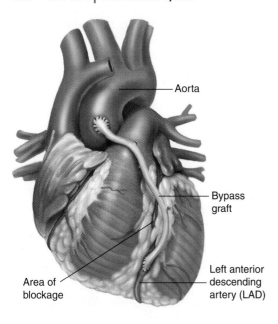

Aorta

Bypass graft

Left anterior descending artery (LAD)

Area of blockage

Figure 5–6. Coronary artery bypass graft (CABG).

defibrillator dē-FĬB-rĭ-lā-tĕr	Device used to administer a defibrillating electric shock to restore normal heart rhythm
automatic implantable cardioverter-defibrillator (AICD) căr-dē-ō-VĔR-tĕr dē-FĬB-rĭ-lā-tĕr	Surgically implanted electrical device that automatically detects and corrects potentially fatal arrhythmias by delivering low-energy shocks to the heart; also called *implantable cardioverter defibrillator* (ICD) (See Figure 5-7.)
automatic external defibrillator (AED) dē-FĬB-rĭ-lā-tĕr	Portable computerized device that analyzes the patient's heart rhythm and delivers an electrical shock to stimulate a heart in cardiac arrest
endarterectomy ĕnd-ăr-tĕr-ĔK-tō-mē	Surgical removal of the lining of an artery
carotid endarterectomy kă-RŎT-ĭd ĕnd-ăr-tĕr-ĔK-tō-mē	Removal of plaque (atherosclerosis) and thromboses from an occluded carotid artery to reduce the risk of stroke (See Figure 5-8.)

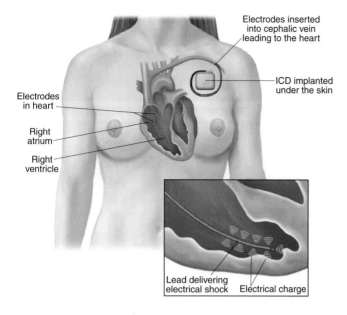

Electrodes inserted into cephalic vein leading to the heart

ICD implanted under the skin

Electrodes in heart

Right atrium

Right ventricle

Lead delivering electrical shock

Electrical charge

Figure 5–7. Automatic implantable cardioverter-defibrillator (AICD).

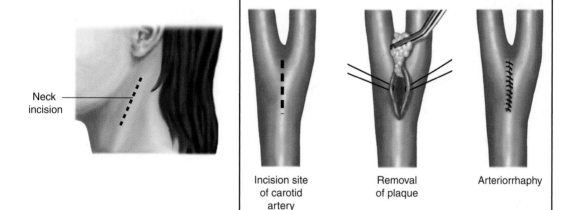

Neck incision

Incision site of carotid artery

Removal of plaque

Arteriorrhaphy

Figure 5–8. Endarterectomy of the common carotid artery.

| **endovenous laser therapy (EVLT)** ĕn-dō-VĒ-nŭs | Treatment of large varicose veins in the legs in which a laser fiber is inserted directly into the affected vein to heat the lining within the vein, causing it to collapse, shrink, and eventually disappear; also called *endovenous laser ablation (EVLA)* |

 Get a closer look at varicose veins, on page 120.

sclerotherapy sklĕr-ō-THĔR-ă-pē *scler/o:* hardening; sclera (white of eye) *-therapy:* treatment	Chemical injection into a varicose vein that causes inflammation and formation of fibrous tissue, which closes the vein Get a closer look at varicose veins, on page 120.
valvuloplasty VĂL-vū-lō-plăs-tē	Insertion of a balloon catheter in a blood vessel in the groin through the aorta and into the heart to widen a stenotic (stiffened) heart valve and increase blood flow; also called *percutaneous valvuloplasty*

Pharmacology

anticoagulants ăn-tĭ-kō-ĂG-ū-lănts	Prevent the clotting or coagulation of blood
beta blockers	Slow the heart rate and reduce the force with which the heart muscle contracts, thereby lowering blood pressure
nitrates NĪ-trāts	Relieve chest pain associated with angina and ease symptoms of heart failure (HF)
statins STĂ-tĭnz	Reduce cholesterol levels in the blood and block production of an enzyme in the liver that produces cholesterol
thrombolytics thrŏm-bō-LĬT-ĭks	Dissolve blood clots in a process known as *thrombolysis*

Pronunciation Help	Long Sound	ā in rāte	ē in rēbirth	ī in īsle	ō in ōver	ū in ūnite
	Short Sound	ă in ălone	ĕ in ĕver	ĭ in ĭt	ŏ in nŏt	ŭ in cŭt

Closer Look

Take a closer look at these cardiovascular disorders to enhance your understanding of the medical terminology associated with them.

Coronary Artery Disease

Coronary artery disease (CAD) is a condition that involves narrowing of the coronary arteries, resulting in failure of the arteries to deliver an adequate supply of oxygenated blood to the heart muscle **(myocardium)**. Narrowing of arterial walls **(arteriostenosis)** usually caused by atherosclerosis, which is a common form of arteriosclerosis. CAD causes the ordinarily smooth lining of the artery to become roughened as the atherosclerotic plaque collects in the artery. This accumulation causes partial and, eventually, total blockage **(occlusion)** of the artery. The illustration below shows a partial occlusion that results in a decreased supply of oxygenated blood to the myocardium, a condition known as *ischemia* (A). The illustration also shows a later stage of atherosclerosis with total occlusion (B). When the occlusion is total or almost total, the affected area of the heart muscle dies (infarction), causing a heart attack, or *myocardial infarction (MI)*. Surgical treatment for CAD includes angioplasty and coronary artery bypass graft (CABG), both of which are discussed above.

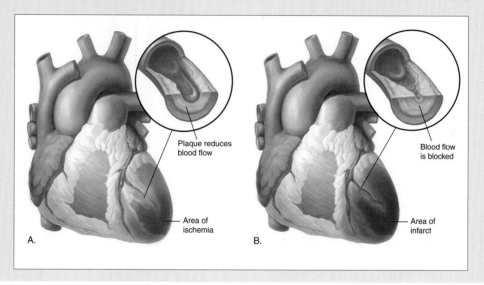

A. Plaque reduces blood flow — Area of ischemia

B. Blood flow is blocked — Area of infarct

(Continued)

Closer Look—cont'd

Varicose Veins

Normal veins have healthy (competent) valves. The venous walls are strong enough to withstand the lateral pressure of blood exerted on them. Blood flows through competent valves in one direction, toward the heart. In **varicose veins,** also known as *varicosities,* dilation of veins from long periods of pressure prevents complete closure of the valves. Unhealthy or damaged **(incompetent)** valves do not close completely. The incompetent valves result in a backflow and pooling of blood in the veins. This pooling causes varicosities that contribute to enlarged, twisted superficial veins, called *varicose veins.* Varicose veins commonly appear blue, bulging, and twisted. If left untreated, varicose veins can cause aching and feelings of fatigue as well as skin changes. Because the blood pools, the risk of **thrombosis** is increased as well. Treatment consists of **sclerotherapy** and such surgical interventions as **endovenous laser ablation (EVLA)** of the greater saphenous (large) veins in the legs and **microphlebectomies** of the lesser saphenous (small) veins. Stripping and ligation of varicose veins is less commonly performed. The illustration below shows valve function in competent and incompetent valves (A) and varicose veins (B).

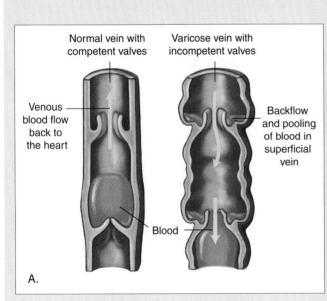

A.

Normal vein with competent valves

Varicose vein with incompetent valves

Venous blood flow back to the heart

Backflow and pooling of blood in superficial vein

Blood

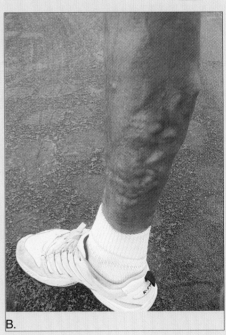

B.

Additional Medical Vocabulary Recall

Match the medical term(s) below with the definitions in the numbered list.

arrhythmia   endarterectomy   HTN   stroke
bruit   fibrillation   nitrate   thrombolytics
DVT   HF   Raynaud disease   statin
embolus   Holter monitor   rheumatic heart disease   varicose veins

1. _____ are swollen, distended veins most commonly seen in the lower legs.

2. _____ means irregular, random contraction of heart fibers.

3. _____ are drugs used to dissolve a blood clot.

4. _____ is a mass of undissolved matter that travels through the bloodstream and becomes lodged in a blood vessel.

5. _____ is a condition in which the heart cannot pump enough blood to meet the metabolic requirement of body tissues.

6. _____ refers to formation of a blood clot in a deep vein of the body.

7. _____ refers to blood pressure that is consistently higher than normal.

8. _____ is irregularity or loss of heart rhythm.

9. _____ is an agent that reduces cholesterol levels in the blood and blocks production of cholesterol in the liver.

10. _____ is a soft blowing sound caused by turbulent blood flow.

11. _____ refers to partial brain damage due to interruption of its blood supply, commonly caused by blockage of an artery.

12. _____ is a streptococcal infection that causes damage to heart valves and heart muscle.

13. _____ is a device worn by a patient that records prolonged electrocardiograph readings, usually for 24 hours, on a portable tape.

14. _____ is numbness in fingers or toes due to intermittent constriction of arterioles in the skin.

15. _____ is the excision of the lining of an artery.

Competency Verification: Check your answers in Appendix B, Answer Key, on page 363. Review material that you did not answer correctly.

Correct Answers _____ × **6.67 =** _____ %

Pronunciation and Spelling

Use the following list to practice correct pronunciation and spelling of medical terms. Practice the pronunciation aloud and then write the correct spelling of the term. The first word is completed for you.

Pronunciation	Spelling
1. ĂN-ū-rĭzm	*aneurysm*
2. ă-RĬTH-mē-ă	
3. ăth-ĕ-rō-sklĕ-RŌ-sĭs	
4. brwē	
5. kăr-dē-ō-MĔG-ă-lē	
6. dī-ĂS-tō-lē	
7. ē-lĕk-trō-kăr-dē-ŎG-ră-fē	
8. fĭ-brĭl-Ā-shŭn	
9. ĭn-FĂRK-shŭn	
10. hī-pĕr-TĔN-shŭn	
11. ĭs-KĒ-mē-ă	
12. mī-ō-KĂR-dē-ăl	
13. tăk-ē-KĂR-dē-ă	
14. THRŎM-bŭs	
15. VĂR-ĭ-kōs	

Competency Verification: Check your answers in Appendix B, Answer Key, on page 364. Review material that you did not answer correctly.

Correct Answers: _____ × 6.67 = _____ %

Abbreviations

The table below introduces abbreviations associated with the cardiovascular system.

Abbreviation	Meaning	Abbreviation	Meaning
AED	automatic external defibrillator	EVLA	endovenous laser ablation; endoluminal laser ablation
AICD	automated implantable cardioverter-defibrillator	EVLT	endovenous laser therapy; endoluminal laser therapy
ASHD	arteriosclerotic heart disease	HDL	high-density lipoprotein
BP	blood pressure	HF	heart failure
CABG	coronary artery bypass graft	HTN	hypertension
CAD	coronary artery disease	ICD	implantable cardioverter-defibrillator
CV	cardiovascular	MI	myocardial infarction
CVA	cerebrovascular accident; costovertebral angle	MVP	mitral valve prolapse
DVT	deep vein thrombosis; deep venous thrombosis	RV	right ventricle
ECHO	echocardiogram; echocardiography; echoencephalogram; echoencephalography	SVC	superior vena cava
ECG, EKG	electrocardiogram; electrocardiography	TIA	transient ischemic attack

Chart Notes

Chart notes comprise part of the medical record and are used in various types of health care facilities. The chart notes that follow were dictated by the patient's physician and reflect common clinical events using medical terminology to document the patient's care. By studying and completing the terminology and chart notes sections below you will learn and understand terms associated with the medical specialty of cardiology.

Terminology

The following terms are linked to chart notes in the specialty of cardiology. Practice pronouncing each term aloud and then use a medical dictionary such as *Taber's Cyclopedic Medical Dictionary, Appendix A: Glossary of Medical Word Elements* on page 337, or other resources to define each term.

Term	Meaning
apnea ăp-NĒ-ă	
desiccated DĔS-ĭ-kā-tĕd	
dyspnea dĭsp-NĒ-ă	
EKG	
fibrillation fĭ-brĭl-Ā-shŭn	
malaise mă-LĀZ	
myocardial infarction mī-ō-KĂR-dē-ăl ĭn-FĂRK-shŭn	
ST segment-T wave	
syncope SĬN-kō-pē	
tachycardia tăk-ē-KĂR-dē-ă	
thyroidectomy thī-royd-ĔK-tō-mē	

Visit *http://davisplus.fadavis.com/gylys-express* for the terminology pronunciation exercise associated with this chart note.

Myocardial Infarction

Read the chart notes below aloud. Underline any term you have trouble pronouncing or cannot define. If needed, refer to the Terminology section above for correct pronunciations and meanings of terms.

This 65-year-old female presents at the hospital for evaluation of a syncopal episode. She states that most recently she has experienced generalized malaise, increased shortness of breath while at rest, and dyspnea followed by periods of apnea and syncope.

Her past history includes recurrent episodes of thyroiditis, which led her to have a thyroidectomy 6 years ago while she was under the care of Dr. Knopp. At the time of surgery, the results of her EKG were interpreted as sinus tachycardia with nonspecific ST segment-T wave changes. The tachycardia was attributed to preoperative anxiety and thyroiditis. Postoperatively, under the direction of Dr. Knopp, the patient was treated with a daily dose of 50 mg of desiccated thyroid and has been symptom-free until this admission.

On clinical examination, the patient's radial pulse was found to be irregular, and the EKG showed uncontrolled atrial fibrillation with evidence of a recent myocardial infarction.

Chart Note Analysis

From the chart note above, select the medical word that means

1. temporary cessation of breathing: _____

2. occurring after an operation: _____

3. feeling of apprehension, worry, uneasiness, or dread: _____

4. inflammation of the thyroid gland: _____

5. fainting: _____

6. dried up: _____

7. extremely rapid, incomplete contractions of the chambers of the heart: _____

8. discomfort or indisposition, commonly indicating infection: _____

9. tachycardia that originates with the SA node: _____

10. abbreviation for a test that provides a recording of electrical impulses of the heart _____

11. difficult breathing: _____

12. abbreviation for metric unit of one one-thousandth of a gram: _____

 Competency Verification: Check your answers in Appendix B, Answer Key, on page 364. Review material that you did not answer correctly.

Correct Answers _____ × 8.34 = _____ %

Demonstrate What You Know!

To evaluate your understanding of how medical terms you have studied in this and previous chapters are used in a clinical environment, complete the numbered sentences by selecting an appropriate term from the list below.

aneurysm	arteriosclerosis	cardiologist	nitrate	statin
angioplasty	arteriostenosis	ischemia	oxygen	tachycardia
arteriole	cardiomegaly	MI	phlebitis	tricuspid

1. The _____ provides nonsurgical treatment to detect, prevent, and treat heart and vascular disease.

2. A small artery is called a(n) _____.

3. An endovascular procedure that reopens a narrowed, blocked vessel by balloon dilation is called _____.

4. To reduce plaque build up in arteries and lower blood cholesterol levels, the cardiologist prescribes a drug called a(n) _____.

5. The valve that contains three leaflets is the _____ valve.

6. Without CV circulation, body tissues are deprived of nutrients and _____.

7. Disorder characterized by thickening and calcification of arterial walls is _____.

8. A patient with an enlarged heart suffers from _____.

9. The diagnosis of inflammation of a vein is charted as _____.

10. A drug that treats chest pain associated with angina is called a(n) _____.

11. Decreased supply of oxygenated blood to a body part or organ is called _____.

12. When performing an angiogram, the surgeon notes a narrowing of an artery, which is charted as _____.

13. A widened, stretched out portion of a blood vessel that forms a bulge is called a(n) _____.

14. A patient arrives at the emergency room with a rapid heart rate, a condition called _____.

15. When heart tissue dies as a result of lack of oxygen, the patient has suffered a(n) _____.

Competency Verification: Check your answers in Appendix B, Answer Key, page 364. Review material that you did not answer correctly.

Correct Answers: _____ × 6.67 = _____ %

Multimedia Review. If you are not satisfied with your retention level of the cardiovascular chapter, go to *http://davisplus.fadavis.com/gylys-express* to complete the website activities linked to this chapter. It is your choice whether or not you want to take advantage of these reinforcement exercises before continuing with the next chapter.

Blood, Lymphatic, and Immune Systems

MULTIMEDIA STUDY TOOLS.
To enrich your medical terminology skills, look for this multimedia icon throughout the text. It will help alert you to when it is best to use the various multimedia resources available with this textbook to enhance your studies.

Objectives

Upon completion of this chapter, you will be able to:

- Describe types of medical treatment provided by hematologists and immunologists.
- Discuss the main components of blood and their functions.
- Understand the four different types of blood groups.
- Name five structures of the lymphatic system.
- List three primary functions of the lymphatic system.
- Explain the relationship between the lymphatic and the immune systems in the immune response.
- Identify combining forms, suffixes, and prefixes associated with the blood, lymphatic, and immune systems.
- Recognize, pronounce, build, and spell medical terms and abbreviations associated with the blood, lymphatic, and immune systems.
- Demonstrate your knowledge by successfully completing the activities in this chapter.

Vocabulary Preview

Term	Meaning

antigen
ĂN-tĭ-jĕn
anti-: against
   gen: forming, producing,
     origin
	Substance that, when entering the body, prompts the generation of antibodies, causing an immune response

autoimmune aw-tō-ĭ-MŪN	Type of immune response by the body against its own cells or tissues
capillaries KĂP-ĭ-lār-ēz	Microscopic blood vessels that connect the ends of the smallest arteries (arterioles) with the smallest veins (venules) of the circulatory system

hematopoiesis
hē-mă-tō-poy-Ē-sĭs
hemat/o: blood
  -poiesis: formation,
     production
	Production and development of blood cells, normally in the bone marrow

immune response ĭm-MŪN	Defense function of the body that protects it against invading pathogens, foreign tissues, and malignancies
immunodeficiency ĭm-ū-nō-dĕ-FĬSH-ĕn-sē	Decreased or compromised ability to fight disease or a condition resulting from a defective immune mechanism
interstitial fluid ĭn-tĕr-STĬSH-ăl	Fluid between cells and in tissue spaces
lymphocyte LĬM-fō-sīt *lymph/o:* lymph *-cyte:* cell	Type of white blood cell (WBC) found in the lymph nodes, spleen, bloodstream, and lymph that functions in the body's immune system by recognizing and deactivating foreign substances (antigens)
monocytes MŎN-ō-sīts *mono-:* one *-cyte:* cell	Large white blood cells formed in the bone marrow that circulate in the bloodstream and destroys pathogenic bacteria through phagocytosis
oncology ŏn-KŎL-ō-jē *onc/o:* tumor *-logy:* study of	Branch of medicine concerned with the study of cancerous growths (malignancies)

Term	Meaning
pathogens PĂTH-ō-jĕns *path/o:* disese *-gen:* forming, producing, origin	Any microorganism capable of producing disease
transfusion trăns-FŪ-zhŭn	Collection of blood or a blood component from a donor followed by its infusion into a recipient

Pronunciation Help	Long Sound	ā in rāte	ē in rēbirth	ī in īsle	ō in ōver	ū in ūnite
	Short Sound	ă in ălone	ĕ in ĕver	ĭ in ĭt	ŏ in nŏt	ŭ in cŭt

Hematology

Hematology is the study of the blood and blood-forming tissues, and the diseases associated with these tissues. Physicians who specialize in the study and treatment of blood and blood disorders are called *hematologists.* Hematologists treat malignant (cancerous) and nonmalignant blood diseases. Historically, they were the first to use chemical therapies (chemotherapy) to treat hematological malignancies. With time, it was discovered that these treatments could also be effective on so-called "solid tumors," such as breast, lung, and stomach cancers (previously only treated with surgery). Consequently, hematology became closely associated with the medical specialty of **oncology.** Oncological terms are included throughout all body system chapters. In addition, *Appendix H, Index of Oncological Terms* provides a summary of these terms.

Immunology

Immunology is the study of the body's protection from invading organisms and its responses to them. These invaders include viruses, bacteria, protozoa, or even larger parasites. Anything that causes an immune response is called an *antigen.* An antigen may be harmless, such as grass pollen, or harmful, such as the flu virus. Disease-causing antigens are called *pathogens.* The immune system is designed to protect the body from pathogens. The body's ability to fight disease and protect itself depends on an adequately functioning **immune response.** An **immunologist** is the medical specialist who studies and treats the body's defense mechanism against invasion of foreign substances that cause disease. The immunologist is consulted when the immune system breaks down and the body loses its ability to recognize **antigens** or its ability to mount an attack against them. Our immune system also has the ability to react in a manner disadvantageous to our own body by way of allergic and **autoimmune** diseases. Thus, immunologists treat patients with **immunodeficiency** diseases, such as acquired immune deficiency syndrome (AIDS); immune complex diseases, such as malaria and viral hepatitis; autoimmune diseases, such as lupus; transplanted cells and organs; allergies; and various cancer types related to the immune system.

Blood, Lymphatic, and Immune Systems Quick Study

Blood

Blood is composed of a clear yellow fluid called *plasma* and various cell types with different functions. The major function of blood is to transport oxygen and nutrients to the cells and remove carbon dioxide and metabolic waste products from the cells. The three main types of cells, also called *formed elements,* found in the blood are erythrocytes (red blood cells), leukocytes (white blood cells), and platelets (clotting cells). Erythrocytes deliver oxygen to the body tissues via the circulatory system. Leukocytes provide a line of defense against **pathogens.** Platelets have a clotting ability that prevents excessive loss of blood. All three cells are produced in the bone marrow by a process called **hematopoiesis.**

Blood Types

The four main blood types, or *groups,* are A, B, AB, and O. The groups are based on the presence or absence of A or B antigens on the red blood cells (RBCs). The antigens, also known as *markers,* stimulate production of antibodies.

Safe administration of blood from donor to recipient requires careful typing and crossmatching to ensure a compatible transfusion. Incompatible transfusions can result in serious, possibly fatal, reactions. For example, antibodies contained in type A blood and type B blood can cause each other to **agglutinate** (clump together). Because type O blood does not contain A or B antigens, type O blood may be given to a person with any of the other blood type. Thus, a person with type O blood is called a *universal donor.* Similarly, a person with type AB blood is a universal recipient, because type AB blood has no antibodies against the other blood types. For a summary of compatible donors and recipients, see Table 6-1 below.

Rh Factor

In addition to ABO antigens, blood may contain other antigens, called *Rh factors.* When these antigens are present on RBCs, the blood type is further classified as *Rh-positive* (Rh+). When these antigens are not present, the blood type is classified as *Rh-negative* (Rh−). Thus, a person with Rh+ blood may receive a transfusion with Rh+ or Rh− blood. However, a person with Rh− blood can receive a transfusion with only Rh− blood.

Table 6-1	**Blood Types, Donors, and Recipients**			
Blood Type	**Antigen on RBC**	**Antigen on Plasma**	**Donate To**	**Receive From**
A	A	anti-B antibodies	A or AB	A or O
B	B	anti-A antibodies	B or AB	B or O
AB (universal recipient)	A and B	none	AB only	A, B, AB, O
O (universal donor)	none	anti-A and anti-B antibodies	A, B, AB, O	O

Lymphatic and Immune Systems

The **lymphatic system** consists of lymph, lymph vessels, lymph nodes, and three organs: the tonsils, thymus, and spleen, as shown in the figure *Lymphatic System* on page xxx. The lymph circulating through the lymphatic system comes from the blood. It contains white blood cells (leukocytes) responsible for immunity as well as **monocytes** and **lymphocytes. Interstitial fluid** is created when certain components of blood plasma filter through tiny capillaries into the spaces between cells, called *interstitial* (or *intercellular*) *spaces*. Thin-walled vessels called *lymph capillaries* absorb most interstitial fluid from the interstitial spaces. At this point of absorption, interstitial fluid becomes lymph and passes through lymphatic tissue called *lymph nodes*. The nodes are located in clusters in such areas as the neck (cervical lymph nodes), under the arm (axillary lymph nodes), pelvis (iliac lymph nodes), and groin (inguinal lymph nodes). These nodes act as filters against foreign materials. Eventually, lymph reaches large lymph vessels in the upper chest and reenters the bloodstream.

The lymphatic and immune systems are closely involved with the **immune response.** They work together to protect the body against invasion of foreign organisms such as viruses and bacteria.

 An extensive anatomy and physiology review is included in *TermPlus,* the powerful, interactive CD-ROM program.

Medical Word Building

Building medical words using word elements related to the blood, lymphatic, and immune system will enhance your understanding of those terms and reinforce your ability to use terms correctly.

Combining Forms

Begin your study of the blood, lymphatic, and immune systems by reviewing their associated combining forms (CFs) and other word elements. These are illustrated in the figures *Blood Components* below and *Lymphatic System* on the next page.

Blood Components

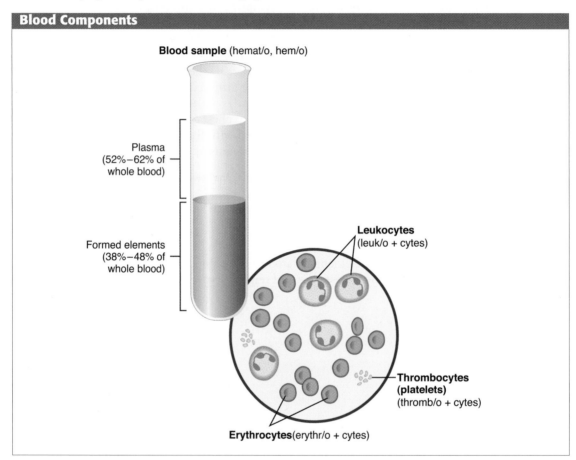

Lymphatic System

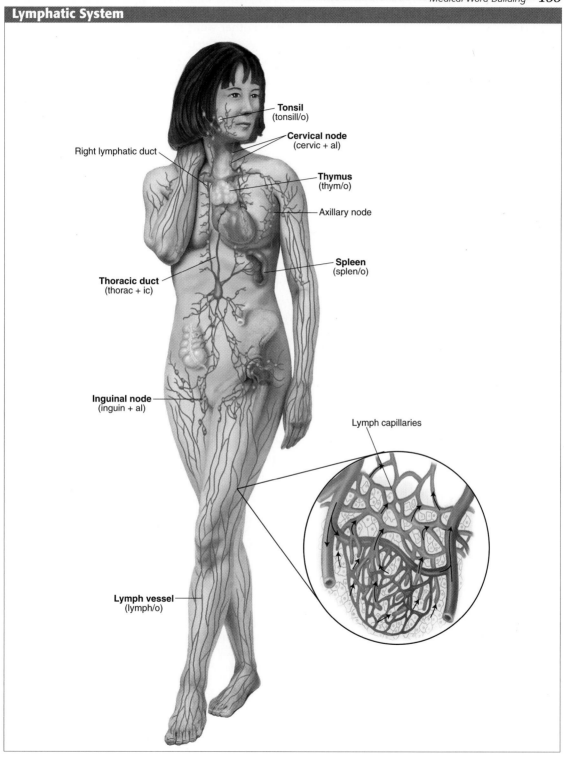

Tonsil
(tonsill/o)

Cervical node
(cervic + al)

Right lymphatic duct

Thymus
(thym/o)

Axillary node

Spleen
(splen/o)

Thoracic duct
(thorac + ic)

Inguinal node
(inguin + al)

Lymph capillaries

Lymph vessel
(lymph/o)

In the table below, CFs are listed alphabetically and other word parts are defined as needed. Review the medical word and study the elements that make up the term. Then complete the meaning of the medical words in the right-hand column. The first one is completed for you. You may also refer to *Appendix A: Glossary of Medical Word Elements* to complete this exercise.

Combining Form	Meaning	Medical Word	Meaning
Blood System			
agglutin/o	clumping, gluing	**agglutin**/ation (ă-gloo-tĭ-NĀ-shŭn) *-ation:* process (of)	*process by which particles are caused to adhere and form into clumps*
embol/o	embolus (plug)	**embol**/ectomy (ĕm-bō-LĔK-tō-mē) *-ectomy:* excision, removal	
erythr/o	red	**erythr**/o/cyte (ĕ-RĬTH-rō-sīt) *-cyte:* cell	
hem/o **hemat/o**	blood	**hem**/o/phobia (hē-mō-FŌ-bē-ă) *-phobia:* fear **hemat**/oma (hēm-ă-TŌ-mă) *-oma:* tumor	
leuk/o	white	**leuk**/o/cyte (LOO-kō-sīt) *-cyte:* cell	
myel/o	bone marrow; spinal cord	**myel**/o/gen/ic (mī-ĕ-lō-JĔN-ĭk) *gen:* forming, producing, origin *-ic:* pertaining to	
thromb/o	blood clot	**thromb**/o/lysis (thrŏm-BŌL-ĭ-sĭs) *-lysis:* separation; destruction; loosening	
ven/o	vein	**ven**/ous (VĒ-nŭs) *-ous:* pertaining to	

Combining Form	Meaning	Medical Word	Meaning
Lymphatic and Immune Systems			
aden/o	gland	**aden/o**/pathy (ă-dĕ-NŎP-ă-thē) *-pathy:* disease	
immun/o	immune, immunity, safe	**immun/o**/gen (ĭ-MŪ-nō-jĕn) *-gen:* forming, producing, origin	
lymph/o	lymph	**lymph/o**/poiesis (lĭm-fō-poy-Ē-sĭs) *-poiesis:* formation, production	
lymphaden/o	lymph gland (node)	**lymphaden**/itis (lĭm-făd-ĕn-Ī-tĭs) *-itis:* inflammation	
lymphangi/o	lymph vessel	**lymphangi**/oma (lĭm-făn-jē-Ō-mă) *-oma:* tumor	
phag/o	swallowing, eating	**phag/o**/cyte (FĂG-ō-sīt) *-cyte:* cell	
splen/o	spleen	**splen/o**/megaly (splĕ-nō-MĔG-ă-lē) *-megaly:* enlargement	
thym/o	thymus gland	**thym**/oma (thī-MŌ-mă) *-oma:* tumor	

Suffixes and Prefixes

In the table below, suffixes and prefixes are listed alphabetically and other word parts are defined as needed. Review the medical word and study the elements that make up the term. Then complete the meaning of the medical words in the right-hand column. You may also refer to *Appendix A: Glossary of Medical Word Elements* to complete this exercise.

Word Element	Meaning	Medical Word	Meaning
Suffixes			
-emia	blood condition	leuk/**emia** (loo-KĒ-mē-ă) *leuk/o:* white	
-phage	swallowing, eating	macro/**phage** (MĂK-rō-făj) macro-: large	
-phylaxis	protection	ana/**phylaxis** (ăn-ă-fĭ-LĂK-sĭs) *ana-:* against; up; back	
-poiesis	formation, production	hem/o/**poiesis** (hē-mō-poy-Ē-sĭs) *hem/o:* blood	
-stasis	standing still	hem/o/**stasis** (hē-mō-STĀ-sĭs) *hem/o:* blood	
Prefixes			
macro-	large	**macro**/cyte (MĂK-rō-sīt) *-cyte:* cell	
micro-	small	**micro**/cyte (MĪ-krō-sīt) *-cyte:* cell	
mono-	one	**mono**/nucle/osis (mŏn-ō-nū-klē-Ō-sĭs) *nucle:* nucleus *-osis:* abnormal condi- tion; increase (used primarily with blood cells)	

 Competency Verification: Check your answers in Appendix B, Answer Key, page 364. If you are not satisfied with your level of comprehension, review the terms in the table and retake the review.

 Listen and Learn, the audio CD-ROM included in this book, will help you master pronunciation of selected medical words. Use it to practice pronunciations of the medical terms in the above "Word Building" tables and for instructions to complete the *Listen and Learn* exercise.

Flash-Card Activity. Enhance your study and reinforcement of this chapter's word elements with the power of DavisPlus flash-card activity. Do so by visiting *http://davisplus.fadavis.com/gylys-express.* We recommend you complete the flash-card activity before continuing with the next section.

Medical Terminology Word Building

In this section, combine the word parts you have learned to construct medical terms related to the blood, lymphatic, and immune systems.

Use *hemat/o* (blood) to build words that mean:

1. tumor (composed) of blood _____

2. production and development of blood cells _____

3. specialist in the study of blood _____

Use *thromb/o* (blood clot) to build words that mean:

4. excision or removal of a thrombus _____

5. resembling a thrombus _____

6. separation, destruction, loosening of a blood clot _____

Use *-cytes* (cells) to build words that mean:

7. cells that are red _____

8. cells that are white _____

9. cells that swallow or eat _____

Use *lymph/o* (lymph) to build words that mean:

10. formation or production of lymph _____

11. lymph cells _____

12. disease of lymph glands _____

Use *immun/o* (immune, immunity, safe) to build words that mean:

13. study of immunity _____

14. producing immunity _____

Use *agglutin/o* (clumping, gluing) to build words that mean:

15. process of cells clumping together _____

16. forming, producing, or origin of clumping or gluing _____

Use *splen/o* (spleen) to build words that mean:

17. enlargement of the spleen _____

18. enlargement of the liver and spleen _____

Use myel/o (bone marrow, spinal cord) to build a word that means:

19. pertaining to forming, producing, or origin in bone marrow _____

Use -*phylaxis* (protection) to build a word that means:

20. against protection _____

> **Competency Verification:** Check your answers in Appendix B, Answer Key, on page 366.
> Review material that you did not answer correctly.
>
> **Correct Answers** _____ × 5 = _____ %

Additional Medical Vocabulary

The following tables list additional terms related to the blood, lymphatic, and immune systems. Recognizing and learning these terms will help you understand the connection between common signs, symptoms, and diseases and their diagnoses. Included are medical and surgical procedures as well as pharmacological agents used to treat diseases.

Signs, Symptoms, and Diseases
Blood System

anemia ă-NĒ-mē-ă *an:* without, not -*emia:* blood condition	Blood disorder characterized by a deficiency of red blood cell production and hemoglobin, increased red blood cell destruction, or blood loss (See Figure 6-1.)
aplastic ā-PLĂS-tĭk	Failure of bone marrow to produce stem cells because it has been damaged by disease, cancer, radiation, or chemotherapy drugs; rare but serious form of anemia
pernicious pĕr-NĬSH-ŭs	Deficiency of erythrocytes due to inability to absorb vitamin B_{12} into the body, which plays a vital role in hematopoiesis
sickle cell SĬK-ăl	Hereditary disorder of anemia characterized by crescent or sickle-shaped erythrocytes; particularly prevalent among persons of African descent
	Get a closer look at sickle cell anemia on pages 143 and 144.

thalassemia
  thăl-ă-SĒ-mē-ă
  thallass/o: sea
    -*emia:* blood
           condition
	Group of hereditary anemias caused by an inability to produce hemoglobin; usually seen in people of Mediterranean origin

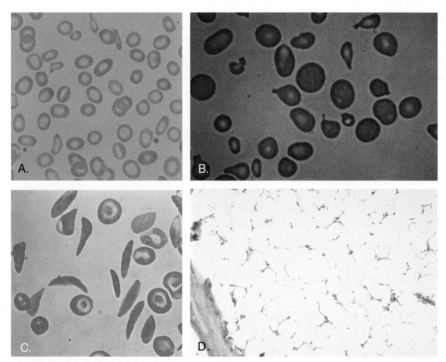

Figure 6–1. Anemias. (A) Iron-deficiency anemia with pale, oval RBCs (magnification x 400). (B) Pernicious anemia with large, misshapen RBCs (magnification x 400). (C) Sickle-cell anemia (magnification x 400). (D) Aplastic anemia in bone marrow (magnification x 200).

(A,B, and C from *Listen, Look and Learn*, Vol 3, *Coagulation, Hematology*. The American Society of Clinical Pathologists Press, Chicago, 1973, with permission; D from Harmening, DM: *Clinical Hematology and Fundamentals of Hemostasis*, ed 3. FA Davis, Philadelphia, 1997, with permission.)

hemophilia hē-mō-FĬL-ē-ă 　*hem/o:* blood 　*-philia:* attraction for	Group of hereditary bleeding disorders characterized by a deficiency of one of the factors necessary for coagulation of blood
leukemia loo-KĒ-mē-ă 　*leuk/o:* white 　*-emia:* blood condition	Malignant disease of the bone marrow characterized by excessive production of leukocytes

Lymphatic and Immune System

acquired immune deficiency syndrome (AIDS) ă-KWĬRD ĭm-ŪN dē-FĬSH-ĕn-sē SĬN-drōm	Deficiency of cellular immunity induced by infection with the human immunodeficiency virus (HIV), characterized by increasing susceptibility to infections, malignancies, and neurological diseases
Hodgkin disease HŎJ-kĭn	Malignant disease characterized by painless, progressive enlargement of lymphoid tissue (usually first evident in cervical lymph nodes), splenomegaly, and the presence of unique Reed-Sternberg cells in the lymph nodes
human immunodeficiency virus (HIV) ĭm-ū-nō-dē-FĬSH-ĕn-sē VĪ-rus	Retrovirus that causes AIDS
immunodeficiency disease ĭm-ū-nō-dĕ-FĬSH-ĕn-sē	Any of a group of diseases caused by a defect in the immune system and generally characterized by susceptibility to infections and chronic diseases
Kaposi sarcoma KĂP-ō-sē săr-KŌ-mă *sarc:* flesh (connective tissue) *-oma:* tumor	Malignancy of connective tissue, including bone, fat, muscle, and fibrous tissue that is commonly fatal (because the tumors readily metastasize to various organs) and closely associated with AIDS
lymphadenitis lĭm-făd-ĕn-Ī-tĭs *lymph:* lymph *aden:* gland *-itis:* inflammation	Inflammation and enlargement of the lymph nodes, usually as a result of infection
lymphedema lĭmf-ĕ-DĒ-mă *lymph:* lymph *-edema:* swelling	Debilitating condition of localized fluid retention and tissue swelling caused by a blockage in the lymphatic system that prevents lymph fluid in the upper limbs from draining adequately

mononucleosis mŏn-ō-nū-klē-Ō-sĭs *mono-:* one *nucle:* nucleus *-osis:* abnormal condition; increase (used primarily with blood cells)	Acute infection caused by the Epstein-Barr virus (EBV) and characterized by a sore throat, fever, fatigue, and enlarged lymph nodes
multiple myeloma mī-ĕ-LŌ-mă	Malignant disease of bone marrow plasma cells (antibody-producing B lymphocytes)
non-Hodgkin lymphoma nŏn-HŎJ-kĭn lĭm-FŌ-mă *lymph:* lymph *-oma:* tumor	Any of a heterogeneous group of malignant tumors involving lymphoid tissue except for Hodgkin disease; previously called *lymphosarcoma*
opportunistic infection	Any infection that results from a defective immune system that cannot defend against pathogens normally found in the environment
stroke	Sudden loss of neurological function, caused by vascular injury (loss of blood flow) to an area of the brain; also known as *CVA*
systemic lupus erythematosus (SLE) LŪ-pŭs ĕr-ĭ-thē-mă-TŌ-sĭs	Chronic autoimmune inflammatory disease with variable features that affect many body systems, particularly the skin, kidneys, heart, and lungs

Diagnostic Procedures

bone marrow aspiration ăs-pĭ-RĀ-shŭn	Removal of a small amount of tissue (bone marrow biopsy) to diagnose blood disorders (such as anemias), cancers, or infectious diseases or to gather cells for later infusion into a patient (bone marrow transplantation) (See Figure 6-2.)

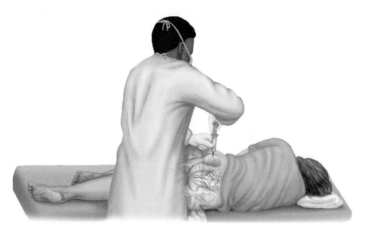

Figure 6–2. Bone marrow aspiration.

ELISA	Test to screen blood for presence of HIV antibodies or for other disease-causing substances

lymphangiography
lĭm-făn-jē-ŎG-ră-fē
   lymph: lymph
   angi/o: vessel (usually blood or lymph)
   -graphy: process of recording
	Radiographic examination of lymph glands and lymphatic vessels after an injection of a contrast medium to view the path of lymph flow as it moves into the chest region

tissue typing	Technique used to determine the histocompatibility of tissues; used in grafts and transplants with the recipient's tissues and cells; also known as *histocompatibility testing*
Western blot	Test to detect presence of viral DNA in the blood and used to confirm the diagnosis of AIDS as well as detecting other viruses

Medical and Surgical Procedures

blood transfusion	Administration of whole blood or a component, such as packed red cells, to replace blood lost through trauma, surgery, or disease

bone marrow transplant	Diseased bone marrow is destroyed by irradiation and chemotherapy, then replaced from a healthy donor to simulate production of normal blood cells; used to treat aplastic anemia, leukemia, and certain cancers
lymphangiectomy lĭm-făn-jē-ĔK-tō-mē *-ectomy:* excision	Removal of a lymph vessel

Pharmacology

anticoagulants ăn-tĭ-kō-ĂG-ū-lăntz	Prevent or delay blood coagulation
immunizations ĭm-ū-nĭ-ZĀ-shŭns	Vaccination or injection of immune globulins to induce immunity to a particular infectious disease
immunosuppressants ĭm-ū-nō-sū-PRĔS-ănts	Suppress the immune response to prevent organ rejection after transplantation or slow the progression of autoimmune disease
thrombolytics thrŏm-bō-LĬT-ĭks	Dissolve a blood clot
vaccinations văk-sĭ-NĀ-shŭnz	Introduction of altered antigens (viruses or bacteria) into the body to produce an immune response and protect against disease

Pronunciation Help	Long Sound	ā in rāte	ē in rēbirth	ī in īsle	ō in ōver	ū in ūnite
	Short Sound	ă in ălone	ĕ in ĕver	ĭ in ĭt	ŏ in nŏt	ŭ in cŭt

Closer Look

Take a closer look at this blood disorder to enhance your understanding of the medical terminology associated with it.

Sickle Cell Anemia

Sickle cell anemia is an inherited form of **anemia**. It is a condition in which there are not enough healthy red blood cells (RBCs) to carry adequate oxygen throughout the body. Normally, RBCs are flexible and round and move easily through blood vessels. In sickle cell anemia, the RBCs

(Continued)

Closer Look—cont'd

become rigid and sticky and are shaped like crescent moons, or sickles. These irregularly shaped cells can get stuck in small blood vessels, which can slow or block blood flow and oxygen to parts of the body. Because sickle cells impair circulation, chronic ill health (**fatigue, dyspnea** on exertion, swollen joints), periodic crises, long-term complications, and premature death can result. The incidence of sickle cell anemia is highest among African Americans and those of Mediterranean ancestry. There is no cure for sickle cell anemia. However, treatment can relieve pain and help prevent further problems associated with this disease. The illustration below shows the most common clinical signs and symptoms of sickle cell anemia.

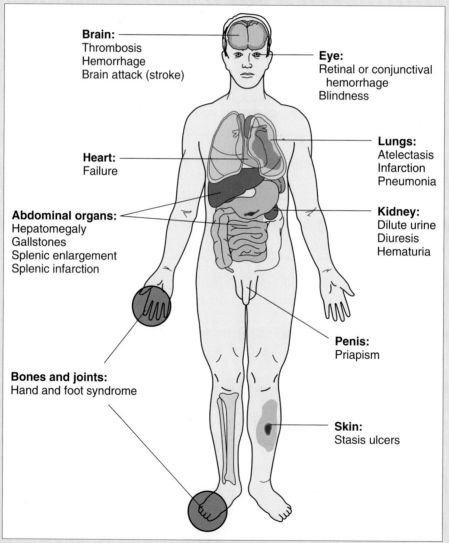

Brain:
Thrombosis
Hemorrhage
Brain attack (stroke)

Eye:
Retinal or conjunctival
hemorrhage
Blindness

Lungs:
Atelectasis
Infarction
Pneumonia

Heart:
Failure

Abdominal organs:
Hepatomegaly
Gallstones
Splenic enlargement
Splenic infarction

Kidney:
Dilute urine
Diuresis
Hematuria

Penis:
Priapism

Bones and joints:
Hand and foot syndrome

Skin:
Stasis ulcers

From Williams and Hopper: *Understanding Medical-Surgical Nursing,* ed 2. FA Davis, 2002, page 381, with permission.

Additional Medical Vocabulary Recall

Match the medical term(s) below with the definitions in the numbered list.

AIDS	HIV	lymphedema
anemia	Hodgkin disease	mononucleosis
anticoagulants	leukemia	SLE
ELISA	lymphadenitis	thrombolytics
hemophilia	lymphangiography	tissue typing

1. _____ is a disease characterized by deficiency of RBCs or hemoglobin.

2. _____ is an acute infection caused by Epstein-Barr virus (EBV) and characterized by a sore throat, fever, fatigue, and enlarged lymph nodes.

3. _____ are drugs that dissolve a blood clot.

4. _____ is a chronic autoimmune inflammatory disease that affects many body systems.

5. _____ is inflammation and enlargement of the lymph nodes.

6. _____ is the retrovirus that causes AIDS.

7. _____ is a radiographic examination of lymph glands and lymphatic vessels after an injection of a contrast medium.

8. _____ is also known as *histocompatibility testing.*

9. _____ refers to malignant solid tumors of the lymphatic system with presence of Reed-Sternberg cells.

10. _____ is induced by infection with the human immunodeficiency virus (HIV).

11. _____ is a malignant disease of the bone marrow characterized by excessive production of leukocytes.

12. _____ is a test to detect HIV antibodies.

13. _____ is a debilitating condition of localized fluid retention and tissue swelling caused by blockage.

14. _____ is a hereditary bleeding disorder.

15. _____ are agents that prevent formation of blood clots.

Competency Verification: Check your answers in Appendix B, Answer Key, on page 366. Review material that you did not answer correctly.

Correct Answers _____ × 5 = _____ %

Pronunciation and Spelling

Use the following list to practice correct pronunciation and spelling of medical terms. Practice the pronunciation aloud and then write the correct spelling of the term. The first word is completed for you.

Pronunciation	Spelling
1. ă-dĕ-NŎP-ă-thē	*adenopathy*
2. ă-gloo-tĭ-NĀ-shŭn	
3. ăn-ă-fĭ-LĂK-sĭs	
4. ăn-tĭ-kō-ĂG-ū-lănt	
5. ĕ-RĬTH-rō-sīt	
6. hēm-ă-TŌ-mă	
7. hē-mō-STĀ-sĭs	
8. ĭ-MŪ-nō-jĕn	
9. loo-KĒ-mē-ă	
10. lĭm-făn-jē-Ŏ-grăf-ē	
11. MĂK-rō-sīt	
12. mŏn-ō-nū-klē-Ō-sĭs	
13. FĂG-ō-sīt	
14. splĕ-nō-MĔG-ă-lē	
15. văk-sĭ-NĀ-shŭn	

Competency Verification: Check your answers in Appendix B, Answer Key, on page 366. Review material that you did not answer correctly.

Correct Answers: _____ × 6.67 = _____ × %

Abbreviations

The table below introduces abbreviations associated with the blood, lymphatic and immune system.

Abbreviation	Meaning	Abbreviation	Meaning
A, B, AB, O	blood types in ABO blood group	KS	Kaposi sarcoma
AIDS	acquired immune deficiency syndrome	lymphos	lymphocytes
CA	cancer	NK	natural killer cell
CBC	complete blood count	PCP	*Pneumocystis* pneumonia; primary care physician; phencyclidine (hallucinogen)
EBV	Epstein-Barr virus	RBC, rbc	red blood cell
ELISA	enzyme-linked immunosorbent assay	SLE	systemic lupus erythematosus
ESR	erythrocyte sedimentation rate	WBC, wbc	white blood cell
Hb, Hgb	hemoglobin	WNL	within normal limits
HIV	human immunodeficiency virus		

Chart Notes

Chart notes comprise part of the medical record and are used in various types of health care facilities. The chart notes that follow were dictated by the patient's physician and reflect common clinical events using medical terminology to document the patient's care. By studying and completing the terminology and chart notes sections below you will learn and understand terms associated with the medical specialty of immunology.

Terminology

The following terms are linked to chart notes in the specialty of immunology. Practice pronouncing each term aloud and then use a medical dictionary such as *Taber's Cyclopedic Medical Dictionary, Appendix A: Glossary of Medical Word Elements* on page 337, or other resources to define each term.

Term	Meaning
AIDS	
antiretroviral ăn-tĭ-rĕt-rō-VĪ-răl	
CD4	
dyspnea dĭsp-NĒ-ă	
hemoglobin HĒ-mō-glō-bĭn	
platelets PLĂT-lĕts	
***Pneumocystis* pneumonia** nū-mō-SĬS-tĭs nū-MŌ-nē-ă	
sputum SPŪ-tŭm	
WNL	

 Visit *http://davisplus.fadavis.com-gylys/express* for the terminology pronunciation exercise associated with this chart note.

Acquired Immune Deficiency Syndrome (AIDS)

Read the chart note on the next page aloud. Underline any term you have trouble pronouncing or cannot define. If needed, refer to the Terminology section above for correct pronunciations and meanings of terms.

SUBJECTIVE: Patient returns to clinic today for continued evaluation and treatment of his AIDS diagnosis. He has completed 2 weeks of antiretroviral therapy. He is tolerating this quite well. Today, he complains of chills, night sweats, and persistent cough with clear productive sputum along with some dyspnea.

OBJECTIVE: Vital Signs: T 99.9°F. P 100. B/P 135/70. WEIGHT: 150 pounds. Lungs: diminished breath sounds in right middle lower lobe.

Laboratory data from today: CD4: 190. White count: 3.3. Hemoglobin: 12.8. Platelets: 123. Liver function tests are WNL.

ASSESSMENT: A 40-year-old man with a 2-year diagnosis of AIDS and possible complications of secondary infection in the lungs, rule out *Pneumocystis* pneumonia.

PLAN:
1. Chest x-ray.
2. Sputum culture.
3. Continue antiretroviral therapy.
4. Tylenol as needed for fever.
5. Return to the clinic in 2 weeks.

Chart Note Analysis

From the chart note above, select the medical word that means

1. difficult breathing: _____

2. drug treatment for a viral infection: _____

3. symptoms of a fever: _____

4. medication used to control fever: _____

5. laboratory test to measure the oxygen carrying capacity of the blood: _____

6. a frequent cough: _____

7. a type of pneumonia seen in AIDs patients: _____

8. abbreviation for a normal test result: _____

9. laboratory test performed on T lymphocytes: _____

10. mucus or phlegm coughed up from the respiratory tract: _____

✓ **Competency Verification:** Check your answers in Appendix B, Answer Key, on page 366. Review material that you did not answer correctly.

Correct Answers: _____ × **10** = _____ %

Demonstrate What You Know!

To evaluate your understanding of how medical terms you have studied in this and previous chapters are used in a clinical environment, complete the numbered sentences by selecting an appropriate term from the list below.

agglutination	HIV	oncology
antigen	Hodgkin	pathogen
aplastic	immunodeficiency	pernicious
hematology	lymphadenitis	phagocytes
hemopoiesis	lymphocytes	splenomegaly

1. _____ is the study of blood and the diseases associated with it.

2. The formation or production of blood is known as _____.

3. The branch of medicine concerned with study of malignancies is _____.

4. Immune cells known as _____ are located in the lymph nodes, spleen, blood, and lymph.

5. _____ are cells that ingest bacteria.

6. _____ anemia is characterized by a failure of bone marrow to produce stem cells.

7. _____ disease is a malignant disease characterized by painless, progressive enlargement of lymphoid tissue.

8. The retrovirus that causes AIDS is known as _____.

9. _____ anemia is characterized by a deficiency of RBCs due to an inability to absorb vitamin B_{12}.

10. A toxin, bacteria, or foreign cell that is introduced into the body and stimulates the production of antibodies is known as a(n) _____.

11. _____ is a pathological condition in which the spleen is enlarged.

12. _____ is an inflammation and enlargement of the lymph nodes.

13. An inability to fight disease is a condition known as _____.

14. _____ refers to any microorganism capable of producing disease.

15. The process of cells clumping together is called _____.

 Competency Verification: Check your answers in Appendix B, Answer Key, on page 366. Review material that you did not answer correctly.

Correct Answers: _____ × 6.67 = _____ × %

Multimedia Review. If you are not satisfied with your retention level of the blood, lymphatic, and immune chapter, visit *http://davisplus.fadavis.com/gylys-express* and complete the website activities linked to this chapter. It is your choice whether or not you want to take advantage of these reinforcement exercises before continuing with the next chapter.

Digestive System

MULTIMEDIA STUDY TOOLS.
To enrich your medical terminology skills, look for this multimedia icon throughout the text. It will help alert you to when it is most advantageous to integrate the various multimedia resources available with this textbook into your studies.

Objectives

Upon completion of this chapter, you will be able to:

- Describe types of medical treatment provided by gastroenterologists.
- Name the primary structures of the digestive system and discuss their functions.
- Identify combining forms, suffixes, and prefixes associated with the digestive system.
- Recognize, pronounce, build, and spell medical terms associated with the digestive system.
- Demonstrate your knowledge of this chapter by successfully completing the activities in this chapter.

Gastroenterology

Gastroenterology is the branch of medicine concerned with diseases of the digestive tract. The **gastroenterologist** diagnoses and treats disorders of the esophagus, stomach, small intestine, large intestine (colon), liver, gallbladder, and pancreas.

To specialize in gastroenterology, a person must first become a licensed physician and then complete an internal medicine residency followed by a 2- to 4-year fellowship in gastroenterology. In this capacity, the gastroenterologist does not perform surgery. However, under the broad classification of surgery, they perform procedures such as liver **biopsy** and **endoscopic examinations.** Endoscopic procedures are commonly used to inspect the esophagus, stomach, and small and large intestines. These procedures help detect pathological conditions, including cancers, at an early stage. Additional diagnostic tests, x-rays, drugs, and medical and surgical procedures are also used to diagnose and treat gastrointestinal diseases.

Digestive System Quick Study

Food is essential for our survival and is required for the chemical reactions that occur in every cell of the body. However, the foods we eat must be broken down physically and chemically into nutrients so that they can be absorbed by cell membranes. This process is known as *digestion,* and the organs of the digestive system collectively perform these functions.

The digestive system consists of the digestive tract, also called the *alimentary canal* or *gastrointestinal (GI) tract,* and the accessory organs of digestion. The digestive tract is a tube starting at the mouth, where food enters the body, and ends at the anus, where solid waste products are excreted from the body. The digestive tube is twisted, swollen, and shaped along its length into several distinct regions: mouth, pharynx (throat), esophagus, stomach, small intestine, large intestine, rectum, and anus. These structures are separated into two sections: the **upper gastrointestinal tract** (mouth, pharynx, esophagus, and stomach) and the **lower gastrointestinal tract** (large and small intestines, rectum, and anus). (See *Digestive system,* page 156.) Food passing through the digestive tract mixes with many chemicals that break it down into nutrient molecules. The digestive system absorbs the molecules into the bloodstream. The body eliminates the indigestible remains after this process of absorption in a process called *defecation.* The accessory organs of digestion, including the liver, gallbladder, and pancreas, help in the absorption process and other processes essential to proper digestion. Although food does not pass through these organs, they play an important role in the processing of food and nutrients.

 An extensive anatomy and physiology is included in *TermPlus*, the powerful, interactive CD-ROM program.

Medical Word Building

Building medical words using word elements related to the digestive system will enhance your understanding of those terms and reinforce your ability to use terms correctly.

Combining Forms

Begin your study of digestive terminology by reviewing the organs and their associated combining forms (CFs), which are illustrated in the figure *Digestive System* on the next page.

Digestive System

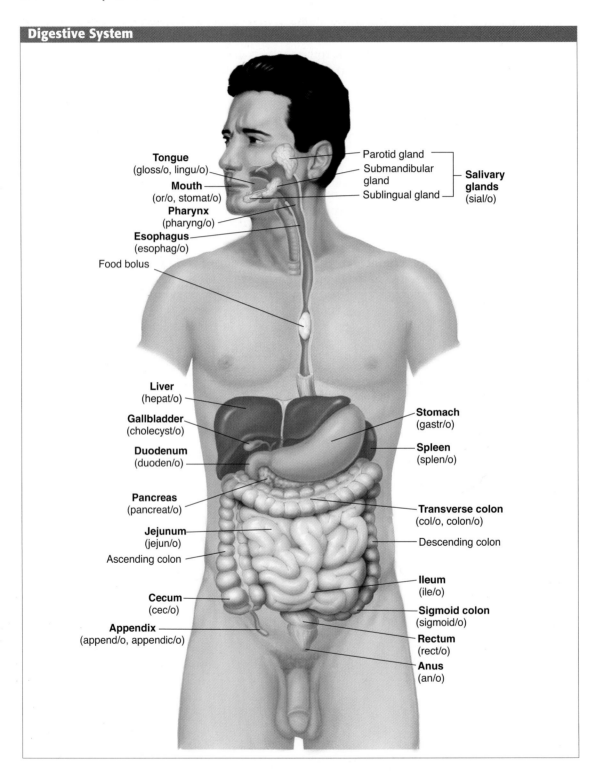

Tongue
(gloss/o, lingu/o)

Mouth
(or/o, stomat/o)

Pharynx
(pharyng/o)

Esophagus
(esophag/o)

Food bolus

Parotid gland

Submandibular gland

Sublingual gland

Salivary glands
(sial/o)

Liver
(hepat/o)

Gallbladder
(cholecyst/o)

Duodenum
(duoden/o)

Pancreas
(pancreat/o)

Jejunum
(jejun/o)

Ascending colon

Cecum
(cec/o)

Appendix
(append/o, appendic/o)

Stomach
(gastr/o)

Spleen
(splen/o)

Transverse colon
(col/o, colon/o)

Descending colon

Ileum
(ile/o)

Sigmoid colon
(sigmoid/o)

Rectum
(rect/o)

Anus
(an/o)

In the table below, CFs are listed alphabetically and highlighted and other word parts are defined as needed. Review the medical word and study the elements that make up the term. Then complete the meaning of the medical words in the right-hand column. The first one is completed for you. You may also refer to *Appendix A: Glossary of Medical Word Elements* to complete this exercise.

Combining Form	Meaning	Medical Word	Meaning
Oral Cavity			
dent/o	teeth	**dent**/ist (DĔN-tĭst) *-ist:* specialist	*specialist in treatment of the teeth*
odont/o		orth/**odont**/ist (ŏr-thō-DŎN-tĭst) *orth:* straight *-ist:* specialist	
gingiv/o	gum(s)	**gingiv**/itis (jĭn-jĭ-VĪ-tĭs) *-itis:* inflammation	
gloss/o	tongue	hypo/**gloss**/al (hī-pō-GLŎS-ăl) *hypo-:* under, below, deficient *-al:* pertaining to	
lingu/o		sub/**lingu**/al (sŭb-LĬNG-gwăl) *sub-:* under, below *-al:* pertaining to	
or/o	mouth	**or**/al (OR-ăl) *-al:* pertaining to	
stomat/o		**stomat**/o/pathy (stō-mă-TŎP-ă-thē) *-pathy:* disease	
ptyal/o	saliva	**ptyal**/ism (TĪ-ă-lĭzm) *-ism:* condition	
sial/o	saliva, salivary gland	**sial**/o/rrhea (sī-ă-lō-RĒ-ă) *-rrhea:* discharge, flow	

(Continued)

Combining Form	Meaning	Medical Word	Meaning
Oral Cavity			
esophag/o	esophagus	**esophag/o**/scope (ē-SŎF-ă-gō-skōp) *–scope:* instrument for examining	
gastr/o	stomach	**gastr/o**/scopy (găs-TRŎS-kō-pē) *–scopy:* visual examination	
pharyng/o	pharynx (throat)	**pharyng/o**/tonsill/itis (fă-rĭng-gō-tŏn-sĭ-LĪ-tĭs) *tonsill:* tonsils *-itis:* inflammation	
pylor/o	pylorus (sphinc-ter in lower portion of the stomach that opens into the duodenum)	**pylor/o**/tomy (pī-lor-ŎT-ō-mē) *-tomy:* incision	
Small Intestine			
duoden/o	duodenum (first part of small intestine)	**duoden/o**/scopy (dū-ŏd-ĕ-NŎS-kō-pē) *–scopy:* visual examination	
enter/o	intestine (usually small intestine)	**enter/o**/pathy (ĕn-tĕr-ŎP-ă-thē) *-pathy:* disease	
jejun/o	jejunum (second part of small intestine)	**jejun/o**/rrhaphy (jĕ-joo-NOR-ă-fē) *-rrhaphy:* suture	
ile/o	ileum (third part of small intestine)	**ile/o**/stomy (ĭl-ē-ŎS-tō-mē) *-stomy**: forming an opening (mouth)	
Large Intestine			
an/o	anus	peri/**an**/al (pĕr-ē-Ā-năl) *peri-:* around *-al:* pertaining to	

*When the suffix –stomy is used with a CF that denotes an organ, it refers to a surgical opening to the outside of the body.

Combining Form	Meaning	Medical Word	Meaning
Large Intestine			
append/o	appendix	**append/**ectomy (ăp-ĕn-DĔK-tō-mē) *-ectomy:* excision, removal	
appendic/o		**appendic/**itis (ă-pĕn-dĭ-SĪ-tĭs) *-itis:* inflammation	
col/o	colon	**col/o/**stomy (kō-LŎS-tō-mē) *-stomy**: forming an opening (mouth)	
colon/o		**colon/o/**scopy (kō-lŏn-ŎS-kō-pē) *-scopy:* visual examination Get a closer look at colonoscopy on pages 172 and 173.	
proct/o	anus, rectum	**proct/o/**logist (prŏk-TŎL-ō-jĭst) *-logist:* specialist in the study of	
rect/o	rectum	**rect/o/**cele (RĔK-tō-sēl) *-cele:* hernia, swelling	
sigmoid/o	sigmoid colon	**sigmoid/o/**tomy (sĭg-moyd-ŎT-ō-mē) *-tomy:* incision	
Accessory Organs of Digestion			
cholangi/o	bile vessel	**cholangi/**ole (kō-LĂN-jē-ōl) *-ole:* small, minute	
chol/e**	bile, gall	**chol/e/**lith (KŌ-lē-lĭth) *-lith:* stone, calculus Get a closer look at gallstones on pages 173 and 174.	

***Using the combining vowel* e *instead of* o *is an exception to the rule.*

(Continued)

Combining Form	Meaning	Medical Word	Meaning
Accessory Organs of Digestion			
cholecyst/o	gallbladder	**cholecyst**/ectomy (kō-lē-sĭs-TĔK-tō-mē) *-ectomy:* excision, removal	
choledoch/o	bile duct	**choledoch/o**/tomy (kō-lĕd-ō-KŎT-ō-mē) *-tomy:* incision	
hepat/o	liver	**hepat**/itis (hĕp-ă-TĪ-tīs) *-itis:* inflammation	
pancreat/o	pancreas	**pancreat/o**/lysis (păn-krē-ă-TŎL-ĭ-sĭs) *-lysis:* separation; destruction; loosening	

Suffixes and Prefixes

In the table below, suffixes and prefixes are listed alphabetically and highlighted and other word parts are defined as needed. Review the medical word and study the elements that make up the term. Then complete the meaning of the medical words in the right-hand column. You may also refer to *Appendix A: Glossary of Medical Word Elements* to complete this exercise.

Word Element	Meaning	Medical Words	Meaning
Suffixes			
-algia	pain	gastr/**algia** (găs-TRĂL-jē-ă) *gastr:* stomach	
-dynia		gastr/o/**dynia** (găs-trō-DĬN-ē-ă) *gastr/o:* stomach	
-emesis	vomiting	hyper/**emesis** (hī-pĕr-ĔM-ĕ-sĭs) *hyper-:* excessive, above normal	
-iasis	abnormal condition (produced by something specified)	chol/e/lith/**iasis** (kō-lē-lĭ-THĪ-ă-sĭs) *chol/e:* bile, gall *lith/o:* stone, calculus	

Word Element	Meaning	Medical Words	Meaning
Suffixes			
-megaly	enlargement	hepat/o/**megaly** (hĕp-ă-tō-MĔG-ă-lē) *hepat/o:* liver	
-orexia	appetite	an/**orexia** (ăn-ō-RĔK-sē-ă) *an-:* without, not	
-osis	abnormal condition; increase (used primarily with blood cells)	cirrh/**osis** (sĭr-RŌ-sĭs) *cirrh:* yellow	
-pepsia	digestion	dys/**pepsia** (dĭs-PĔP-sē-ă) *dys-:* bad; painful; difficult	
-phagia	swallowing, eating	dys/**phagia** (dĭs-FĀ-jē-ă) *dys-:* bad; painful; difficult	
-prandial	meal	post/**prandial** (pōst-PRĂN-dē-ăl) *post-:* after, behind	
-rrhea	discharge, flow	dia/**rrhea** (dī-ă-RĒ-ă) *dia-:* through, across	
Prefixes			
endo-	in, within	**endo**/scopy (ĕn-DŎS-kō-pē) *-scopy:* visual examination Get a closer look at endoscopy on page 172 and page 173.	
hemat-	blood	**hemat**/emesis (hĕm-ăt-ĔM-ĕ-sĭs) *-emesis:* vomiting	
hypo-	under, below, deficient	**hypo**/gastr/ic (hī-pō-GĂS-trĭk) *gastr/o:* stomach *-ic:* pertaining to	

Get a closer look at endoscopy on page 172 and page 173.

Competency Verification: Check your answers in Appendix B, Answer Key, page 366. If you are not satisfied with your level of comprehension, review the terms in the table and retake the review.

 Listen and Learn, the audio CD-ROM included in this book, will help you master pronunciation of selected medical words. Use it to practice pronunciations of the medical terms in the above "Word Building" tables and for instructions to complete the Listen and Learn exercise.

 Flash-Card Activity. Enhance your study and reinforcement of this chapter's word elements with the power of DavisPlus flash-card activity. Do so by visiting http://davisplus.fadavis.com/ gylys-express. We recommend you complete the flash-card activity before continuing with the next section.

Medical Terminology Word Building

In this section, combine the word parts you have learned to construct medical terms related to the digestive system.

Use *esophag/o* (esophagus) to build words that mean:

1. spasm of the esophagus _____
2. stricture or narrowing of the esophagus _____

Use *gastr/o* (stomach) to build words that mean:

3. inflammation of the stomach _____
4. pain in the stomach _____
5. disease of the stomach _____

Use *duoden/o* (duodenum), *jejun/o* (jejunum), or *ile/o* (ileum) to build words that mean:

6. excision of all or part of the jejunum _____
7. inflammation of the ileum _____
8. pertaining to the jejunum and ileum _____

Use *enter/o* (usually small intestine) to build words that mean:

9. inflammation of the small intestine _____
10. disease of the small intestine _____

Use *col/o* (colon) to build words that mean:

11. pertaining to the colon and rectum _____
12. prolapse or downward displacement of the colon _____

Use *proct/o* (anus, rectum) or *rect/o* (rectum) to build words that mean:

13. narrowing or constriction of the rectum _____

14. herniation of the rectum _____

15. paralysis of the anus (anal muscles) _____

Use *chol/e* (bile, gall) to build words that mean:

16. inflammation of the gallbladder _____

17. abnormal condition of a gallstone _____

Use *hepat/o* (liver) or *pancreat/o* (pancreas) to build words that mean:

18. tumor of the liver _____

19. enlargement of the liver _____

20. inflammation of the pancreas _____

Competency Verification: Check your answers in Appendix B, Answer Key, on page 369. Review material that you did not answer correctly.

Correct Answers _____ × 5 = _____ %

Additional Medical Vocabulary

The following tables list additional terms related to the digestive system. Recognizing and learning these terms will help you understand the connection between common signs, symptoms, and diseases and their diagnoses. Included are medical and surgical procedures as well as pharmacological agents used to treat diseases.

Signs, Symptoms, and Diseases

appendicitis ă-pĕn-dĭ-SĪ-tĭs *appendic:* appendix *-itis:* inflammation	Inflammation of the appendix, typically an acute condition caused by blockage of the appendix followed by infection that is treated with surgical removal of the inflamed appendix and antibiotic therapy (See Figure 7-1.)
ascites ă-SĪ-tēz	Pathological build up of fluid in the abdominal (peritoneal) cavity due to liver disease, cancer, heart failure, or kidney failure
borborygmus bŏr-bō-RĬG-mŭs	Gurgling or rumbling sound heard over the large intestine that is caused by gas moving through the intestines

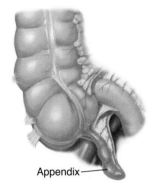

Appendix

A. Diseased appendix

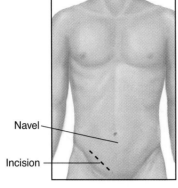

Navel

Incision

B. Incision site

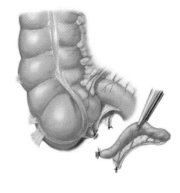

C. Excision of diseased appendix

Figure 7–1. Appendectomy.

cirrhosis
sĭ-RŌ-sĭs
  cirrh: yellow
  -osis: abnormal condition; increase (used primarily with blood cells)
	Chronic liver disease characterized by destruction of liver cells that eventually leads to ineffective liver function and jaundice

diverticular disease dī-věr-TĬK-ū-lăr	Formation of bulging pouches (diverticula) throughout the colon, but most commonly in the lower portion of the colon (includes diverticulosis, diverticular bleeding, and diverticulitis) (See Figure 7-2.)

dysentery
DĬS-ěn-těr-ē
  dys-: bad; painful; difficult
  enter: intestine (usually small intestine)
  -y: condition; process
	Inflammation of the intestine, especially of the colon, caused by chemical irritants, bacteria, or parasites and characterized by diarrhea, colitis, and abdominal cramps

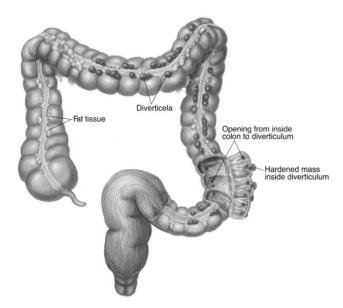

Figure 7–2. Diverticular disease.

fistula FĬS-tū-lă	Abnormal tunnel connecting two body cavities such as the rectum and the vagina (rectovaginal fistula) or a body cavity to the skin (such as the rectum to the outside of the body) caused by an injury, infection, or inflammation
gastroesophageal reflux disease (GERD) găs-trō-ē-sŏf-ă-JĒ-ăl RĒ-flŭks dĭ-ZĒZ *gastr/o:* stomach *esophag:* esophagus *-eal:* pertaining to	Backflow (reflux) of gastric contents into the esophagus due to malfunction of the lower esophageal sphincter (LES)
hematochezia hĕm-ă-tō-KĒ-zē-ă	Passage of bright red, bloody stools (usually an indication that the colon is bleeding somewhere) commonly caused by diverticulitis or hemorrhoids but may be a symptom of CA
hemorrhoid HĔM-ō-royd *hem/o:* blood *-oid:* resembling	Mass of enlarged, twisted varicose veins in the mucous membrane inside (internal) or just outside (external) the rectum; also called *piles*

hernia HĔR-nē-ă	Protrusion or projection of an organ or a part of an organ through the wall of the cavity that normally contains it (See Figure 7-3.)
strangulated	Hernia in which the protruding viscus is so tightly trapped that it leads to necrosis with gangrene results, requiring immediate surgery

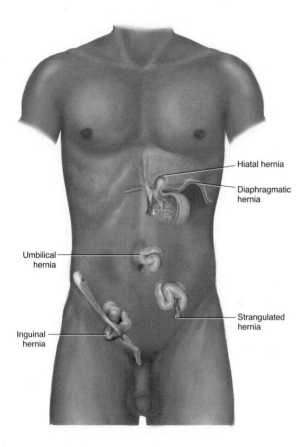

Hiatal hernia

Diaphragmatic hernia

Umbilical hernia

Strangulated hernia

Inguinal hernia

Figure 7–3. Common locations of hernia.

inflammatory bowel disease (IBD) ĭn-FLĂM-ă-tŏr-ē BŌ-wăl	Disorder that causes inflammation of the intestines
Crohn disease krōn	Chronic IBD that may affect any portion of the intestinal tract (usually the ileum) and is distinguished from closely related bowel disorders by its inflammatory pattern, which tends to be patchy or segmented; also called *regional colitis*

ulcerative colitis
  ŬL-sĕr-ā-tĭv kō-LĪ-tĭs
   col: colon
   -itis: inflammation
	Chronic IBD of the colon characterized by ulcers, constant diarrhea mixed with blood, and pain

irritable bowel syndrome (IBS) ĬR-ĭ-tă-bl BŌ-wăl	Common colon disorder characterized by constipation, diarrhea, gas, and bloating that does not cause permanent damage to the colon; also called *spastic colon*

jaundice
JAWN-dĭs
  jaund: yellow
   -ice: noun ending
	Yellow discoloration of the skin, mucous membranes, and sclerae of the eyes caused by excessive levels of bilirubin in the blood; also called *hyperbilirubinemia*

obesity	Condition in which body weight exceeds the range of normal or healthy, which is characterized as a body mass index (BMI) greater than 25
morbid obesity	More severe obesity in which a person has a body mass index (BMI) of 40 or greater, which is generally 100 lb or more over ideal body weight
ulcer ŬL-sĕr	Open sore that may result from a perforation or lesion of the skin or mucous membrane accompanied by sloughing of inflamed necrotic (pathological death of a cell) tissue
volvulus VŎL-vū-lŭs	Twisting of the bowel on itself, causing obstruction

Diagnostic Procedures

barium enema (BE) BĂ-rē-ŭm ĔN-ĕ-mă	Radiographic examination of the rectum and colon after administration of barium sulfate (radiopaque contrast medium) into the rectum. BE is used for diagnosis of obstructions, tumors, or other abnormalities, such as ulcerative colitis. (See Figure 7-4.)
barium swallow BĂ-rē-ŭm	Radiographic examination of the esophagus, stomach, and small intestine after oral administration of barium sulfate (radiopaque contrast medium); also called *upper GI series*
cholangiography kō-lăn-jē-ŎG-ră-fē	Radiographic examination of the bile ducts with a contrast medium to reveal gallstones or other obstruction in the bile ducts

esophagogastroduodenoscopy (EGD)
ĕ-sŏf-ă-gō-găs-trō-doo-ō-dĕn-ŎS-kō-pē
  endo-: in, within
  -scopy: visual
         examination
	Visual examination of the esophagus (esophagoscopy), stomach (gastroscopy), and duodenum (duodenoscopy) using an endoscope; also called *upper GI endoscopy*

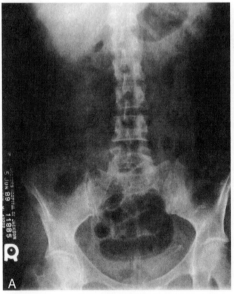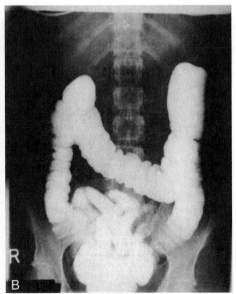

Figure 7–4. Barium enema done poorly (A) and correctly (B).

stool guaiac GWĪ-ăk	Test performed on feces using the reagent gum guaiac to detect presence of blood in feces that is not apparent on visual inspection; also called *hemoccult test*

Medical and Surgical Procedures

bariatric surgery BĂR-ē-ă-trĭk	Any of a group of procedures used to treat morbid obesity (See Figure 7-5.)
vertical banded gastroplasty GĂS-trō-plăs-tē *gastr/o:* stomach *-plasty:* surgical repair	Bariatric surgery in which the upper stomach near the esophagus is stapled vertically to reduce it to a small pouch and a band is inserted that restricts and delays food from leaving the pouch, causing a feeling of fullness (See Figure 7-5A.)
Roux-en-Y gastric bypass (RGB) rū-ĕn-WĪ GĂS-trĭk	Bariatric surgery in which the stomach is first stapled to decrease it to a small pouch and then the jejunum is shortened and connected to the small stomach pouch, causing the base of the duodenum leading from the nonfunctioning portion of the stomach to form a Y configuration, which decreases the pathway of food through the intestine, thus reducing absorption of calories and fats (See Figure 7-5B.)

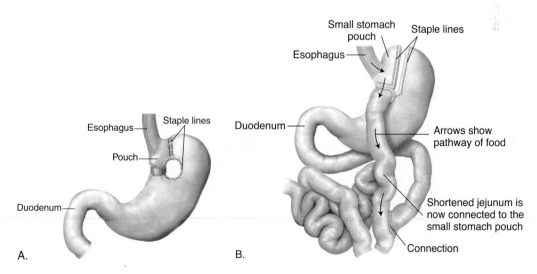

Figure 7–5. Bariatric surgery. (A) Vertical banded gastroplasty. (B) Roux-en-Y gastric bypass.

colostomy kō-LŎS-tō-mē	Excision of a diseased part of the colon and relocation of the remaining end of the healthy colon through the abdominal wall to divert fecal flow to a colostomy bag (See Figure 7-6.)

lithotripsy
LĬTH-ō-trĭp-sē
  lith/o: stone, calculus
  -tripsy: crushing
extracorporeal shock-
wave lithotripsy
(ESWL)
ĕks-tră-kor-POR-ē-ăl
LĬTH-ō-trĭp-sē
  extra-: outside
  corpor: body
    -eal: pertaining to
  lith/o: stone, calculus
  -tripsy: crushing
	Eliminating a stone within the gallbladder or urinary system by crushing it surgically or using a noninvasive method, such as ultra-sonic shock waves, to shatter it
	
	Use of shock waves as a noninvasive method to destroy stones in the gallbladder and biliary ducts

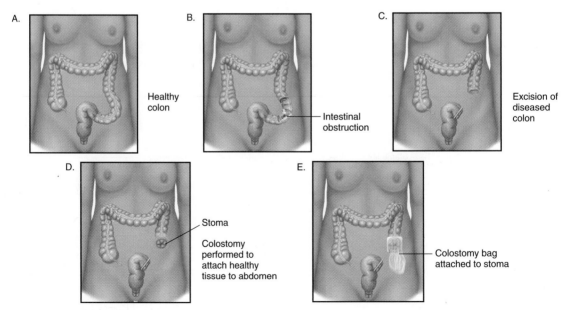

Figure 7–6. Colostomy.

nasogastric intubation
nā-zō-GĂS-trĭk ĭn-tū-BĀ-shŭn
  nas/o: nose
  gastr: stomach
    -ic: pertaining to
	Insertion of a soft plastic nasogastric tube through the nostrils, past the pharynx, and down the esophagus into the stomach to remove substances from the stomach; deliver medication, food, or fluids; or obtain a specimen for laboratory analysis

polypectomy
pŏl-ĭ-PĔK-tō-mē
  polyp: small growth
  -ectomy: excision,
      removal
	Excision of small, tumorlike, benign growths (polyps) that project from a mucous membrane surface (See Figure 7-7.)

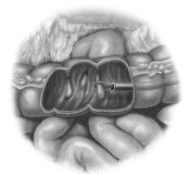

Polyps are removed from
colon for examination

Figure 7–7. Polypectomy.

Pharmacology

antacids ănt-ĂS-ĭds	Neutralize acids in the stomach
antidiarrheals ăn-tĭ-dī-ă-RĒ-ăls	Control loose stools and relieve diarrhea by absorbing excess water in the bowel or slowing peristalsis in the intestinal tract
antiemetics ăn-tĭ-ē-MĔT-ĭks	Control nausea and vomiting by blocking nerve impulses to the vomiting center of the brain

laxatives LĂK-să-tĭvz	Relieve constipation and facilitate passage of feces through the lower GI tract

Pronunciation Help	Long Sound	ā in rāte	ē in rēbirth	ī in īsle	ō in ōver	ū in ūnite
	Short Sound	ă in ălone	ĕ in ĕver	ĭ in ĭt	ŏ in nŏt	ŭ in cŭt

Closer Look

Take a closer look at the diagnostic procedures and disorders to enhance your understanding of the medical terminology associated with them.

Endoscopy

Endoscopy is a minimally invasive diagnostic procedure that utilizes an endoscope (rigid or flexible fiberoptic tube and a lighted optical system) to visually examine the gastrointestinal tract. Endoscopy can also be used to obtain samples for cytologic and histologic examination and to follow the course of a disease, such as the assessment of the healing of gastric and duodenal ulcers. A camera or video recorder is commonly used during endoscopic procedures to provide a permanent record for later reference. The organ being examined dictates the name of the endoscopic procedure. For example, visual examination of the esophagus is known as *esophagoscopy*, visual examination of the stomach is known as *gastroscopy*, and visual examination of the duodenum is known as *duodenoscopy*.

In the digestive system, endoscopies can be grouped into upper and lower GI endoscopies. An **upper GI endoscopy** uses an endoscope inserted through the nose or mouth. It includes endoscopy of the esophagus (**esophagoscopy**), stomach (**gastroscopy**), duodenum (**duodenoscopy**), and the esophagus, stomach, and duodenum (**esophagogastroduodenoscopy**). Upper GI endoscopies help identify tumors, **esophagitis, gastroesophageal varices** (varicose veins or varicosities), peptic ulcers, and the source of upper GI bleeding. Endoscopy is also used to confirm the presence and extent of varices in the lower esophagus and stomach in patients with liver disease. Lower GI endoscopies consist of endoscopy of the colon (**colonoscopy**), sigmoid colon (**sigmoidoscopy**), and rectum and anal canal (**proctoscopy**). A **lower GI endoscopy** employs the use of an endoscope inserted through the rectum. Endoscopy of the lower GI tract helps identify pathological conditions of the colon, such as colorectal cancer. In the lower GI, endoscopy may be combined with a **polypectomy**. Detection of polyps in the colon requires their retrieval and testing for cancer. The illustration below shows the location of a colonoscopy and a sigmoidoscopy.

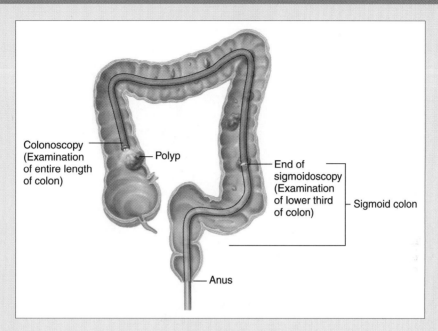

Most endoscopic procedures are considered relatively painless, but may be associated with moderate discomfort. For example, in esophagogastroduodenoscopy, most patients tolerate the procedure with only topical anesthesia of the oropharynx using lidocaine spray. Complications are rare but can include perforation of an organ under inspection with the endoscope or biopsy instrument. If such a complication occurs, surgery may be required to repair the injury.

Gallstones

The gallbladder is usually the site where gallstones **(choleliths),** or calculi form **(cholelithiasis).** When calculi are present in the common bile duct, the condition is known as *choledocholithiasis.* These stones may be formed of cholesterol or calcium-based compounds and range from a microscopic size to more than an inch. The cause of cholelithiasis is not well understood. Any factors that cause the bile to become overloaded with cholesterol may increase the likelihood of the formation of cholesterol-based gallstones. Such factors include obesity, high-calorie diets, certain drugs, oral contraceptives, multiple pregnancies, and increasing age.

Asymptomatic gallstones are neither removed nor treated. If a gallstone travels and obstructs the common bile duct or the cystic duct, pain can develop in the **epigastric** region, right upper quadrant, or both and sometimes radiates to the upper right back area. This discomfort is generally accompanied by **nausea** and vomiting. Symptomatic gallstone disease is treated by **laparoscopic cholecystectomy.** Surgery involves incisions in the abdomen through which pass a tiny video camera and surgical instruments. Surgeons view video pictures on a monitor and remove the gallbladder by manipulating the surgical instruments. The illustration below shows various sites of gallstones.

(Continued)

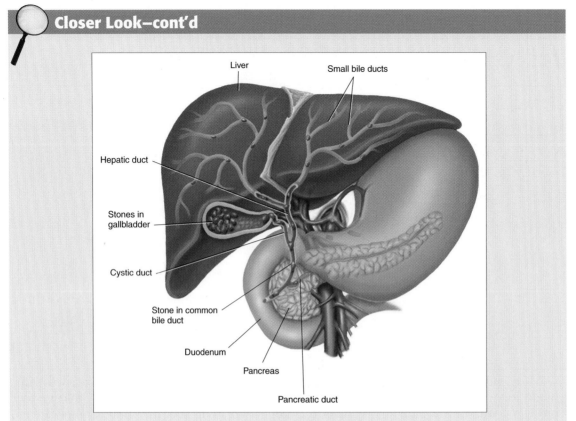

Additional Medical Vocabulary Recall

Match the medical term(s) below with the definitions in the numbered list.

ascites	fistula	lithotripsy
barium enema	hematochezia	nasogastric intubation
barium swallow	IBD	polyp
cirrhosis	IBS	stool guaiac
Crohn disease	jaundice	volvulus

1. _____ is a test performed on feces that detects the presence of blood that is not apparent on visual inspection.

2. _____ refers to insertion of a tube through the nose into the stomach for therapeutic and diagnostic purposes.

3. _____ is a small benign growth that projects from the mucous membrane.

4. _____ is an abnormal accumulation of serous fluid in the peritoneal cavity.

5. _____ refers to chronic inflammatory bowel disease, which usually affects the ileum.

6. _____ refers to surgically crushing a stone.

7. _____ is an abnormal passageway between two body cavities that normally do not connect.

8. _____ is a yellow discoloration of the skin caused by hyperbilirubinemia.

9. _____ is a radiographic examination of the rectum and colon after administration of barium sulfate.

10. _____ refers to an inflammatory bowel disease, as seen in Crohn disease.

11. _____ refers to passage of stools containing red blood.

12. _____ means twisting of the bowel on itself, causing obstruction.

13. _____ refers to a chronic liver disease characterized by destruction of liver cells and jaundice.

14. _____ is a radiographic examination of the esophagus, stomach, and small intestine after oral administration of a contrast medium.

15. _____ is a colon disorder characterized by constipation, diarrhea, gas, and bloating; also called *spastic colon*.

Competency Verification: Check your answers in Appendix B, Answer Key, on page 369. Review material that you did not answer correctly.

Correct Answers _____ × **6.67** = _____ %

Pronunciation and Spelling

Use the following list to practice correct pronunciation and spelling of medical terms. First practice the pronunciation aloud. Then write the correct spelling of the term. The first word is completed for you.

Pronunciation	Spelling
1. ă-pĕn-dĭ-SĪ-tĭs	*appendicitis*
2. ă-SĪ-tēz	
3. bĭl-ĭ-ROO-bĭn	
4. bōr-bō-RĬG-mŭs	
5. kŏ-lăn-jē-ō-păn-krē-ă-TŎG-ră-fē	
6. kō-lē-sĭs-TĔK-tō-mē	
7. kō-LĔD-ō-kō-plăs-tē	
8. kō-lē-lĭ-THĪ-ă-sĭs	
9. sĭr-RŌ-sĭs	
10. kō-LŎS-tō-mē	
11. krōn dĭ-ZĒZ	
12. dū-ŏd-ĕ-NĪ-tĭs	
13. ĕn-tĕr-ŎP-ă-thē	
14. ĕ-sŏf-ă-gō-găs-trō-doo-ō-dĕn-ŎS-kō-pē	
15. găs-trō-ĕ-sŏf-ă-JĔ-ăl	
16. glŏs-ĔK-tō-mē	
17. hĕp-ă-TĪ-tĭs	
18. ĭl-ē-ō-RĔK-tăl	
19. JAWN-dĭs	
20. sĭg-moyd-ŎT-ō-mē	

Competency Verification: Check your answers in Appendix B, Answer Key, on page 369. Review material that you did not answer correctly.

Correct Answers: _____ × 5 = _____ %

Abbreviations

The table below introduces abbreviations associated with the digestive system.

Abbreviation	Meaning	Abbreviation	Meaning
BE	barium enema; below the elbow	GERD	gastroesophageal reflux disease
BM	bowel movement	GI	gastrointestinal
CA	cancer; chronological age; cardiac arrest	HAV	hepatitis A virus
Ca	calcium; cancer	HBV	hepatitis B virus
EGD	esophagogastroduodenoscopy	IBD	inflammatory bowel disease
ERCP	endoscopic retrograde cholangiopancreatography	IBS	irritable bowel syndrome
ESWL	extracorporeal shock-wave lithotripsy	RGB	Roux-en-Y gastric bypass
FBS	fasting blood sugar	UGI	upper gastrointestinal

Chart Notes

Chart notes comprise part of the medical record and are used in various types of health care facilities. The chart notes that follow were dictated by the patient's physician and reflect common clinical events using medical terminology to document the patient's care. By studying and completing the terminology and chart notes sections below you will learn and understand terms associated with the medical specialty of gastroenterology medicine.

Terminology

The following terms are linked to chart notes in the specialty of gastroenterology. First, practice pronouncing each term aloud. Then, use a medical dictionary such as *Taber's Cyclopedic Medical Dictionary*, *Appendix A: Glossary of Medical Word Elements* on page 337, or other resources to define each term.

Term	Meaning
angulation ăng-ū-LĀ-shŭn	
anorectal ā-nō-RĔK-tăl	

(Continued)

Term	Meaning
carcinoma kăr-sĭ-NŌ-mă	
cm	
diarrhea dī-ă-RĒ-ă	
diverticulum dī-vĕr-TĬK-ū-lŭm	
dysphagia dĭs-FĀ-jē-ă	
emesis ĔM-ĕ-sĭs	
enteritis ĕn-tĕr-Ī-tĭs	
hematemesis hĕm-ăt-ĔM-ĕ-sĭs	
ileostomy ĭl-ē-ŎS-tō-mē	
nausea NAW-sē-ă	
polyp PŎL-ĭp	
postprandial pōst-PRĂN-dē-ăl	
sigmoidoscopy sĭg-moy-DŎS-kō-pē	

 Visit *http://davisplus.fadavis.com/gylys-express* for the terminology pronunciation exercise associated with this chart note.

Rectal Bleeding

Read the chart note below aloud. Underline any term you have trouble pronouncing and any terms that you cannot define. If needed, refer to the Terminology section above for correct pronunciations and meanings of terms.

> This 50-year-old white man has lost approximately 40 pounds since his last examination. The patient says he has had no dysphagia or postprandial distress, and there is no report of diarrhea, nausea, emesis, hematemesis, or constipation. The patient has had a history of regional enteritis, appendicitis, and colonic bleeding.
>
> The regional enteritis resulted in an ileostomy with appendectomy about 6 months ago. On 5/30/XX, a sigmoidoscopy using a 10-cm scope showed no evidence of bleeding at the anorectal area. A 35-cm scope was then inserted to a level of 13 cm. At this point, angulation prevented further passage of the scope. No abnormalities had been encountered, but there was dark blood noted at that level.
>
> Impression: Rectal bleeding due to a polyp, bleeding diverticulum, or rectal carcinoma.

Chart Note Analysis

From the chart note above, select the medical word that means

1. following a meal: _____

2. pertaining to the anus and rectum: _____

3. abnormal formation of an angle: _____

4. tumor on a small stem: _____

5. sac or pouch on the wall of a canal: _____

6. painful or difficult swallowing: _____

7. inflammation of the small intestine: _____

8. creation of a surgical passage through the abdominal wall to the last portion of the small intestine:

_____

9. vomiting blood: _____

10. malignant tumor: _____

 Competency Verification: Check your answers in Appendix B, Answer Key, on page 369. Review material that you did not answer correctly.

Correct Answers _____ **× 10 =** _____ **%**

Demonstrate What You Know!

To evaluate your understanding of how medical terms you have studied in this and previous chapters are used in a clinical environment, complete the numbered sentences by selecting an appropriate term from the list below.

bariatric	gastroesophagitis	hemorrhoids	pylorotomy	stones
bile ducts	GERD	nausea	sigmoidoscopy	stool
constipation	hematemesis	orthodontist	stomach	sublingually

1. When medication is placed under the tongue, it is administered _____.

2. A specialist who straightens teeth is called a(n) _____.

3. A patient suffering from inflammation of the stomach and esophagus has a condition known as _____.

4. A patient with obesity who has failed to lose weight by numerous other means may consider _____ surgery.

5. During a(n) _____, the patient's last section of the colon is under direct visual examination.

6. A diagnosis of _____ indicates a mass of dilated, tortuous veins in the anorectal area.

7. When the surgeon makes an incision into the upper sphincter of the stomach, the surgical procedure is known as _____.

8. A person suffering from _____ has infrequent passage of hard, dry feces.

9. A patient who vomits blood is diagnosed with a condition known as _____.

10. Cholangiography is a radiographic examination of the _____ to reveal gallstones or other obstructions.

11. _____ is an unpleasant sensation that precedes vomiting.

12. Test performed using the reagent "guaiac" requires a _____ sample.

13. ESWL uses shock waves to destroy _____ in the gallbladder and biliary ducts.

14. A nasogastric tube is inserted through the nose into the _____.

15. _____ is a chronic condition which may cause heartburn due to malfunction of the lower esophageal sphincter, which allows gastric acid to reflux into the esophagus.

Competency Verification: Check your answers in Appendix B, Answer Key, on page 369. Review material that you did not answer correctly.

Correct Answers: _____ × **6.67** = _____ %

Multimedia Review. If you are not satisfied with your retention level of the digestive chapter, visit *http://davisplus.fadavis.com/gylys-express* to complete the website activities linked to this chapter. It is your choice whether or not you want to take advantage of these reinforcement exercises before continuing with the next chapter.

Urinary System

MULTIMEDIA STUDY TOOLS.
To enrich your medical terminology skills, look for
this multimedia icon throughout the text. It will help
alert you to when it is most advantageous to integrate
the various multimedia resources available with this
textbook into your studies.

Objectives

*Upon completion of this chapter, you will
be able to:*

- Describe types of medical treatment provided by
  urologists and nephrologists.
- Name the primary structures of the urinary
  system and discuss their functions.
- Identify combining forms, suffixes, and prefixes
  associated with the urinary system.
- Recognize, pronounce, build, and spell medical
  terms and abbreviations associated with the
  urinary system.
- Demonstrate your knowledge by successfully
  completing the activities in this chapter.

Vocabulary Preview

Term	Meaning
cystoscopy sĭs-TŎS-kō-pē *cyst/o:* bladder *-scopy:* visual examination	Visual examination of the urinary bladder and urethra using a cystoscope (thin, tubelike instrument with a light and lens for viewing) inserted through the urethra
dialysis dī-ĂL-ĭ-sĭs *dia-:* through, across *-lysis:* separation; destruction; loosening	Mechanical filtering process used to remove metabolic waste products from blood, draw off excess fluids, and regulate body chemistry when kidneys fail to function properly
electrolytes ē-LĔK-trō-līts	Solutions that conduct electricity, such as acids, bases, and salts (sodium, potassium)
metabolism mě-TĂB-ō-lĭzm	Sum of all physical and chemical changes that take place within an organism
pH	Symbol for the measure of hydrogen ion concentration in a solution or the acidity or alkalinity of a substance
transurethral resection of the prostate (TURP)	Surgical procedure that removes part of an enlarged prostate via an instrument inserted through the urethra

Pronunciation Help	Long Sound	ā in rāte	ē in rēbirth	ī in īsle	ō in ōver	ū in ūnite
	Short Sound	ă in ălone	ĕ in ĕver	ĭ in ĭt	ŏ in nŏt	ŭ in cŭt

Urology and Nephrology

Urology

The medical specialty of **urology** is associated with the urinary system. Physicians who specialize in female and male urinary disorders are called *urologists*. Because some male urinary structures perform urinary and reproductive functions, urologists also diagnose and treat male reproductive disorders, such as infertility and sexual dysfunction. Urologists also specialize in surgeries, such as transurethral **resection of the prostate,** as well as **cystoscopy** and various other types of procedures to treat urinary tract disorders.

Nephrology

Nephrologists specialize in diagnosis and management of kidney disease, kidney transplantation, and **dialysis** therapies. The medical specialty of **nephrology** is a subspecialty of internal medicine. After completing a residency, the internist is required to complete additional training, or a fellowship, as a nephrologist.

Urinary System Quick Study

The primary function of the **urinary system** is to remove waste products of **metabolism** from the blood by excreting them in the urine. Organs of the urinary system are the kidneys, ureters, bladder, and urethra. Formation of urine is performed by the function of the kidneys. Other important functions of the kidneys include regulating the body's tissue fluid and maintaining a balance of **electrolytes** and an acid-base balance **(pH)** in the blood. The other urinary structures store and eliminate urine. (See *Urinary System*, page 186.)

 An extensive anatomy and physiology review is included in *TermPlus*, the powerful, interactive CD-ROM program.

Medical Word Building

Building medical words using word elements related to the urinary system will enhance understanding of those terms and reinforce the ability to use terms correctly.

Combining Forms

Begin the study of urology terminology by reviewing the organs of the urinary system and their associated combining forms (CFs). These are illustrated in the figure *Urinary System* on next page.

Urinary System

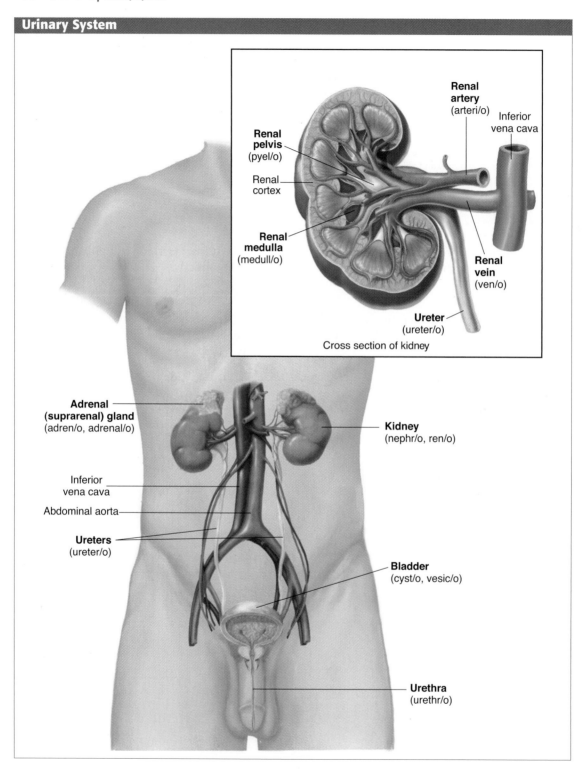

Renal
artery
(arteri/o)

Inferior
vena cava

Renal
pelvis
(pyel/o)

Renal
cortex

Renal
medulla
(medull/o)

Renal
vein
(ven/o)

Ureter
(ureter/o)

Cross section of kidney

Adrenal
(suprarenal) gland
(adren/o, adrenal/o)

Kidney
(nephr/o, ren/o)

Inferior
vena cava

Abdominal aorta

Ureters
(ureter/o)

Bladder
(cyst/o, vesic/o)

Urethra
(urethr/o)

In the table below, CFs are listed alphabetically and other word parts are defined as needed. Review the medical word and study the elements that make up the term. Then complete the meaning of the medical word in the right-hand column. The first one is completed for you. You may also refer to *Appendix A: Glossary of Medical Word Elements* to complete this exercise.

Combining Form	Meaning	Medical Word	Meaning
cyst/o	bladder	**cyst/o**/scopy (sĭs-TŎS-kō-pē) *-scopy:* visual examination	*visual examination of the bladder*
vesic/o		**vesic/o**/cele (VĚS-ĭ-kō-sēl) *-cele:* hernia, swelling	
glomerul/o	glomerulus	**glomerul/o**/pathy (glō-mĕr-ū-LŎP-ă-thē) *-pathy:* disease	
meat/o	opening, meatus	**meat/**us (mē-Ā-tŭs) *-us:* condition, structure	
nephr/o	kidney	hydr/o/**nephr/**osis (hī-drō-nĕf-RŌ-sĭs) *hydr/o:* water *-osis:* abnormal condition (used primarily with blood cells) Get a closer look at hydronephrosis on pages 199 and 200.	
ren/o		**ren/**al (RĒ-năl) *-al:* pertaining to	
pyel/o	renal pelvis	**pyel/o**/plasty (PĪ-ĕ-lō-plăs-tē) *-plasty:* surgical repair	
ur/o	urine, urinary tract	**ur/**emia (ū-RĒ-mē-ă) *-emia:* blood condition	
urin/o		**urin/**ary (Ū-rĭ-nār-ē) *-ary:* pertaining to	

(Continued)

Combining Form	Meaning	Medical Word	Meaning
ureter/o	ureter	**ureter/o**/stenosis (ū-rē-tĕr-ō-stĕ-NŌ-sĭs) *–stenosis:* narrowing, stricture	
urethr/o	urethra	**urethr/o**/cele (ū-RĒ-thrō-sēl) *–cele:* hernia, swelling	

Suffixes and Prefixes

In the table below, suffixes and prefixes are listed alphabetically and other word parts are defined as needed. Review the medical word and study the elements that make up the term. Then complete the meaning of the medical word in the right-hand column. You may also refer to *Appendix A: Glossary of Medical Word Elements* to complete this exercise.

Word Element	Meaning	Medical Word	Meaning
Suffixes			
-emia	blood condition	azot/**emia** (ăz-ō-TĒ-mē-ă) *azot:* nitrogenous compounds	
-iasis	abnormal condition (produced by something specified)	lith/**iasis** (lĭth-Ī-ă-sĭs) *lith:* stone, calculus	
-lysis	separation; destruction; loosening	dia/**lysis** (dī-ĂL-ĭ-sĭs) *dia-:* through, across Get a closer look at dialysis on pages 200 and 201.	
-pathy	disease	nephr/o/**pathy** (ně-FRŎP-ă-thē) *nephr/o:* kidney	
-pexy	fixation (of an organ)	nephr/o/**pexy** (NĚF-rō-pěks-ē) *nephr/o:* kidney	

Word Element	Meaning	Medical Word	Meaning
Suffixes			
-ptosis	prolapse, downward displacement	nephr/o/**ptosis** (nĕf-rŏp-TŌ-sĭs) *nephr/o:* kidney	
-tripsy	crushing	lith/o/**tripsy** (LĬTH-ō-trĭp-sē) *lith/o:* stone, calculus	
-uria	urine	olig/uria (ōl-ĭg-Ū-rē-ă) *olig:* scanty	
Prefixes			
an-	without, not	**an**/uria (ăn-Ū-rē-ă) *-uria:* urine	
poly-	many, much	poly/**uria** (pŏl-ē-Ū-rē-ă) *-uria:* urine	
supra-	above; excessive; superior	**supra**/ren/al (soo-pră-RĒ-năl) *ren:* kidney *-al:* pertaining to	

 Competency Verification: Check your answers in Appendix B, Answer Key, page 369. Review material that you did not answer correctly.

 Listen and Learn, the audio CD-ROM included in this book, will help you master pronunciation of selected medical words. Use it to practice pronunciations of the medical terms in the above "Word Building" tables and for instructions to complete the *Listen and Learn* exercise.

 Flash-Card Activity. Enhance your study and reinforcement of this chapter's word elements with the power of DavisPlus flash-card activity. Do so by visiting *http://davisplus.fadavis.com/gylys-express.* We recommend you complete the flash-card activity before continuing with the next section.

Medical Terminology Word Building

In this section, combine the word parts you have learned to construct medical terms related to the urinary system.

Use *nephr/o* (kidney) to build words that mean:

1. stone or calculus in the kidney _____

2. disease of the kidney _____

3. abnormal condition of water in the kidney _____

Use *pyel/o* (renal pelvis) to build words that mean:

4. dilation of the renal pelvis _____

5. disease of the renal pelvis _____

Use *ureter/o* (ureter) to build words that mean:

6. hernia or swelling of the ureter _____

7. surgical repair of the ureter _____

Use *cyst/o* (bladder) to build words that mean:

8. inflammation of the bladder _____

9. instrument to view the bladder _____

Use *azot/o* (nitrogenous compounds) to build words that mean:

10. nitrogenous compounds in the urine _____

11. nitrogenous compounds in the blood _____

Use *urethr/o* (urethra) to build words that mean:

12. narrowing or stricture of the urethra _____

13. instrument used to incise the urethra _____

Use *ur/o* (urine, urinary tract) to build words that mean:

14. radiography of the urinary tract _____

15. disease of the urinary tract _____

Competency Verification: Check your answers in Appendix B, Answer Key, on page 371. Review material that you did not answer correctly.

Correct Answers _____ **× 6.67 =** _____ **%**

Additional Medical Vocabulary

The following table lists additional terms related to the urinary system. Recognizing and learning these terms will help you understand the connection between common signs, symptoms, and diseases and their diagnoses. Included are medical and surgical procedures as well as pharmacological agents used to treat diseases.

Signs, Symptoms, and Diseases

azoturia
ăz-ō-TŪ-rē-ă
 	
  azot: nitrogenous
          compounds
  -uria: urine
	Increase of nitrogenous substances, especially urea, in urine

diuresis
dī-ū-RĒ-sĭs
 	
  di-: double
  ur: urine
  -esis: condition
	Increased formation and secretion of urine

dysuria
dĭs-Ū-rē-ă
 	
  dys-: bad; painful;
       difficult
  -uria: urine
	Painful or difficult urination, typically due to a urinary tract condition, such as cystitis

edema ĕ-DĒ-mă	Abnormal accumulation of fluids in the cells, tissues, or other parts of the body that may be a sign of kidney failure or other disease

end-stage renal disease (ESRD)
RĒ-năl
 	
  ren: kidney
  -al: pertaining to
	Kidney disease that has advanced to the point that the kidneys can no longer adequately filter blood and eventually requires dialysis or renal transplantation for survival; also called *chronic renal failure* (CRF)
	
	 Get a closer look at dialysis, on pages 200 and 201.

enuresis
ĕn-ū-RĒ-sĭs
   en-: in, within
   ur: urine
   -esis: condition
	Involuntary discharge of urine after the age at which bladder control should be established; also called *night-time bed-wetting* or *nocturnal enuresis*

hypospadias
hī-pō-SPĀ-dē-ăs
   hyp/o: under, below, deficient
   -spadias: slit, fissure
	Abnormal congenital opening of the male urethra on the undersurface of the penis

interstitial nephritis
ĭn-tĕr-STĬSH-ăl
nĕf-RĪ-tĭs
   nephr: kidney
   -itis: inflammation
	Pathological changes in renal interstitial tissue that result in destruction of nephrons and severe impairment in renal function

nephrolithiasis
nĕf-rō-lĭth-Ī-ă-sĭs
   nephr/o: kidney
   lith: stone, calculus
   -iasis: abnormal condition (produced by something specified)
	Formation of stones, or *calculi,* in the kidney that results when substances that are normally dissolved in the urine (such as calcium and acid salts) solidify (See Figure 8-1.)

renal hypertension
RĒ-năl hī-pĕr-TĔN-shŭn
   ren: kidney
   -al: pertaining to
   hyper-: excessive, above normal
   -tension: to stretch
	High blood pressure that results from kidney disease

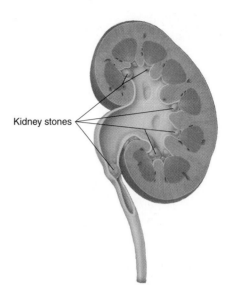

Kidney stones

Figure 8–1. Kidney stones in the calyces and ureter.

uremia ū-RĒ-mē-ă *ur:* urine *-emia:* blood	Elevated level of urea and other nitrogenous waste products in the blood; also called *azotemia*
urinary tract infection (UTI)	Infection of the kidneys, ureters, or bladder by microorganisms that either ascend from the urethra or that spread to the kidney from the bloodstream
Wilms tumor vĭlmz TOO-mŏr	Malignant neoplasm of the kidney that occurs in young children, usually before age 5, and includes such common early signs as hypertension, a palpable mass, pain, and hematuria

Diagnostic Procedures

blood urea nitrogen (BUN) ū-RĒ-ă NĪ-trō-jĕn	Laboratory test that measures the amount of urea (nitrogenous waste product) in the blood and demonstrates the kidneys' ability to filter urea from the blood for excretion in urine
kidney, ureter, bladder (KUB)	Radiographic examination to determine the location, size, shape, and possible malformation of the kidneys, ureters, and bladder

pyelography pī-ĕ-LŎG-ră-fē *pyel/o:* renal pelvis *-graphy:* process of recording	Radiographic study of the kidney, ureters and, usually, the bladder after injection of a contrast agent
intravenous pyelography (IVP) ĭn-tră-VĒ-nŭs pī-ĕ-LŎG-ră-fē *intra-:* in, within *ven:* vein *-ous:* pertaining to *pyel/o:* renal pelvis *-graphy:* process of recording	Radiographic imaging in which a contrast medium is injected intravenously and serial x-ray films are taken to provide visualization of the entire urinary tract; also called *intravenous urography* (IVU) or *excretory urography* (EU)
retrograde pyelography (RP) RĔT-rō-grād pī-ĕ-LŎG-ră-fē *retro-:* backward, behind *-grade:* to go *pyel/o:* renal pelvis *-graphy:* process of recording	Radiographic imaging in which a contrast medium is introduced through a cystoscope directly into the bladder and ureters to provide detailed visualization of the urinary structures and also to locate urinary tract obstruction
renal scan RĒ-năl *ren:* kidney *-al:* pertaining to	Nuclear medicine imaging procedure that determines renal function and shape through measurement of a radioactive substance injected intravenously that concentrates in the kidney
urinalysis (UA) ū-rĭ-NĂL-ĭ-sĭs	Physical, chemical, and microscopic analysis of urine

voiding cystourethrog-raphy (VCUG)
sĭs-tō-ū-rē-THRŎG-ră-fē
 	
   cyst/o: bladder
 urethr/o: urethra
  -graphy: process of
        recording
	Radiography of the bladder and urethra during the process of voiding urine after filling the bladder with a contrast medium

Medical and Surgical Procedures

catheterization kăth-ĕ-tĕr-ĭ-ZĀ-shŭn	Insertion of a catheter (hollow flexible tube) into a body cavity or organ to instill a substance or remove fluid, most commonly through the urethra into the bladder to withdraw urine (See Figure 8-2.)

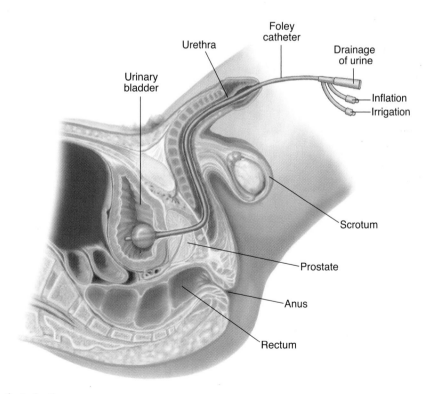

Figure 8–2. Catheterization.

cystoscopy sĭs-TŎS-kō-pē *cyst/o:* bladder *-scopy:* visual examination	Insertion of a rigid or flexible cystoscope through the urethra to examine the urinary bladder, obtain biopsies of tumors or other growths, and remove polyps (See Figure 8-3.)

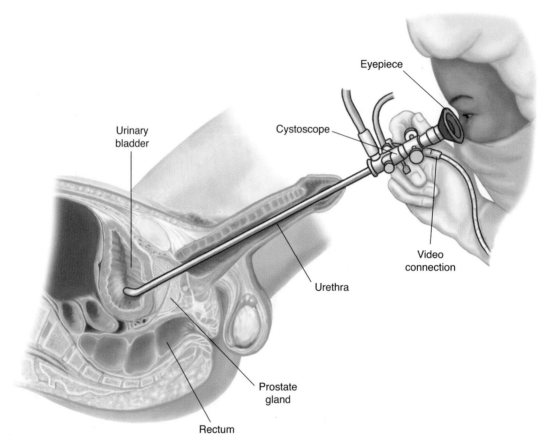

Figure 8–3. Cystoscopy.

lithotripsy
LĬTH-ō-trĭp-sē
  lith/o: stone, calculus
  -tripsy: crushing

extracorporeal shock-wave lithotripsy (ESWL)
ĕks-tră-kor-POR-ē-ăl SHŎK-wāv
  extra: outside
  corpor: body
   -eal: pertaining to
  lith/o: stone, calculus
  -tripsy: crushing

Method of removing stones that crushes them into smaller pieces so they can be expelled in the urine

Use of powerful sound wave vibrations to break up stones in the kidney (See Figure 8-4.)

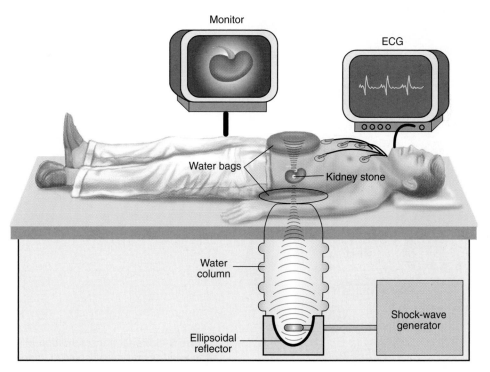

Figure 8–4. Extracorporeal shock-wave lithotripsy.

nephrolithotomy něf-rō-lĭth-ŎT-ō-mē *nephr/o:* kidney *lith/o:* stone, calculus *-tomy:* incision	Surgical procedure that involves a small incision in the skin and insertion of an endoscope into the kidney to remove a renal calculus
renal transplantation RĒ-năl trăns-plăn-TĀ-shŭn *ren:* kidney *-al:* pertaining to	Organ transplant of a kidney in a patient with end-stage renal disease; also called *kidney transplantation* (See Figure 8-5.)

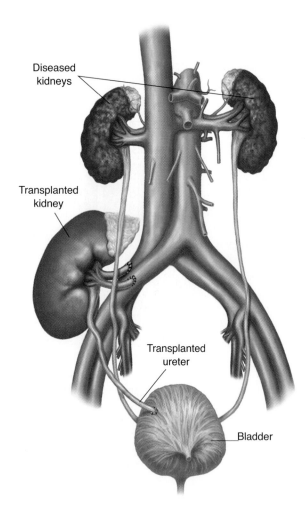

Figure 8–5. Renal transplantation in which the donor kidney is typically placed inferior to the normal anatomical location and the patient's kidneys are usually left in place.

Pharmacology

antibiotics ăn-tĭ-bī-ŎT-ĭks	Treat bacterial infections of the urinary tract by acting on the bacterial membrane or one of its metabolic processes
antispasmodics ăn-tē-spăz-MŎD-ĭks	Decrease spasms in the urethra and bladder (caused by UTIs and catheterization) by relaxing the smooth muscles lining their walls, thus allowing normal emptying of the bladder
diuretics dī-ū-RĔT-ĭks	Block reabsorption of sodium by the kidneys, thereby increasing the amount of salt and water excreted in the urine (causes reduction of fluid retained in the body and prevents edema)

Pronunciation Help	Long Sound	ā in rāte	ē in rēbirth	ī in īsle	ō in ōver	ū in ūnite
	Short Sound	ă in ălone	ĕ in ĕver	ĭ in ĭt	ŏ in nŏt	ŭ in cŭt

Closer Look

Take a closer look at these urological procedures and conditions to enhance your understanding of the medical terminology associated with them.

Hydronephrosis

Hydronephrosis is an excessive accumulation of urine in the renal pelvis due to obstruction of a ureter. Because urine is blocked from flowing into the bladder, it flows backward (**refluxes**) into the renal pelvis and calyces. This reflux causes hydronephrosis and results in abnormal dilation of the renal pelvis and the calyces of one or both kidneys. The main causes of urinary tract obstructions leading to hydronephrosis include a stone or **stricture.** Other causes include tumor growth, thickening of the bladder wall, and **prostatomegaly.**

The illustration on the next page depicts urinary obstruction in the proximal part of the ureter due to a stone (**calculus**), a condition called *hydroureter*. The illustration also shows the enlarged right kidney, which is caused by pressure from urine reflux, a condition called *hydronephrosis*.

Although a partial obstruction and hydronephrosis may not produce symptoms initially, the pressure built up behind the area of obstruction eventually results in symptoms of renal dysfunction.

(Continued)

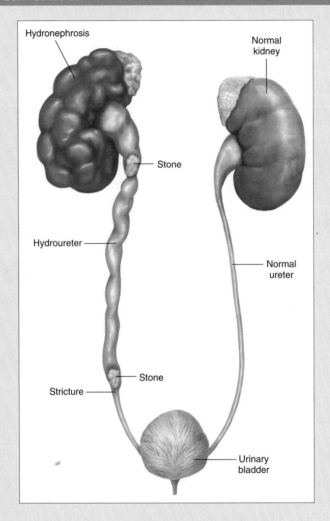

Dialysis

Dialysis is the process of removing waste products from the blood when the kidneys are unable to do so. There are two types of dialysis: hemodialysis and peritoneal dialysis.

Hemodialysis involves passing the blood through an artificial kidney for filtering out impurities. The illustration at the top of the next page shows the process of hemodialysis.

Peritoneal dialysis involves introducing fluid into the abdomen through a catheter. Dialysate fluid flows through the catheter and remains in the abdominal cavity for several hours. During that time, the fluid pulls body wastes from the blood into the abdominal cavity. The fluid is then removed from the abdomen via a catheter. The illustration at the bottom of the next page shows the introduction of dialysis fluid into the peritoneal cavity (A) and draining the fluid with waste products from the peritoneal cavity (B).

Closer Look—cont'd

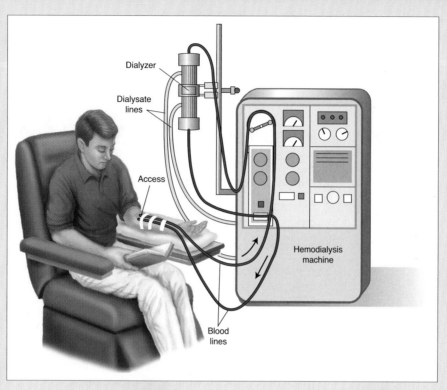

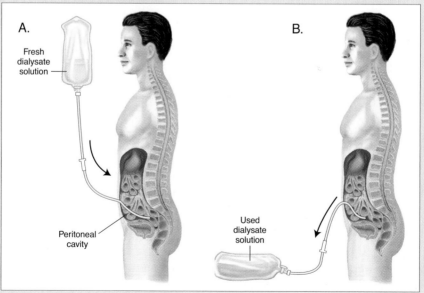

Additional Medical Vocabulary Recall

Match the medical term(s) below with the definitions in the numbered list.

azoturia	diuresis	interstitial nephritis	uremia
BUN	dysuria	renal hypertension	VCUG
catheterization	enuresis	retrograde pyelography	Wilms tumor
dialysis	hydronephrosis	UA	

1. _____ refers to physical, chemical, and microscopic examination of urine.

2. _____ is a malignant neoplasm in the kidney that occurs in young children.

3. _____ is an increase in nitrogenous compounds in urine.

4. _____ means painful or difficult urination, which is a symptom of numerous conditions.

5. _____ means increased formation and secretion of urine.

6. _____ is a radiologic technique in which a contrast medium is introduced through a cystoscope to provide detailed visualization of urinary collecting system.

7. _____ accumulation of urine in the kidney due to an obstruction in the ureter.

8. _____ is associated with pathological changes in the renal interstitial tissue, which may be primary or due to a toxic agent.

9. _____ is a test that measures the amount of urea excreted by kidneys into the blood.

10. _____ means urinary incontinence, including bed-wetting.

11. _____ refers to insertion of a hollow, flexible tube into a body cavity or organ to instill a substance or remove fluid.

12. _____ is radiography of the bladder and urethra after introduction of a contrast medium and during the process of urination.

13. _____ refers to an elevated level of urea and other nitrogenous waste products in blood.

14. _____ refers to high blood pressure that results from kidney disease.

15. _____ is the mechanical filtering process used to cleanse blood of high concentrations of metabolic waste products.

 Competency Verification: Check your answers in Appendix B, Answer Key, on page 371. Review material that you did not answer correctly.

Correct Answers _____ × **6.67 =** _____ %

Pronunciation and Spelling

Use the following list to practice correct pronunciation and spelling of medical terms. Practice the pronunciation aloud and then write the correct spelling of the term. The first word is completed for you.

Pronunciation	Spelling
1. ăz-ō-TĒ-mē-ă	*azotemia*
2. kăth-ĕ-tĕr-ĭ-ZĀ-shŭn	
3. sĭs-TŎS-kō-pē	
4. sĭs-tō-ū-RĒ-thrō-skōp	
5. glō-mĕr-ū-lō-nĕ-FRĪ-tĭs	
6. ĭn-KŎN-tĭ-nĕns	
7. LĬTH-ō-trĭp-sē	
8. nĕf-rō-lĭth-ŎT-ō-mē	
9. nĕf-rŏp-TŌ-sĭs	
10. nĕf-rō-sklĕ-RŌ-sĭs	
11. ŏl-ĭg-Ū-rē-ă	
12. pŏl-ē-Ū-rē-ă	
13. prō-tēn-Ū-rē-ă	
14. PĪ-ĕ-lō-plăs-tē	
15. pī-ō-nĕf-RŌ-sĭs	
16. RĔT-rō-grād pī-ĕ-LŎG-ră-fē	
17. ū-rē-tĕr-ĔK-tă-sĭs	
18. ū-rē-tĕr-ō-stĕ-NŌ-sĭs	
19. ū-RĒ-thrō-sēl	
20. ū-RŎL-ō-jĭst	

Competency Verification: Check your answers in Appendix B, Answer Key, on page 371.
Review material that you did not answer correctly.

Correct Answers: _____ × 5 = _____ %

Abbreviations

The table below introduces abbreviations associated with the urinary system.

Abbreviation	Meaning	Abbreviation	Meaning
ARF	acute renal failure	KUB	kidney, ureter, bladder
BNO	bladder neck obstruction	RP	retrograde pyelography
BUN	blood urea nitrogen	TURP	transurethral resection of the prostate
cysto	cystoscopy	UA	urinalysis
ESRD	end-stage renal disease	US	ultrasound, ultrasonography
ESWL	extracorporeal shock-wave lithotripsy	UTI	urinary tract infection
IVP	intravenous pyelography	VCUG	voiding cystourethrography
		WBC, wbc	white blood cell

Chart Notes

Chart notes make up part of the medical record and are used in various types of health care facilities. The chart notes below were dictated by the patient's physician and reflect common clinical events using medical terminology to document the patient's care. By studying and completing the terminology and chart note analysis sections below you will learn and understand terms associated with the medical specialty of urology.

Terminology

The following terms are linked to chart notes in the medical specialty of urology and nephrology. Practice pronouncing each term aloud and then use a medical dictionary such as *Taber's Cyclopedic Medical Dictionary, Appendix A: Glossary of Medical Word Elements,* page 337, or other resources to define each term.

Term	Meaning
cholecystectomy kō-lē-sĭs-TĔK-tō-mē	
choledocholithiasis kō-lĕd-ō-kō-lĭ-THĪ-ă-sĭs	
choledocholithotomy kō-lĕd-ō-kō-lĭth-ŎT-ō-mē	

Term	Meaning
cholelithiasis kō-lē-lĭ-THĪ-ă-sĭs	
cystitis sĭs-TĪ-tĭs	
cystoscopy sĭs-TŎS-kō-pē	
epigastric ĕp-ĭ-GĂS-trĭk	
hematuria hĕm-ă-TŪ-rē-ă	
nocturia nŏk-TŪ-rē-ă	
polyuria pŏl-ē-Ū-rē-ă	
incontinence ĭn-KŎNT-ĭn-ĕns	
urinary ŪR-ĭ-nār-ē	

 Visit *http://davisplus.fadavis.com/gylys-express* for the terminology pronunciation exercise associated with this chart note.

Cystitis

Read the chart note below aloud. Underline any term you have trouble pronouncing and any terms that you cannot define. If needed, refer to the Terminology section above for correct pronunciations and meanings of terms.

> This 50-year-old white woman has been complaining of diffuse pelvic pain with urinary bladder spasm since cystoscopy 10 days ago, at which time marked cystitis was noted. She reports nocturia three to four, urinary frequency, urgency, and epigastric discomfort. The patient has a history of polyuria, hematuria, and urinary incontinence. There is a history of numerous stones, large and small, in the gallbladder. In 19xx she was admitted to the hospital with cholecystitis, chronic and acute; cholelithiasis; and choledocholithiasis. Subsequently, cholecystectomy, choledocholithotomy, and incidental appendectomy were performed.
>
> Impression: Urinary incontinence due to cystitis and is temporary in nature.

Chart Note Analysis

From the chart note above, select the medical word that means

1. inflammation of the bladder: _____

2. urination at night: _____

3. blood in the urine: _____

4. visual examination of the bladder: _____

5. region above the stomach: _____

6. frequent urge to urinate: _____

7. excision of the appendix: _____

8. abnormal condition of gallstones: _____

9. inflammation of the gallbladder: _____

10. abnormal condition of stones in the bile duct: _____

11. excessive urination: _____

12. uncontrolled loss of urine from the bladder: _____

13. incision into the bile duct to remove stones: _____

14. excision of the gallbladder: _____

15. organ that stores bile: _____

Competency Verification: Check your answers in Appendix B, Answer Key, on page 371. Review material that you did not answer correctly.

Correct Answers: _____ × **6.67** = _____ %

Demonstrate What You Know!

To evaluate your understanding of how medical terms you have studied in this and previous chapters are used in a clinical environment, complete the numbered sentences by selecting an appropriate term from the list below.

anuria	edema	intravenous	nephromegaly	pyuria
continence	hematuria	lithotomy	pus	urinary
diuretic	hernia	nephrologist	pyelopathy	urologist

1. A person who suffers from nephrosis exhibits swelling, or _____, around the ankles, feet and eyes.

2. To stimulate the flow of urine, a patient would be prescribed a _____.

3. A Dx of hydronephrosis would indicate an obstruction in the _____ tract.

4. Any disease of the renal pelvis is known as _____.

5. Medication administered into a vein is said to be given by an _____ method.

6. _____ is evident in a urine sample that contains red blood cells.

7. A patient with cystitis will usually show pus in the urine. This condition is called _____.

8. A person who is not forming urine has a condition called _____.

9. A physician who treats disorders of the urinary tract is a _____.

10. When a person has the ability to control their bladder it is known as urinary _____.

11. A diseased kidney can lead to _____, also called *enlarged kidney*.

12. The rupture or protrusion of an organ through a wall of a body cavity is called a _____.

13. In pyonephrosis, there is an accumulation of _____ in the kidneys.

14. When an incision is performed for the purpose of removing a calculus, the surgical procedure is called a _____.

15. A physician who manages kidney transplants and dialysis therapies is a _____.

Competency Verification: Check your answers in Appendix B, Answer Key, on page 371. Review material that you did not answer correctly.

Correct Answers: _____ × 6.67 = _____ %

Multimedia Review. If you are not satisfied with your retention level of the urinary chapter, visit *http://davisplus.fadavis.com/gylys-express* to complete the website activities linked to this chapter. It is your choice whether or not you want to take advantage of these reinforcement exercises before continuing with the next chapter.

Reproductive System

MULTIMEDIA STUDY TOOLS.
To enrich your medical terminology skills, look for this multimedia icon throughout the text. It will help alert you to when it is best to use the various multimedia resources available with this textbook to enhance your studies.

Objectives

Upon completion of this chapter, you will be able to:

- Describe types of medical treatment provided by gynecologists, obstetricians, and urologists.
- Name the primary structures of the female and male reproductive systems and discuss their functions.
- Identify combining forms, suffixes, and prefixes associated with the female and male reproductive systems.
- Recognize, pronounce, build, and spell medical terms and abbreviations associated with the female and male reproductive systems.
- Demonstrate your knowledge of this chapter by successfully completing the activities in this chapter.

Vocabulary Preview

Term	Meaning
neonate NĒ-ō-nāt	Infant from birth to 28 days of age
infertility ĭn-fĕr-TĬL-ĭ-tē	Persistent inability to conceive a child
gamete GĂM-ēt	Reproductive cell (spermatozoon in the male and ovum in the female)
fertilization FĔR-tĭ-lĭ-zā-shŭn	Union of the male and female gametes to form a zygote, leading to the development of a new individual
ova Ō-văh	Female reproductive cells (plural of *ovum*)
postpartum pōst-PĂR-tĕm 　*post-:* after, behind 　*-partum:* childbirth; labor	Occurring after childbirth

Pronunciation Help	Long Sound	ā in rāte	ē in rēbirth	ī in īsle	ō in ōver	ū in ūnite
	Short Sound	ă in ălone	ĕ in ĕver	ĭ in ĭt	ŏ in nŏt	ŭ in cŭt

Gynecology and Obstetrics and Urology

Gynecology and Obstetrics

Gynecology is the medical specialty concerned with diagnosis and treatment of female reproductive disorders, including the breasts. The **gynecologist** is a physician who specializes in gynecology. Unlike most medical specialties, gynecology includes the surgical and nonsurgical expertise of the physician. Because obstetrics is studied in conjunction with gynecology, the physician's medical practice commonly includes both areas of expertise. This branch of medicine is called *obstetrics and gynecology (OB-GYN)*. The obstetrician and gynecologist possess knowledge of endocrinology because hormones play an important role in the functions of the female reproductive system, especially the process of secondary sex characteristics, menstruation, pregnancy, and menopause. Therefore **infertility,** birth control, and hormone imbalance are all part of the treatment provided by an OB-GYN physician.

Obstetrics is the branch of medicine concerned with pregnancy and childbirth, including the study of the physiological and pathological functions of the female reproductive tract. It also involves the care of the mother and fetus throughout pregnancy, childbirth, and the immediate **postpartum** period. An **obstetrician** is a physician who specializes in obstetrics. The branch of medicine that concentrates on the care of the **neonate** and in the diagnosis and treatment of disorders of the neonate is known as *neonatology*. When an infant is born, physicians called *neonatologists* specialize in providing their medical care.

Urology

Urology is the branch of medicine specializing in treating disorders of the male reproductive system. Thus, the **urologist** is a specialist who diagnosis and manages various male reproductive dysfunctions. The urologist utilizes diagnostic tests, medical and surgical procedures, and drugs to treat diseases as well as sexual dysfunctions and **infertility** in the male. In addition, the urologist diagnoses and treats diseases that affect the urinary system of men and women.

Reproductive Systems Quick Study

Although anatomical structures of the female and male reproductive systems differ, both have a common purpose. They are specialized to produce and unite **gametes** and transport them to sites of **fertilization.** Reproductive systems of both sexes are designed specifically to perpetuate the species and pass genetic material from generation to generation. In addition, both sexes produce hormones, which are vital in development and maintenance of sexual characteristics and regulation of reproductive physiology. In women, the reproductive system includes the ovaries, fallopian tubes, uterus, vagina, clitoris, and vulva. In men, the reproductive system includes the testes, epididymis, vas deferens, seminal vesicles, ejaculatory duct, prostate, and penis.

Female Reproductive System

The female reproductive system is composed of internal organs of reproduction and external genitalia. The internal organs are the ovaries, fallopian tubes (oviducts, uterine tubes), uterus, and vagina. External organs are known collectively as the *vulva* or *genitalia.* Included in the vulva are the mons pubis, labia majora, labia minora, clitoris, and Bartholin glands. The combined organs of the female reproductive system are designed to produce and transport **ova,** discharge ova from the body if fertilization does not occur. It also nourishes and provides a place for the developing fetus throughout pregnancy if fertilization occurs. The ovaries of the female reproductive system also produce the female sex hormones estrogen and progesterone, which are responsible for development of secondary sex characteristics, such as breast development and regulation of the menstrual cycle.

Male Reproductive System

The primary sex organs of the male are called *gonads,* specifically the *testes* (singular, *testis*). Gonads produce gametes (sperm) and secrete sex hormones. The remaining accessory reproductive organs are structures that are essential in caring for and transporting sperm. These organs and structures are designed to accomplish the male's reproductive role of producing and delivering sperm to the female reproductive tract, where fertilization can occur.

These structures can be divided into three categories:

1. sperm-transporting ducts, which include the epididymis, ductus deferens, ejaculatory duct, and urethra
2. accessory glands, which include the seminal vesicles, prostate gland, and bulbourethral glands
3. copulatory organ, the penis, which contains erectile tissue.

 An extensive anatomy and physiology review is included in *TermPlus,* the powerful, interactive CD-ROM program.

Medical Word Building

Building medical words using word elements related to the female and male reproductive systems will enhance your understanding of those terms and reinforce your ability to use terms correctly.

Combining Forms

Begin your study of female and male reproductive terminology by reviewing the organs and their associated combining forms (CFs), which are illustrated in the figure, *Female Reproductive System* below and *Male Reproductive System* on the next page.

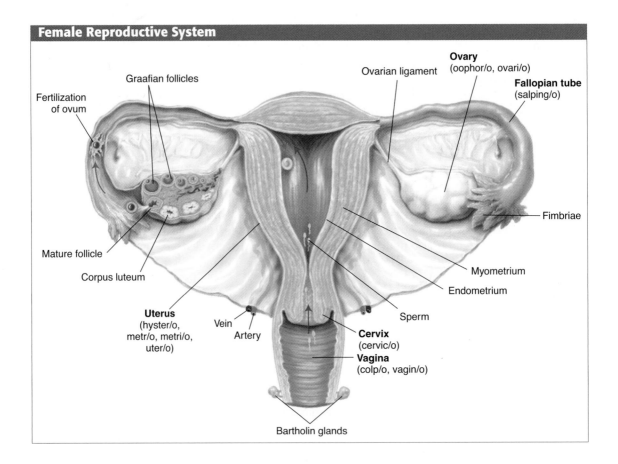

Female Reproductive System

Male Reproductive System

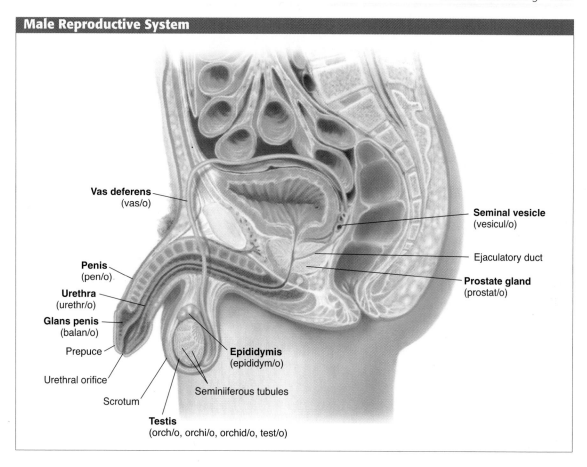

Vas deferens
(vas/o)

Seminal vesicle
(vesicul/o)

Ejaculatory duct

Penis
(pen/o)

Prostate gland
(prostat/o)

Urethra
(urethr/o)

Glans penis
(balan/o)

Prepuce

Epididymis
(epididym/o)

Urethral orifice

Scrotum

Seminiiferous tubules

Testis
(orch/o, orchi/o, orchid/o, test/o)

In the table below, CFs are listed alphabetically and other word parts are defined as needed. Review the medical word and study the elements that make up the term. Then complete the meaning of the medical words in the right-hand column. The first one is completed for you. You may also refer to *Appendix A: Glossary of Medical Word Elements* to complete this exercise.

Combining Form	Meaning	Medical Word	Meaning
Female Reproductive System			
amni/o	amnion (amniotic sac)	**amni/o**/centesis (ăm-nē-ō-sĕn-TĒ-sĭs) *–centesis:* surgical puncture	*surgical puncture of the amniotic sac (to remove fluid for laboratory analysis)*
		Get a closer look at amniocentesis on pages 233 and 234.	

(Continued)

Combining Form	Meaning	Medical Word	Meaning
Female Reproductive System			
cervic/o	neck; cervix uteri (neck of uterus)	**cervic**/itis (sĕr-vĭ-SĪ-tĭs) *-itis:* inflammation	
colp/o	vagina	**colp/o**/scopy (kŏl-PŎS-kō-pē) *-scopy:* visual examination	
vagin/o		**vagin/o**/cele (VĂJ-ĭn-ō-sēl) *-cele:* hernia, swelling	
galact/o	milk	**galact/o**/rrhea (gă-lăk-tō-RĒ-ă) *-rrhea:* discharge, flow	
lact/o		**lact/o**/gen (LĂK-tō-jĕn) *-gen:* forming, producing, origin	
gynec/o	woman, female	**gynec/o**/logist (gī-nĕ-KŎL-ō-jĭst) *-logist:* specialist in study of	
hyster/o	uterus (womb)	**hyster**/ectomy (hĭs-tĕr-ĔK-tō-mē) *-ectomy:* excision, removal	
uter/o		**uter/o**/vagin/al (ū-tĕr-ō-VĂJ-ĭ-năl) *vagin:* vagina *-al:* pertaining to	
mamm/o	breast	**mamm/o**/gram (MĂM-ō-grăm) *-gram:* record, writing	
mast/o		**mast/o**/pexy (MĂS-tō-pĕks-ē) *-pexy:* fixation (of an organ)	
men/o	menses, menstruation	**men/o**/rrhagia (mĕn-ō-RĂ-jē-ă) *-rrhagia:* bursting forth (of)	

Combining Form	Meaning	Medical Word	Meaning
Female Reproductive System			
metr/o	uterus (womb); measure	endo/**metr**/itis (ĕn-dō-mē-TRĪ-tĭs) *endo-:* in, within *-itis:* inflammation	
nat/o	birth	pre/**nat**/al (prē-NĀ-tl) *pre-:* before, in front of *-al:* pertaining to	
oophor/o	ovary	**oophor**/oma (ō-ŏf-ōr-Ō-mă) *-oma:* tumor	
ovari/o		**ovari**/o/rrhexis (ō-văr-rē-ō-RĔK-sĭs) *-rrhexis:* rupture	
perine/o	perineum	**perine**/o/rrhaphy (pĕr-ĭ-nē-OR-ă-fē) *-rrhaphy:* suture	
salping/o	tube (usually fallopian or eustachian [auditory] tubes)	**salping**/ectomy (săl-pĭn-JĔK-tō-mē) *-ectomy:* excision, removal	
vulv/o	vulva	**vulv**/o/pathy (vŭl-VŎP-ă-thē) *-pathy:* disease	
episi/o		**episi**/o/tomy (ĕ-pĭs-ē-ŎT-ō-mē) *-tomy:* incision	
Male Reproductive System			
andr/o	male	**andr**/o/gen (ĂN-drō-jĕn) *-gen:* forming, producing, origin	
balan/o	glans penis	**balan**/itis (băl-ă-NĪ-tĭs) *-itis:* inflammation	
gonad/o	gonads, sex glands	**gonad**/o/tropin (gŏn-ă-dō-TRŌ-pĭn) *-tropin:* stimulate	

(Continued)

Combining Form	Meaning	Medical Word	Meaning
Male Reproductive System			
olig/o	scanty	olig/o/sperm/ia (ŏl-ĭ-gō-SPĔR-mē-ă) *sperm:* spermatozoa, sperm cells *–ia:* condition	
orch/o	testis (plural, testes)	crypt/**orch**/ism (krĭpt-OR-kĭzm) *crypt:* hidden *–ism:* condition	
orchi/o		**orchi/o**/pexy (ŌR-kē-ō-pĕk-sē) *-pexy:* fixation (of an organ)	
orchid/o		**orchid**/ectomy (or-kĭ-DĔK-tō-mē) *-ectomy:* excision, removal	
test/o		**test**/algia (tĕs-TĂL-jē-ă) *-algia:* pain	
prostat/o	prostate gland	**prostat**/itis (prŏs-tă-TĬ-tĭs) *-itis:* inflammmation	
spermat/o	spermatozoa, sperm cells	**spermat/o**/cide (SPĔR-mă-tō-sīd) *-cide:* killing	
sperm/i*		**sperm/i**/cide (SPĔR-mĭ-sīd) *-cide:* killing	
sperm/o		a/**sperm**/ia (ă-SPĔR-mē-ă) *a-:* without, not *-ia:* condition	
varic/o	dilated vein	**varic/o**/cele (VĂR-ĭ-kō-sēl) *-cele:* hernia, swelling	

*Using the combining vowel i instead of o is an exception to the rule.

Combining Form	Meaning	Medical Word	Meaning
Male Reproductive System			
vas/o	vessel; vas deferens; duct	**vas**/ectomy (văs-ĔK-tō-mē) *-ectomy:* excision, removal	
		Get a closer look at vasectomy on pages 234 and 235.	
vesicul/o	seminal vesicle	**vesicul**/itis (vĕ-sĭk-ū-LĬ-tĭs) *-itis:* inflammation	

Suffixes and Prefixes

In the table below, suffixes and prefixes are listed alphabetically and other word parts are defined as needed. Review the medical word and study the elements that make up the term. Then complete the meaning of the medical words in the right-hand column. You may also refer to *Appendix A: Glossary of Medical Word Elements* to complete this exercise.

Word Element	Meaning	Medical Word	Meaning
Suffixes			
-arche	beginning	men/**arche** (mĕn-ĂR-kē) *men:* menses, menstruation	
-cyesis	pregnancy	pseudo/**cyesis** (soo-dō-sī-Ē-sĭs) *pseudo-:* false	
-gravida	pregnant woman	primi/**gravida** (prī-mĭ-GRĂV-ĭ-dă) *primi-:* first	
-para	to bear (offspring)	multi/**para** (mŭl-TĬP-ă-ră) *multi-:* many, much	
-salpinx	tube (usually fallopian or eustachian [auditory] tubes)	hemat/o/**salpinx** (hĕm-ă-tō-SĂL-pinks) *hemat/o:* blood	

(Continued)

Word Element	Meaning	Medical Word	Meaning
Suffixes			
-tocia	childbirth, labor	dys/**tocia** (dĭs-TŌ-sē-ā) *dys-:* bad; painful; difficult	
Prefix			
retro-	backward, behind	**retro**/version (rĕt-rō-VĔR-shŭn) *–version:* turning	

 Competency Verification: Check your answers in Appendix B, Answer Key, page 372. If you are not satisfied with your level of comprehension, review the terms in the table and retake the review.

 Listen and Learn, the audio CD-ROM included in this book, will help you master pronunciation of selected medical words. Use it to practice pronunciations of the medical terms in the above "Word Building" tables and for instructions to complete the Listen and Learn exercise.

 Flash-Card Activity. Enhance your study and reinforcement of this chapter's word elements with the power of DavisPlus flash-card activity. Do so by visiting *http://davisplus.fadavis.com/gylys-express.* We recommend you complete the flash-card activity before continuing with the next section.

Medical Terminology Word Building

In this section, combine the word parts you have learned to construct medical terms related to the male and female reproductive systems.

Use *gynec/o* (woman, female) to build words that mean:

1. disease (specific to) women _____

2. physician who specializes in diseases of the female _____

Use *cervic/o* (neck; cervix uteri) to build words that mean:

3. inflammation of cervix uteri and vagina _____

4. excision of cervix uteri _____

Use *colp/o* (vagina) to build words that mean:

5. instrument used to examine the vagina _____

6. visual examination of the vagina _____

Use *hyster/o* (uterus) to build words that mean:

7. rupture of the uterus _____

8. disease of the uterus _____

Use *metr/o* (uterus) to build words that mean:

9. hemorrhage from the uterus _____

10. inflammation of the uterus _____

Use *salping/o* (tube [usually fallopian or eustachian tube]) to build words that mean:

11. herniation of the fallopian tube _____

12. inflammation of the fallopian tube _____

13. fixation of a fallopian tube _____

Use *prostat/o* (prostate gland) to build words that mean:

14. enlargement of the prostate gland _____

15. pain in the prostate gland _____

Use *orchid/o* or *orchi/o* (testes) to build words that mean:

16. disease of testes _____

17. pain in testes _____

Use *balan/o* (glans penis) to build a word that means:

18. discharge from the glans penis _____

19. inflammation of the glans penis _____

20. surgical repair of the glans penis _____

Competency Verification: Check your answers in Appendix B, Answer Key, on page 374. Review material that you did not answer correctly.

Correct Answers _____ **× 5 =** _____ **%**

Additional Medical Vocabulary

The following tables list additional terms related to the reproductive system. Recognizing and learning these terms will help you understand the connection between common signs, symptoms, and diseases and their diagnoses. Included are medical and surgical procedures as well as pharmacological agents used to treat diseases.

Signs, Symptoms, and Diseases
Female Reproductive System

candidiasis kăn-dĭ-DĪ-ă-sĭs	Vaginal fungal infection caused by *Candida albicans* and characterized by a curdy or cheeselike discharge and extreme itching

cervicitis
sĕr-vĭ-SĪ-tĭs
  cervic: neck; cervix uteri
       (neck of uterus)
  -itis: inflammation
	Inflammation of the uterine cervix, which is usually the result of infection or a sexually transmitted disease

ectopic pregnancy ĕk-TŎP-ik	Implantation of the fertilized ovum outside of the uterine cavity, most commonly in the oviducts (tubal pregnancy) (See Figure 9-1.)

endometriosis
ĕn-dō-mē-trē-Ō-sĭs
  endo-: in, within
  metri: uterus (womb)
  -osis: abnormal condition; increase (used primarily with blood cells)
	Presence of endometrial tissue outside (ectopic) the uterine cavity, such as the pelvis or abdomen (See Figure 9-2.)

fibroid
FĪ-broyd
  fibr: fiber, fibrous tissue
  -oid: resembling
	Benign neoplasm in the uterus that is composed largely of fibrous tissue; also called *leiomyoma*

fistula
FĬS-tū-lă
 	
  vesicovaginal
  vĕs-ĭ-kō-VĂJ-ĭ-năl
  vesic/o: bladder
  vagin: vagina
    -al: pertaining to
	Abnormal tunnel connecting two body cavities (such as the rectum and the vagina) or a body cavity to the skin (such as the rectum to the outside of the body) caused by an injury, infection, or inflammation
	
	    Abnormal duct between the bladder and vagina that results in severe urine loss from the vagina (See Figure 9-3.)

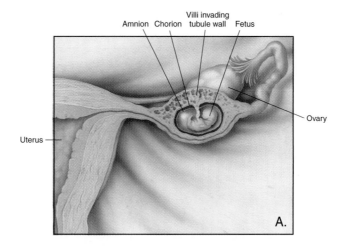

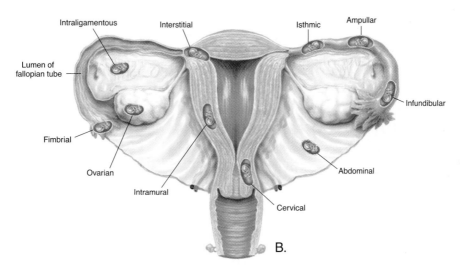

Figure 9–1. (A) Ectopic pregnancy. (B) Various sites of ectopic pregnancy.

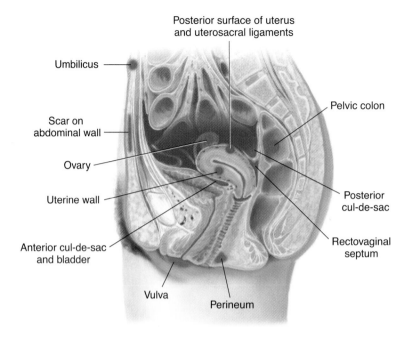

Posterior surface of uterus
and uterosacral ligaments

Umbilicus

Scar on
abdominal wall

Ovary

Uterine wall

Anterior cul-de-sac
and bladder

Vulva

Perineum

Pelvic colon

Posterior
cul-de-sac

Rectovaginal
septum

Figure 9–2. Endometriosis.

pregnancy-induced hypertension (PIH)	Potentially life-threatening disorder that usually develops after the 20th week of pregnancy and is characterized by edema and proteinuria
preeclampsia prē-ē-KLĂMP-sē-ă	Nonconvulsive form of PIH that, if left untreated, may progress to eclampsia
eclampsia ē-KLĂMP-sē-ă	Convulsive form of PIH that may become life threatening
sterility stĕr-ĬL-ĭ-tē	Inability of a woman to become pregnant or for a man to impregnate a woman
toxic shock syndrome (TSS) TŎK-sĭk shŏk *tox:* poison *-ic:* pertaining to	Rare and sometimes fatal staphylococcal infection that generally occurs in menstruating women, most of whom use vaginal tampons

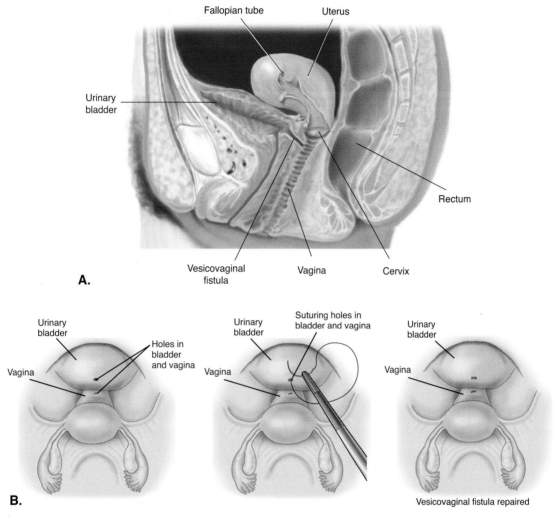

Figure 9–3. Vesicovaginal fistula. (A) Lateral view of female reproductive system with vesicovaginal fistula. (B) Frontal view of the urinary bladder and vagina with vesicovaginal fistula repair.

Male Reproductive System

anorchism
ăn-ŎR-kĭzm
   an: without, not
   orch: testis (plural,
      testes)
   -ism: condition
	Congenital absence of one or both testes; also called *anorchia*

balanitis băl-ă-NĪ-tĭs *balan:* glans penis *-itis:* inflammation	Inflammation of the skin covering the glans penis caused by irritation and invasion of microorganisms and commonly associated with inadequate hygiene of the prepuce and phimosis

cryptorchidism
krĭpt-OR-kĭd-ĭzm
 	
crypt: hidden
orchid: testis (plural,
     testes)
   -ism: condition
	Failure of one or both testicles to descend into the scrotum

epispadias ĕp-ĭ-SPĀ-dē-ăs *epi-:* above, upon *-spadias:* slit, fissure	Congenital defect in which the urethra opens on the upper side of the penis near the glans penis instead of the tip

hypospadias
hī-pō-SPĀ-dē-ăs
 	
  hyp/o: under, below,
     deficient
-spadias: slit, fissure
	Congenital defect in which the male urethra opens on the under-surface of the penis instead of the tip

impotence ĬM-pŏ-tĕns	Inability of a man to achieve or maintain a penile erection; also called *erectile dysfunction*

phimosis
fĭ-MŌ-sĭs
 	
phim: muzzle
   -osis: abnormal condition; increase
     (used primarily
     with blood cells)
	Stenosis or narrowing of the preputial orifice so that the foreskin cannot be pushed back over the glans penis

sexually transmitted disease (STD)	Any disease affecting the male or female reproductive system that is acquired as a result of sexual intercourse or other intimate contact with an infected individual; also called *venereal disease*
chlamydia klă-MĬD-ē-ă	One of the most damaging STDs caused by the bacterium *Chlamydia trachomatis,* causing cervicitis in women and urethritis in men
genital warts JĔN-ĭ-tăl WORTZ *genit:* genitalia *-al:* pertaining to	Wart(s) in the genitalia caused by human papillomavirus (HPV) and possibly associated with cervical cancer in women
gonorrhea gŏn-ō-RĒ-ă *gon/o:* seed (ovum or spermatozoon) *-rrhea:* discharge, flow	Contagious bacterial infection caused by the organism *Neisseria gonorrhoeae* and most commonly affecting the genitourinary tract and, occasionally, the pharynx or rectum
herpes genitalis HĔR-pēz jĕn-ĭ- TĂL-ĭs	Infection with herpes simplex virus type 2 of the male or female genital and anorectal skin and mucosa that may be transmitted through the placenta to the fetus during delivery
syphilis SĬF-ĭ-lĭs	Infectious, chronic STD characterized by lesions that change to a chancre and may involve any organ or tissue
trichomoniasis trĭk-ō-mō-NĪ-ă-sĭs	Protozoal infestation of the vagina, urethra, or prostate and the most common STD affecting men and women, although symptoms are more common in women

Diagnostic Procedures
Female Reproductive System

colposcopy kŏl-PŎS-kō-pē *colp/o:* vagina *-scopy:* visual examination	Examination of the vagina and cervix with an optical magnifying instrument (colposcope)

hysterosalpingography hĭs-tĕr-ō-săl-pĭn-GŎG-ră-fē *hyster/o:* uterus (womb) *salping/o:* tube (usually fallopian or eustachian [auditory] tube) *-graphy:* process of recording	Radiography of the uterus and oviducts after injection of a contrast medium
laparoscopy lăp-ăr-ŎS-kō-pē *lapar/o:* abdomen *-scopy:* visual examination	Visual examination of the abdominal cavity with a laparoscope through one or more small incisions in the abdominal wall, usually at the umbilicus (See Figure 9-4.)
mammography măm-ŎG-ră-fē *mamm/o:* breast *-graphy:* process of recording	Radiography of the breasts used to diagnose benign and malignant tumors
Papanicolaou (Pap) test pă-pă-NĬ-kō-lŏw	Microscopic analysis of a small tissue sample obtained from the cervix and vagina using a swab in order to detect carcinoma

Male Reproductive System

digital rectal examination (DRE) DĬJ-ĭ-tăl RĔK-tăl *rect:* rectum *-al:* pertaining to	Examination of the prostate gland by finger palpation through the anal canal and the rectum (See Figure 9-5.)

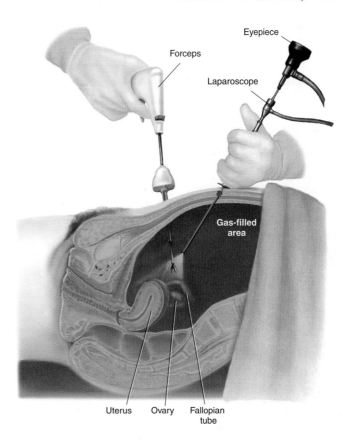

Figure 9–4. Laparoscopy.

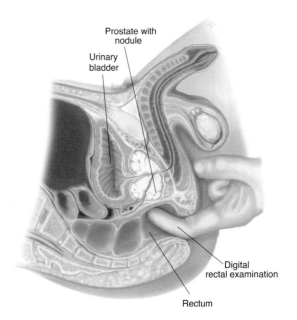

Figure 9–5. Digital rectal examination.

prostate-specific antigen (PSA) test PRŎS-tāt ĂN-tĭ-jĕn	Blood test used to screen for prostate cancer in which elevated levels of PSA are associated with prostate enlargement and cancer

Medical and Surgical Procedures
Female Reproductive System

cerclage sĕr-KLĂZH	Obstetric procedure in which a nonabsorbable suture is used for holding the cervix closed to prevent spontaneous abortion in a woman who has an incompetent cervix
dilatation and curettage (D&C) DĬ-lā-shŭn, kū-rĕ-TĂZH	Surgical procedure that widens the cervical canal of the uterus (dilatation) so that the endometrium of the uterus can be scraped (curettage) to stop prolonged or heavy uterine bleeding, diagnose uterine abnormalities, and obtain tissue for microscopic examination (See Figure 9-6.)
hysterosalpingo-oophorectomy hĭs-tĕr-ō-săl-pĭng-gō-ō-ŏ-for-ĔK-tō-mē *hyster/o:* uterus (womb) *salping/o:* tube (usually fallopian or eustachian [auditory] tube) *oophor:* ovary *-ectomy:* excision	Surgical removal of a uterus, a fallopian tube, and an ovary
lumpectomy lŭm-PĔK-tō-mē	Excision of a small primary breast tumor ("lump") and some of the normal tissue that surrounds it (See Figure 9-7.)

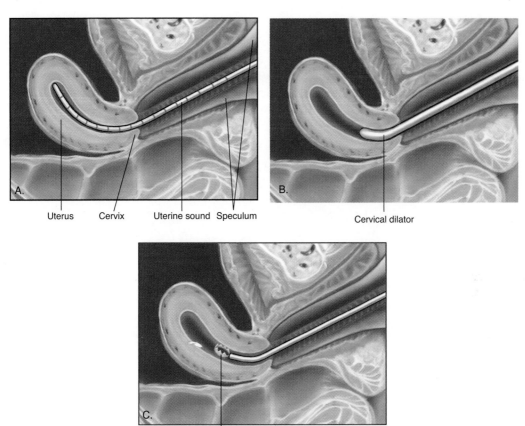

Uterus   Cervix   Uterine sound   Speculum

Cervical dilator

Serrated curet

Figure 9–6. Dilatation and curettage. (A) Examination of the uterine cavity with a uterine sound. (B) Dilatation of the cervix with a series of cervical dilators. (C) Curettage (scraping) of the uterine lining with a serrated uterine curet.

mastectomy măs-TĔK-tō-mē *mast:* breast *-ectomy:* excision, removal	Complete or partial excision of one or both breasts, most commonly performed to remove a malignant tumor
total	Mastectomy that involves excision of an entire breast, nipple, areola, and the involved overlying skin; also called *simple mastectomy*
modified radical	Mastectomy that involves excision of an entire breast, including lymph nodes in the underarm (axillary dissection) (See Figure 9-7.)
radical	Mastectomy that involves excision of an entire breast, all underarm lymph nodes, and chest wall muscles under the breast

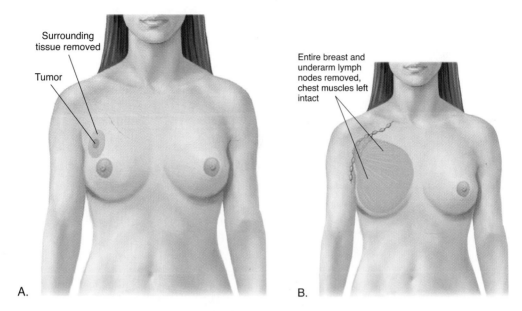

Figure 9–7. Lumpectomy and mastectomy. (A) Lumpectomy with primary tumor in red and surrounding tissue removed in pink. (B) Modified radical mastectomy.

reconstructive breast surgery	Reconstruction of a breast that has been removed due to cancer or other disease and commonly possible immediately following mastectomy so the patient awakens from anesthesia with a breast mound already in place
tissue (skin) expansion	Common breast reconstruction technique in which a balloon expander is inserted beneath the skin and chest muscle, saline solution is gradually injected to increase size, and the expander is then replaced with a more permanent implant (See Figure 9-8.)
transverse rectus abdominis muscle (TRAM) flap	Surgical creation of a skin flap (using skin and fat from the lower half of the abdomen), which is passed under the skin to the breast area, shaped into a natural-looking breast, and sutured into place (See Figure 9-9.)
tubal ligation TŪ-băl lī-GĀ-shŭn	Sterilization procedure that involves blocking both fallopian tubes by cutting or burning them and tying them off

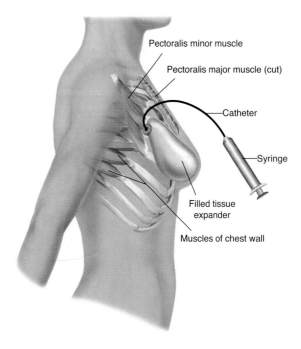

Figure 9–8. Tissue expander for breast reconstruction.

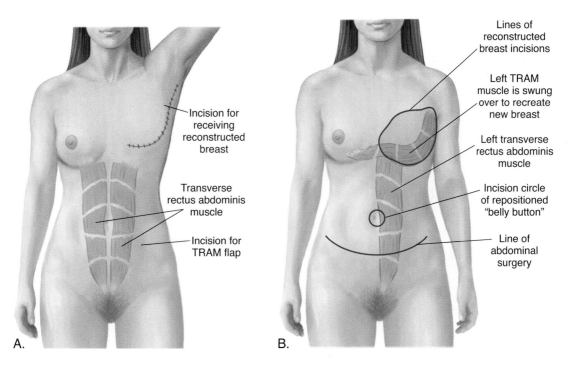

Figure 9–9. TRAM flap. (A) After mastectomy. (B) Process of TRAM reconstruction.

Male Reproductive System

circumcision sĕr-kŭm-SĬ-zhŭn	Surgical removal of the foreskin or prepuce of the penis and usually performed on the male as an infant
transurethral resection of the prostate (TURP) trăns-ū-RĒ-thrăl PRŎS-tāt	Surgical procedure to relieve obstruction caused by benign prostatic hyperplasia (excessive overgrowth of normal tissue) by insertion of a resectoscope into the penis and through the urethra to "chip away" at prostatic tissue and flush out chips using an irrigating solution (See Figure 9-10.)

Pharmacology
Female Reproductive System

antifungals ăn-tĭ-FŬN-gălz	Treat vaginal fungal infection, such as candidiasis
estrogens ĔS-trō-jĕnz	Treat symptoms of menopause (hot flashes, vaginal dryness) through hormone replacement therapy (HRT)

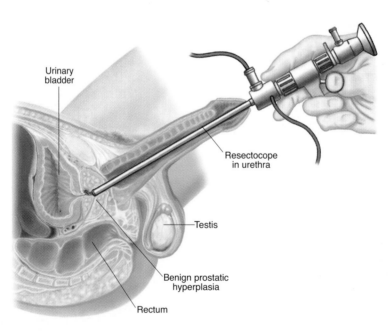

Figure 9–10. Transurethral resection of the prostate (TURP).

hormone replacement therapy (HRT)	Synthetic hormone used to correct a deficiency of estrogen, progesterone, testosterone, or testosterone hormone, relieve symptoms of menopause, and prevent osteoporosis in women
oral contraceptives (OCPs) kŏn-tră-SĔP-tĭvz	Prevent ovulation in order to avoid pregnancy; also known as *birth control pills*

Male Reproductive System

gonadotropins gŏn-ă-dō-TRŌ-pĭns	Hormonal preparation used to increase sperm count in infertility cases
spermicides SPĔR-mĭ-sīdz	Method of birth control that destroy sperm by creating a highly acidic environment in the uterus

Pronunciation Help	Long Sound	ā in rāte	ē in rēbirth	ī in īsle	ō in ōver	ū in ūnite
	Short Sound	ă in ălone	ĕ in ĕver	ĭ in ĭt	ŏ in nŏt	ŭ in cŭt

Closer Look

Take a closer look at these female and male reproductive procedures to enhance your understanding of the medical terminology associated with them.

Amniocentesis

Amniocentesis, also referred to as *amniotic fluid test,* is an obstetric procedure. It is used in prenatal diagnosis of abnormalities and fetal infections. It involves a surgical puncture of the amniotic sac to remove amniotic fluid, which contains fetal cells. After the amniotic fluid is extracted, the fetal cells are separated from the sample. The cells are grown in a culture medium, then fixed and stained. Under a microscope, fetal DNA is examined for genetic abnormalities. The most common abnormalities detected are *Down syndrome, Edward syndrome* (trisomy 18), and *Turner syndrome* (monosomy X).

Although amniocentesis is a routine procedure, possible complications include infection of the amniotic sac from the needle and failure of the puncture to heal properly, which can result in leakage or infection. Serious complications can result in miscarriage. Otherwise, the puncture heals and the amniotic sac replenishes the liquid over the next 24 to 48 hours. The illustration on the next page shows how amniocentesis is performed.

(Continued)

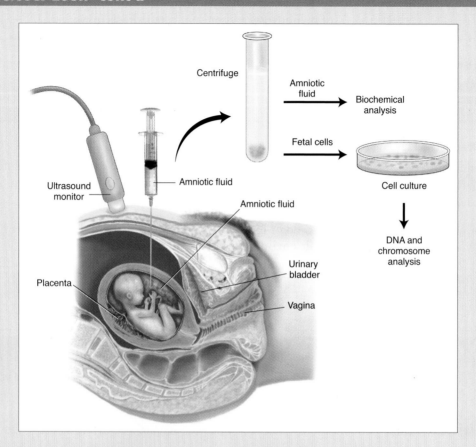

Vasectomy and Its Reversal

During a **vasectomy,** the urologist makes an incision through the scrotal sac with the patient under local anesthesia. The urologist cuts the vas deferens from each testicle, removes a small segment, and ties and binds off **(ligates)** the ends with sutures.

This procedure prevents sperm from mixing with the semen that is ejaculated from the penis, thus preventing fertilization of an egg. The testicles continue to produce sperm, which are reabsorbed by the body. Because the tubes are blocked before the prostate and seminal vesicle, there is still semen release during ejaculation. Vasectomy is considered a permanent method of birth control, but advances in **microsurgery** have made it possible for vasectomy reversal. A urologist will perform vasectomy reversal, also called *vasovasostomy,* if a man wants to regain his fertility. Vasovasostomy is more complicated than a vasectomy and is typically an outpatient procedure with the patient under spinal or general anesthesia. Vasovasostomy has the greatest chance of success within the first 3 years after vasectomy. The illustration below shows the vasectomy procedure and its reversal.

Closer Look—cont'd

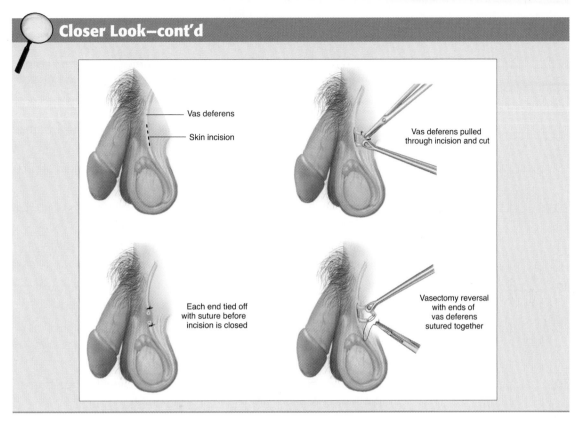

Vas deferens

Skin incision

Vas deferens pulled through incision and cut

Each end tied off with suture before incision is closed

Vasectomy reversal with ends of vas deferens sutured together

Additional Medical Vocabulary Recall

Match the medical terms below with the definitions in the numbered list.

anorchism	cryptorchidism	impotence	PSA
candidiasis	D&C	lumpectomy	sterility
cerclage	endometriosis	mammography	syphilis
chlamydia	fistula	phimosis	TSS
circumcision	gonorrhea	preeclampsia	trichomoniasis

1. _____ refers to failure of the testicles to descend into the scrotum.

2. _____ blood test to screen for prostate cancer.

3. _____ refers to a woman's inability to become pregnant or a man's inability to impregnate a woman.

4. _____ refers to congenital absence of one or both testes.

5. _____ is a vaginal fungal infection caused by *Candida albicans* and marked by a curdy discharge and extreme itching.

6. _____ is caused by infection with the bacterium *Chlamydia trachomatis* and occurs in both sexes.

7. _____ is surgical removal of the foreskin or prepuce of the penis.

8. _____ is an obstetric procedure to prevent spontaneous abortion in a woman who has an incompetent cervix.

9. _____ excision of a small primary breast tumor and some of the normal surrounding tissue.

10. _____ is a condition in which endometrial tissue is found in various abnormal sites throughout the pelvis or in the abdominal wall.

11. _____ refers to radiography of the breast and is used to diagnose benign and malignant tumors.

12. _____ is a sexually transmitted bacterial infection that most commonly affects the genitourinary tract and, occasionally, the pharynx or rectum.

13. _____ is a sexually transmitted disease that is characterized by lesions that change to a chancre, may involve any organ or tissue, and usually exhibits cutaneous manifestations.

14. _____ is a rare and sometimes fatal staphylococcal infection that occurs in menstruating women who use vaginal tampons.

15. _____ is a protozoal infestation of the vagina, urethra, or prostate.

16. _____ refers to widening of the uterine cervix so that the surface lining of the uterus can be scraped.

17. _____ means stenosis of the preputial orifice so that the foreskin does not retract over the glans penis.

18. _____ refers to the inability of a man to achieve a penile erection.

19. _____ nonconvulsive form of PIH that includes treatment of bed rest and blood pressure monitoring.

20. _____ is an abnormal passageway between two body cavities.

 Competency Verification: Check your answers in Appendix B, Answer Key, on page 374. Review material that you did not answer correctly.

Correct Answers _____ × 5 = _____ %

Pronunciation and Spelling

Use the following list to practice correct pronunciation and spelling of medical terms. Practice the pronunciation aloud and then write the correct spelling of the term. The first word is completed for you.

Pronunciation	Spelling
1. sĕr-KLĂZH	*cerclage*
2. sĕr-vĭ-SĪ-tĭs	
3. klă-MĬD-ē-ă	
4. sĕr-kŭm-SĬ-zhŭn	
5. ĕp-ĭ-SPĀ-dē-ăs	
6. gŏn-ă-dō-TRŌ-pĭn	
7. gī-nĕ-KŎL-ō-jĭst	
8. hĭs-tĕr-ō-săl-pĭng-gō-ō-ŏ-for-ĔK-tō-mē	
9. măm-ŎG-ră-fē	
10. ō-ŏf-ōr-Ō-mă	
11. ŌR-kē-ō-pĕk-sē	
12. pă-pă-NĬ-kō-lŏw	
13. pĕr-ĭ-nē-OR-ă-fē	
14. fī-MŌ-sĭs	
15. prŏs-tă-TĪ-tĭs	
16. soo-dō-sī-Ē-sĭs	
17. SPĔR-mĭ-sīd	
18. SĬF-ĭ-lĭs	
19. trĭk-ō-mō-NĪ-ă-sĭs	
20. VĂR-ĭ-kō-sēl	

 Competency Verification: Check your answers in Appendix B, Answer Key, on page 374. Review material that you did not answer correctly.

Correct Answers: _____ × 5 = _____ %

Abbreviations

The table below introduces abbreviations associated with the female and male reproductive systems.

Abbreviation	Meaning	Abbreviation	Meaning
Female Reproductive System			
CS, C-section	cesarean section	Pap	Papanicolaou (test)
D&C	dilatation (dilation) and curettage	para 1, 2, 3	unipara, bipara, tripara (number of viable births)
G	gravida (pregnant)	PID	pelvic inflammatory disease
HRT	hormone replacement therapy	PIH	pregnancy-induced hypertension
US	ultrasound	TAH	total abdominal hysterectomy
IVF	in vitro fertilization	TRAM	transverse rectus abdominis muscle
LMP	last menstrual period	TSS	toxic shock syndrome
OB-GYN	obstetrics and gynecology	TVH	total vaginal hysterectomy
Male Reproductive System			
BPH	benign prostatic hyperplasia, benign prostatic hypertrophy	PSA	prostate-specific antigen
DRE	digital rectal examination	TURP	transurethral resection of the prostate
GU	genitourinary		
Sexually Transmitted Diseases			
GC	gonorrhea	STD	sexually transmitted disease
HPV	human papillomavirus	VD	venereal disease
HSV	herpes simplex virus		

Chart Notes

Chart notes make up part of the medical record and are used in various types of health care facilities. The chart notes that follow were dictated by the patient's physician and reflect common clinical events using medical terminology to document the patient's care. By studying and completing the terminology and chart note analysis sections below you will learn and understand terms associated with the medical specialty of obstetrics-gynecology.

Terminology

The following terms are linked to chart notes in the medical specialty of obstetrics-gynecology. Practice pronouncing each term aloud and then use a medical dictionary such as *Taber's Cyclopedic Medical Dictionary, Appendix A: Glossary of Medical Words Elements* on page 337, or other resources to define each term.

Term	Definition
axilla ăk-SĬL-ă	
D&C dĭl-ă-TĀ-shŭn, kū-rĕ-TĂZH	
gravida 4 GRĂV-ĭ-dă	
laparoscopy lăp-ăr-ŎS-kō-pē	
lesion LĒ-zhŭn	
mastectomy măs-TĔK-tŏ-mē	
menstrual MĔN-stroo-ăl	
metastases mĕ-TĂS-tă-sēz	
neoplastic nē-ō-PLĂS-tĭk	
para 4 PĂR-ă	
postmenopausal pōst-mĕn-ō-PAW-zăl	
Premarin PRĔM-ă-rĭn	
preulcerating prē-ŬL-sĕr-āt-ĭng	

Visit *http://davisplus.fadavis.com/gylys-express* for the supplemental terminology pronunciation exercise associated with these chart notes.

Postmenopausal Bleeding

Read the chart note below aloud. Underline any term you have trouble pronouncing and any terms that you cannot define. If needed, refer to the Terminology section above for correct pronunciations and meanings of terms.

A 52-year-old gravida 4, para 4 woman had her last menstrual period at age 48. She was in our office last month for an evaluation because of postmenopausal bleeding. She has been taking Premarin and has had vaginal bleeding. Patient is currently admitted for gynecological laparoscopy and diagnostic D&C to rule out the possibility of a neoplastic process.

Last year this patient was admitted to the hospital for a simple mastectomy. Patient had a large preulcerating lesion of the left breast with metastases to the axilla, liver, and bone. Further medical evaluation will be performed next week.

Chart Note Analysis

From the chart note above, select the medical word that means

1. movement of cancer cells from one part of the body to another part: _____

2. occurring after menopause: _____

3. an injury or wound that alters tissue: _____

4. pertaining to new tissue formation: _____

5. trade name for estrogen pills: _____

6. removal of a breast: _____

7. pertaining to menstruation: _____

8. visual examination of the abdomen: _____

9. four pregnancies: _____

10. four live births: _____

Competency Verification: Check your answers in Appendix B, Answer Key, page 374. Review material that you did not answer correctly.

Correct Answers _____ × 10 = _____ %

Demonstrate What You Know!

To evaluate your understanding of how medical terms you have studied in this and previous chapters are used in a clinical environment, complete the numbered sentences by selecting an appropriate term from the list below.

aspermia	fertilization	ovaries
colpocystocele	galactorrhea	prostatitis
cryptorchidism	hysterectomy	sperm
dystocia	infertility	spermicide
fallopian tube	obstetrics	urologists

1. The _____ produce estrogen and progesterone.

2. Discharge or flow of milk is known as_____.

3. _____ is the surgical procedure to remove the uterus.

4. _____ is the branch of medicine concerned with pregnancy and childbirth.

5. After giving birth, some women develop a condition in which the bladder herniates into the vaginal wall. This condition is known as _____.

6. When a woman has difficulty achieving pregnancy, she is experiencing a condition known as

_____.

7. Hematosalpinx is a collection of blood in the _____.

8. _____ is a condition of a woman who is experiencing painful childbirth.

9. When an ovum and a sperm unite, the outcome is called _____, or *pregnancy*.

10. When testicles are retained in the abdomen, it is a condition called _____.

11. _____ is an effective agent that destroys spermatozoa.

12. _____ treat male reproductive disorders, such as sexual dysfunction and infertility.

13. A male who has an inflammation of the prostate is suffering from _____.

14. A male who is unable to form sperm has a condition called _____.

15. The male gonads produce _____ and secrete sex hormones.

 Competency Verification: Check your answers in Appendix B, Answer Key, on page 374. Review material that you did not answer correctly.

Correct Answers: _____ × 6.67 = _____ %

Multimedia Review. If you are not satisfied with your retention level of the reproductive chapter, go to *http://davisplus.fadavis.com/gylys-express* and complete the website activities linked to this chapter. It is your choice whether or not you want to take advantage of these reinforcement exercises before continuing with the next chapter.

Endocrine System

MULTIMEDIA STUDY TOOLS.
To enrich your medical terminology skills, look for this multimedia icon throughout the text. It will help alert you to when it is best to use the various multimedia resources available with this textbook to enhance your studies.

Objectives

Upon completion of this chapter, you will be able to:

- Describe types of medical treatment provided by endocrinologists.
- Name the primary structures of the endocrine system.
- Discuss the primary function of the endocrine system.
- Identify combining forms, suffixes, and prefixes associated with the endocrine system.
- Recognize, pronounce, build, and spell medical terms and abbreviations associated with the endocrine system.
- Demonstrate your knowledge by successfully completing the activities in this chapter.

Vocabulary Preview

Term	Meaning
homeostasis hō-mē-ō-STĀ-sĭs *home/o-:* same, alike *-stasis:* standing still	Body's ability to maintain a state of equilibrium within its internal environment, regardless of changing conditions in the outside environment
hormone HOR-mōn	Chemical substance produced by specialized cells of the body that works slowly and affects many different processes, including growth and development, sexual function, mood, and metabolism
metabolism mĕ-TĂB-ō-lĭzm	Sum of all chemical and physical processes occurring within living cells

Pronunciation Help	Long Sound	ā in rāte	ē in rēbirth	ī in īsle	ō in ōver	ū in ūnite
	Short Sound	ă in ălone	ĕ in ĕver	ĭ in ĭt	ŏ in nŏt	ŭ in cŭt

Endocrinology

Endocrinology is the branch of medicine concerned with diagnosis and treatment of **hormone** imbalances and diseases that affect the endocrine glands. Endocrine disorders include:

- diabetes
- thyroid diseases
- metabolic disorders
- over- or underproduction of hormones
- menopause
- osteoporosis
- hypertension
- cholesterol (lipid) disorders
- infertility
- lack of growth (short stature)
- cancers of the endocrine glands.

    Endocrinologists also conduct basic research to learn the ways glands work, and clinical research to learn the best methods to treat patients with a hormone imbalance. Through research, endocrinologists develop new drugs and treatments for hormone problems.

Endocrine System Quick Study

The endocrine system consists of a network of ductless glands with a rich blood supply that enables the hormones these glands produce to enter the bloodstream. The hormones influence almost every cell, organ, and function of the body. In general, the endocrine system controls body processes that occur slowly, such as cell growth. In addition, the endocrine system is also instrumental in regulating mood, growth and development, tissue function, and **metabolism** as well as sexual function and reproductive processes.

 An extensive anatomy and physiology review is included in *TermPlus,* the powerful, interactive CD-ROM program.

Medical Word Building

Building medical words using word elements related to the endocrine and nervous systems will enhance your understanding of those terms and reinforce your ability to use terms correctly.

Combining Forms

Begin your study of endocrine terminology by reviewing their associated combining forms (CFs), which are illustrated in the figure *Endocrine System* on the next page.

Endocrine System

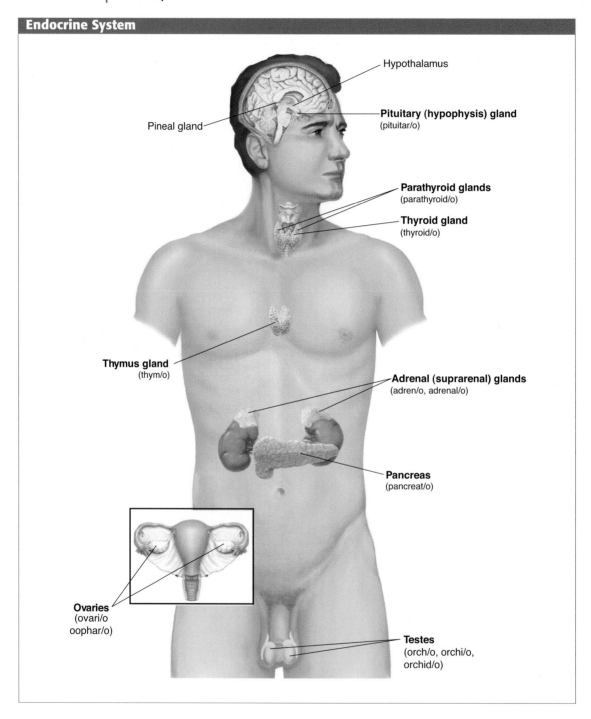

Hypothalamus

Pituitary (hypophysis) gland
(pituitar/o)

Pineal gland

Parathyroid glands
(parathyroid/o)

Thyroid gland
(thyroid/o)

Thymus gland
(thym/o)

Adrenal (suprarenal) glands
(adren/o, adrenal/o)

Pancreas
(pancreat/o)

Ovaries
(ovari/o
oophar/o)

Testes
(orch/o, orchi/o,
orchid/o)

In the table below, CFs are listed alphabetically and other word parts are defined as needed. Review the medical word and study the elements that make up the term. Then complete the meaning of the medical words in the right-hand column. The first one is completed for you. You may also refer to *Appendix A: Glossary of Medical Word Elements* to complete this exercise.

Combining Form	Meaning	Medical Word	Meaning
aden/o	gland	**aden**/oma (ăd-ĕ-NŌ-mă) *-oma:* tumor	*tumor composed of glandular tissue*
adrenal/o	adrenal glands	**adrenal**/ectomy (ăd-rē-năl-ĔK-tō-mē) *-ectomy:* excision, removal	
adren/o		**adren**/al (ăd-RĒ-năl) *-al:* pertaining to	
calc/o	calcium	hypo/**calc**/emia (hī-pō-kăl-SĒ-mē-ă) *hypo-:* under, below, deficient *-emia:* blood condition	
gluc/o	sugar, sweetness	**gluc/o**/genesis (gloo-kō-JĔN-ĕ-sĭs) *-genesis:* forming, producing, origin	
glyc/o		hyper/**glyc**/emia (hī-pĕr-glī-SĒ-mē-ă) *hyper-:* excessive, above normal *-emia:* blood condition	
pancreat/o	pancreas	**pancreat**/itis (păn-krē-ă-TĪ-tĭs) *-itis:* inflammation	
parathyroid/o	parathyroid glands	**parathyroid**/ectomy (păr-ă-thī-royd-ĔK-tō-mē) *-ectomy:* excision, removal	

(Continued)

Combining Form	Meaning	Medical Word	Meaning
pituitar/o	pituitary gland	hypo/**pituitar**/ism (hī-pō-pĭ-TŪ-ĭ-tă-rĭzm) *hypo-:* under, below, deficient *-ism:* condition	
thym/o	thymus gland	**thym**/oma (thī-MŌ-mă) *-oma:* tumor	
thyr/o	thyroid gland	**thyr**/o/megaly (thī-rō-MĔG-ă-lē) *-megaly:* enlargement Get a closer look at thyroid disorders on page 254.	
thyroid/o		**thyroid**/ectomy (thī-royd-ĔK-tō-mē) *-ectomy:* excision, removal	
toxic/o	poison	**toxic**/o/logist (tŏks-ĭ-KŎL-ō-jĭst) *-logist:* specialist in the study of	

Suffixes and Prefixes

In the table below, suffixes and prefixes are listed alphabetically and other word parts are defined as needed. Review the medical word and study the elements that make up the term. Then complete the meaning of the medical words in the right-hand column. You may also refer to *Appendix A: Glossary of Medical Word Elements* to complete this exercise.

Word Element	Meaning	Medical Word	Meaning
Suffixes			
-crine	to secrete	endo/**crine** (ĔN-dō-krĭn) *endo:* in, within	
-ism	condition	hirsut/**ism** (HŬR-sūt-ĭzm) *hirsut:* hairy	

Word Element	Meaning	Medical Word	Meaning
Suffixes			
-toxic	poison	thyr/o/**toxic** (thī-rō-TŎKS-ĭk) *thyr/o:* thyroid gland	
Prefixes			
hyper-	excessive, above normal	**hyper**/thyroid/ism (hī-pĕr-THĪ-royd-ĭzm) *thyroid:* thyroid gland *–ism:* condition Get a closer look at thyroid disorders on page 254.	
poly-	many, much	**poly**/dipsia (pŏl-ē-DĬP-sē-ă) *–dipsia:* thirst	

Competency Verification: Check your answers in Appendix B, Answer Key, page 374. If you are not satisfied with your level of comprehension, review the terms in the table and retake the review.

Listen and Learn, the audio CD-ROM included in this book, will help you master pronunciation of selected medical words. Use it to practice pronunciations of the medical terms in the above "Word Building" tables and for instructions to complete the *Listen and Learn* exercise.

Flash-Card Activity. Enhance your study and reinforcement of this chapter's word elements with the power of the DavisPlus flash-card activity. Do so by visiting *http://davisplus.fadavis.com/gylys-express.* We recommend you complete the flash-card activity before continuing with the next section.

Medical Terminology Word Building

In this section, combine the word parts you have learned to construct medical terms related to the endocrine system.

Use *glyc/o* (sugar) to build words that mean:

1. blood condition of excessive glucose _____

2. blood condition of glucose deficiency _____

3. forming, producing, or orgin of glycogen _____

Use *pancreat/o* (pancreas) to build words that mean:

4. inflammation of the pancreas _____

5. destruction of the pancreas _____

6. disease of the pancreas _____

Use *thyr/o* or *thyroid/o* (thyroid gland) to build words that mean:

7. inflammation of the thyroid gland _____

8. enlargement of the thyroid _____

Build surgical words that mean:

9. excision of a parathyroid gland _____

10. removal of the adrenal gland _____

Competency Verification: check your answers in Appendix B, Answer Key, page 375. Review material that you did not answer correctly.

Correct Answers _____ × 10 = _____ %

Additional Medical Vocabulary

The following tables list additional terms related to the endocrine system. Recognizing and learning these terms will help you understand the connection between common signs, symptoms, and diseases and their diagnoses. Included are medical and surgical procedures as well as pharmacological agents used to treat diseases.

Signs, Symptoms, and Diseases

Endocrine System

Addison disease Ă-dĭ-sŭn	Hypofunctioning of the adrenal cortex that results in generalized malaise, weakness, muscle atrophy, severe loss of fluids and electrolytes, low blood pressure, hypoglycemia, and hyperpigmentation of the skin
Cushing syndrome KOOSH-ing	Cluster of symptoms caused by excessive amounts of cortisol (glucocorticoid) or adrenocorticotropic hormone (ACTH) circulating in the blood; may be due to the use of oral corticosteroid medication or by tumors that produce cortisol or ACTH (See Figure 10-1.)

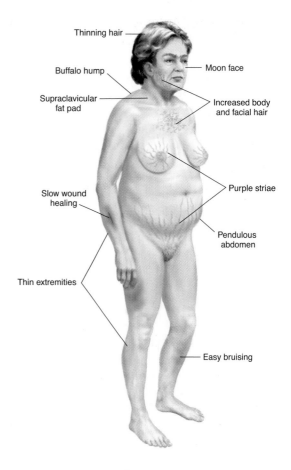

Figure 10–1. Physical manifestations of Cushing syndrome.

diabetes mellitus (DM) dī-ă-BĒ-tēz MĚ-lĭ-tŭs	Group of metabolic diseases characterized by high glucose levels that result from defects in insulin secretion, action, or both and occur in two primary forms: type 1 and type 2
type 1 diabetes	Abrupt onset of DM, usually in childhood, caused by destruction of beta islet cells of the pancreas with complete deficiency of insulin secretion
type 2 diabetes	Gradual onset of DM, usually appearing in middle age and caused by a deficiency in production of insulin or a resistance to the action of insulin by the cells of the body
insulinoma ĭn-sū-lĭn-Ō-mā *insulin:* insulin *-oma:* tumor	Tumor of the islets of Langerhans in the pancreas

panhypopituitarism păn-hī-pō-pĭ-TŪ-ĭ- tăr-ĭzm 　*pan-:* all 　*hyp/o:* under, below, 　　　deficient 　*pituitar:* pituitary gland 　*-ism:* condition	Total pituitary impairment that brings about a progressive and general loss of hormone activity
pheochromocytoma fē-ō-krō-mō-sī-TŌ-mă	Rare adrenal gland tumor that causes excessive release of epinephrine (adrenaline) and norepinephrine (hormones that regulate heart rate and blood pressure) and induces severe blood pressure elevation
pituitarism pĭ-TŪ-ĭ-tăr-ĭzm 　*pituitar:* pituitary gland 　*-ism:* condition	Any disorder of the pituitary gland and its function

Diagnostic Procedures

fasting blood glucose (FBG) GLOO-kōs	Measures the level of glucose in the blood after a 12-hour fast with increased levels that may indicate DM, diabetic acidosis, or some other disorder and decreased levels that may indicate hypoglycemia, hyperinsulinism, or some other disorder; also called *fasting blood sugar (FBS)*
glucose tolerance test (GTT) GLOO-kōs	Administration of glucose after a 12-hour fast to measure blood glucose levels at regular intervals (usually over a period of 3 hours) and used to diagnose diabetes mellitus with higher accuracy than other blood glucose tests
radioactive iodine uptake test (RAIU)	Test that involves oral administration of radioactive iodine (RAI) and measurement of how quickly the thyroid gland takes up (uptake) iodine from the blood to determine thyroid function
thyroid function test (TFT)	Blood test that measures thyroid hormone levels to detect an increase or decrease in thyroid function

total calcium	Blood test that measures calcium to detect parathyroid and bone disorders

Medical and Surgical Procedures

adrenalectomy ăd-rē-năl-ĔK-tō-mē *adrenal:* adrenal glands *-ectomy:* excision, removal	Excision of the adrenal gland to remove an adenoma or a carcinoma
lobectomy lō-BĔK-tō-mē *lob:* lobe *-ectomy:* excision, removal	Removal of one lobe in treatment of endocrine diseases such as hyperthyroidism
thymectomy thī-MĔK-tō-mē *thym:* thymus gland *-ectomy:* excision, removal	Excision of the thymus gland in cases of myasthenia gravis or a tumor
thyroidectomy thī-royd-ĔK-tō-mē *thyroid:* thyroid gland *-ectomy:* excision, removal	Excision of all or part (one lobe) of the thyroid gland

Pharmacology

hormone replacement therapy (HRT)	Synthetic hormone used to correct a deficiency of estrogen, progesterone, testosterone, or testosterone hormone, relieve symptoms of menopause, and prevent osteoporosis in women
insulins ĬN-sū-lĭns	Replace insulin in patients with type 1 diabetes or severe type 2 diabetes

Pronunciation Help	Long Sound	ā in rāte	ē in rēbirth	ī in īsle	ō in ōver	ū in ūnite
	Short Sound	ă in ălone	ĕ in ĕver	ĭ in ĭt	ŏ in nŏt	ŭ in cŭt

Closer Look

Take a closer look at these endocrine disorders to enhance your understanding of the medical terminology associated with them.

Thyroid Disorders

Diseases of the thyroid include thyroid hormone deficiency **(hypothyroidism)** or overproduction **(hyperthyroidism)** and gland inflammation and enlargement **(thyromegaly)**. They are common and may develop at any age. These disorders may be the result of a developmental problem, injury, disease, or dietary deficiency. With treatment, most of these conditions have a good prognosis. However, if untreated, they progress to medical emergencies or irreversible disabilities.

One form of hypothyroidism, called *cretinism*, develops in infants. If not treated, this disorder leads to mental retardation, impaired growth, low body temperatures, and abnormal bone formation. These symptoms usually do not appear at birth because the infant has received thyroid hormones from the mother's blood during fetal development.

When hypothyroidism develops during adulthood, it is called *myxedema*. The characteristics of myxedema are **edema**, low blood levels of thyroid hormones, weight gain, cold intolerance, fatigue, depression, muscle or joint pain, and sluggishness. Recovery may be complete if thyroid hormone is administered soon after symptoms appear.

Hyperthyroidism results from excessive secretions of thyroid hormones that results in a metabolic imbalance. The most common form of hyperthyroidism is **Graves disease**. Graves disease is an autoimmune disease that increases production of thyroid hormones, enlarges the thyroid gland **(goiter)**, and causes multiple system changes. Graves disease is characterized by an elevated metabolic rate, abnormal weight loss, excessive perspiration, muscle weakness, and emotional instability. Also, the eyes are likely to protrude **(exophthalmos)** because of edematous swelling in the tissues behind them. The illustrations below show exophthalmos caused by Graves disease and enlargement of the thyroid gland in goiter.

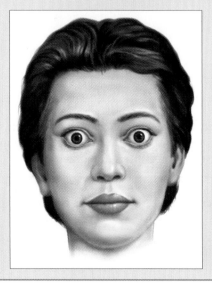
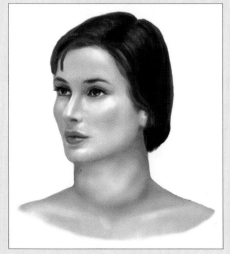

Additional Medical Vocabulary Recall

Match the medical term(s) below with the definitions in the numbered list.

cretinism	insulinoma	total calcium
Cushing syndrome	myxedema	type 1 diabetes
exophthalmos	panhypopituitarism	
HRT	TFT	

1. _____ is a blood test to detect bone and parathyroid abnormalities.

2. _____ is a disease caused by failure of the pancreas to produce insulin.

3. _____ is a congenital condition characterized by severe hypothyroidism commonly associated with other endocrine disorders.

4. _____ is abnormal protrusion of eyeball possibly due to thyrotoxicosis.

5. _____ is a tumor of the pancreas.

6. _____ hypothyroidism that develops during adulthood.

7. _____ measures thyroid hormone levels in the blood.

8. _____ is caused by excessive amounts of cortisol or ACTH circulating in the blood.

9. _____ brings about a progressive and general loss of hormone activity.

10. _____ is used to correct hormone deficiencies.

 Competency Verification: Check your answers in Appendix B, Answer Key, on page 375. Review material that you did not answer correctly.

Correct Answers _____ **× 10 =** _____ **%**

Pronunciation and Spelling

Use the following list to practice correct pronunciation and spelling of medical terms. First practice the pronunciation aloud. Then, write the correct spelling of the term. The first word is completed for you.

Pronunciation	Spelling
1. ăd-ĕ-NŌ-mă	*adenoma*
2. ăd-rē-năl-ĔK-tō-mē	
3. dī-ă-BĒ-tēz	

(Continued)

Pronunciation	Spelling
4. ĕks-ŏf-THĂL-mŏs	
5. GLOO-kōs	
6. hī-pō-kăl-SĒ-mē-ă	
7. hī-pĕr-glī-SĒ-mē-ă	
8. ĭn-sū-lĭn-Ō-mă	
9. MĔ-lĭ-tŭs	
10. mĭks-ĕ-DĒ-mă	
11. păn-krē-ă-TĪ-tĭs	
12. pĕr-ĬF-ĕr-ăl	
13. pĭ-TŪ-ĭ-tă-rĭzm	
14. pŏl-ē-DĬP-sē-ă	
15. tŏks-ĭ-KŎL-ō-jĭst	

 Competency Verification: Check your answers in Appendix B, Answer Key, page 376. Review material that you did not answer correctly.

Correct Answers: _____ × 6.67 = _____ %

Abbreviations

The table below introduces abbreviations associated with the endocrine system.

Abbreviation	Meaning	Abbreviation	Meaning
ADH	antidiuretic hormone	IV	intravenously
BS	blood sugar	LH	luteinizing hormone
DM	diabetes mellitus	PGH	pituitary growth hormone
FBG	fasting blood glucose	PTH	parathyroid hormone
FBS	fasting blood sugar	RAIU	radioactive iodine uptake
GH	growth hormone	RIA	radioimmunoassay
GTT	glucose tolerance test	TFT	thyroid function test
HRT	hormone replacement therapy	TSH	thyroid-stimulating hormone

Chart Notes

Chart notes comprise part of the medical record and are used in various types of health care facilities. The chart notes that follow were dictated by the patient's physician and reflect common clinical events using medical terminology to document the patient's care. By studying and completing the terminology and chart notes sections below, you will learn and understand terms associated with the medical specialty of cardiology.

Terminology

The following terms are linked to chart notes in the specialty of endocrinology. Practice pronouncing each term aloud and then use a medical dictionary such as *Taber's Cyclopedic Medical Dictionary, Appendix A: Glossary of Medical Word Elements* on page 337, or other resources to define each term.

Term	Meaning
aerobic ĕr-Ō-bĭk	
anaerobic ĂN-ĕr-ō-bĭk	
calcaneal kăl-KĀ-nē-ăl	
erythema ĕr-ĭ-THĒ-mă	
malleolus măl-Ē-ŏ-lŭs	
peripheral diabetic neuropathy pĕr-ĬF-ĕr-ăl dī-ă-BĔT-ĭk nū-RŎP-ă-thē	
trophic TRŌF-ĭk	
type I diabetes mellitus dī-ă-BĒ-tēz MĔ-lĭ-tŭs	
ulceration ŬL-sĕr-ā-shŭn	
vascular VĂS-kŭ-lăr	

Visit *http://davisplus.fadavis.com/gylys-express* for the terminology pronunciation exercise associated with this chart note.

Infected Foot

Read the chart note below aloud. Underline any term you have trouble pronouncing or cannot define. If needed, refer to the Terminology section above for correct pronunciations and meanings of terms.

SUBJECTIVE: The patient is a 59-year-old individual with long-term type 1 diabetes mellitus never well controlled. He complains of a hot, swollen left heel and came in through the emergency room.

OBJECTIVE: Physical examination revealed trophic changes in the feet bilaterally with amputation of the right great toe. There is a significant ulceration with early infection in the right heel. In the left heel, there is erythema to the level of the upper malleolus bilaterally and there is marked erythema at the entire calcaneal bed. There is an open foul ulceration of the heel. There are no palpable pulses in either foot. No reflexes and no sensation to deep palpation.

ASSESSMENT: Non-salvageable anaerobic/aerobic infection of the left heel in the context of peripheral diabetic neuropathy and poor circulation.

PLAN:
1. Vascular consultation for amputation.
2. Infectious disease consultation for appropriate antibiotic coverage.

Chart Note Analysis

From the chart note above, select the medical word that means

1. redness of skin: _____

2. agent used to treat infection: _____

3. composed of blood vessels: _____

4. pertaining to the heel: _____

5. nonhealing lesion on the surface of the skin or mucous membrane: _____

6. nerve damage to extremities from diabetes: _____

7. bony prominence on both sides of the ankle joint: _____

8. pertaining to development or nourishment: _____

9. insulin-dependent diabetes: _____

10. without oxygen: _____

Competency Verification: Check your answers in Appendix B, Answer Key, on page 376. Review material that you did not answer correctly.

Correct Answers _____ × **10 =** _____ %

Demonstrate What You Know!

To evaluate your understanding of how medical terms you have studied in this and previous chapters are used in a clinical environment, complete the numbered sentences by selecting an appropriate term from the list below.

aerobic	GTT	hyperglycemia	insulin	thymoma
FBG	homeostasis	hypersecretion	pancreas	toxicologist
Graves	hormones	hypocalcemia	RAIU	ulceration

1. If a patient has an abnormally low level of blood calcium, this condition is diagnosed as
   _____.

2. The term used to describe excessive secretion of a hormone by a gland is _____.

3. Treatment for type 1 diabetes includes _____ injections to maintain a normal level of glucose in the blood.

4. _____ is a condition that requires oxygen for respiration.

5. A(n) _____ is an open lesion on the surface of the skin or mucous membrane.

6. _____ are chemical substances produced by specialized cells of the body that travel in the bloodstream to tissues and organs.

7. _____ is a test in which radioactive iodine is administered to determine thyroid function.

8. _____ disease is characterized by an enlarged thyroid gland and exophthalmos (bulging eyes).

9. _____ measures blood glucose levels at specified intervals (usually over a period of 3 hours) after administration of glucose.

10. _____ is relative equilibrium in the internal environment of the body.

11. A specialist who studies poisons and their effects on the human body is called a(n) _____.

12. The gland responsible for production of insulin is the _____.

13. Results of a blood test show a greater than normal amount of glucose in the blood. This condition is charted as _____.

14. _____ measures the level of circulating glucose in the blood after a 12-hour fast.

15. A tumor of the thymus gland is indicated in the chart as a(n) _____.

Competency Verification: Check your answers in Appendix B, Answer Key, on page 376. Review material that you did not answer correctly.

Correct Answers: _____ × 6.67 = _____ %

Multimedia Review. If you are not satisfied with your retention level of the endocrine chapter, go to *http://davisplus.fadavis.com/gylys-express* and complete the website activities linked to this chapter. It is your choice whether or not you want to take advantage of these reinforcement exercises before continuing with the next chapter.

CHAPTER

Nervous System

11

 MULTIMEDIA STUDY TOOLS.
To enrich your medical terminology skills, look for this multimedia icon throughout the text. It will help alert you to when it is best to use the various multimedia resources available with this textbook to enhance your studies.

Objectives

Upon completion of this chapter, you will be able to:

- Describe types of medical treatment provided by neurologists.
- Name the primary structures of the nervous system and discuss their functions.
- Identify combining forms, suffixes, and prefixes associated with the nervous system.
- Recognize, pronounce, build, and spell medical terms and abbreviations associated with the nervous system.
- Demonstrate your knowledge of this chapter by successfully completing the activities.

Vocabulary Preview

Term	Meaning
cognition kŏg-NĬSH-ŭn	Process of thought—including, reasoning, judgement, and perception
nerve impulse	Electrical signal transmitted along the nerve fiber in response to a stimulus
neurotransmitters nū-rō-TRĂNS-mĭt-ĕrz	Chemicals in the brain that transmit messages between nerve cells (neurons)
peripheral pĕr-ĬF-ĕr-ăl	Pertaining to the outside, surface, or surrounding area of an organ or structure or occurring away from the center
traumatic traw-MĂT-ĭk	Caused by or pertaining to an injury
vascular VĂS-kū-lăr *vascul:* vessel (usually blood or lymph) *-ar:* pertaining to	Pertaining to or composed of blood vessels

Pronunciation Help	Long Sound	ā in rāte	ē in rēbirth	ī in īsle	ō in ōver	ū in ūnite
	Short Sound	ă in ălone	ĕ in ĕver	ĭ in ĭt	ŏ in nŏt	ŭ in cŭt

Neurology

Neurology is the branch of medicine concerned with diagnosis and treatment of diseases of the nervous system, which include the brain, spinal cord, and **peripheral** nerves. The nervous system controls voluntary and involuntary movements as well as some organ and gland functioning. It also controls all the processes of **cognition,** such as thinking, feeling, and remembering. The **neurologist** attempts to detect, diagnose, and treat symptoms and disorders that indicate an impairment of any of these functions. These disorders can include but are not limited to **vascular** problems that affect the brain, infections or inflammations of the brain or the spinal cord tissue, nervous tissue tumors, degenerative neuromuscular disorders, and **traumatic** brain or spinal cord injury. The branch of surgery involving the nervous system, including the brain and spinal cord, is called **neurosurgery.** The physician who specializes in neurosurgery is a **neurosurgeon.**

Nervous System Quick Study

The nervous system controls all critical body activities and reactions and is one of the most complicated systems of the body. In contrast to the endocrine system, which slowly discharges hormones into the bloodstream, the nervous system is designed to act instantaneously by transmitting electrical impulses to specific body locations. The nervous system coordinates voluntary (conscious) activities, such as walking, talking, and eating. It also controls involuntary (unconscious) functions, such as reflexes to pain, body changes related to stress, and processes related to thought and emotions.

The nervous system can be grouped into two main divisions: the **central nervous system (CNS)** and the **peripheral nervous system (PNS).** The **CNS** consists of the brain and spinal cord and is the control center of the body. The **PNS** consists of the peripheral nerves, which include the cranial nerves (emerging from the base of the skull) and the spinal nerves (emerging from the spinal cord). The PNS connects the CNS to remote body parts to relay and receive messages, and its autonomic nerves regulate involuntary functions of the internal organs. (See *Nervous System: Brain and Spinal Cord,* page 264.)

Despite the complex organization of the nervous system, it consists of only two principal types of cells, *neurons* and *neuroglia. Neurons* are the basic structural and functional units of the nervous system. They are grouped into bundles of nerves or nerve tracts that carry electrical messages throughout the body while **neurotransmitters** assist in transmitting messages between neurons. Neurons perform such functions as perception of sensory stimuli, learning, memory, and control of muscles and glands. *Neuroglia* do not carry messages, but perform the functions of support and protection. Many neuroglial, or *glial,* cells form a supporting network by twining around nerve cells or lining certain structures in the brain and spinal cord. Others bind nervous tissue to supporting structures and attach the neurons to their blood vessels. Certain small glial cells are phagocytic. In other words, they protect the CNS from disease by engulfing invading microbes and clearing away debris. *Neuroglia* are of clinical interest because they are a common source of tumors (gliomas) of the nervous system.

 An extensive anatomy and physiology review is included in *TermPlus,* the powerful, interactive CD-ROM program.

Medical Word Building

Building medical words using word elements related to the nervous system will enhance your understanding of those terms and reinforce your ability to use terms correctly.

Combining Forms

Begin your study of nervous system terminology by reviewing the organs and their associated combining forms (CFs), which are illustrated in the figure *Nervous System: Brain and Spinal Cord* on the next page.

Nervous System: Brain and Spinal Cord

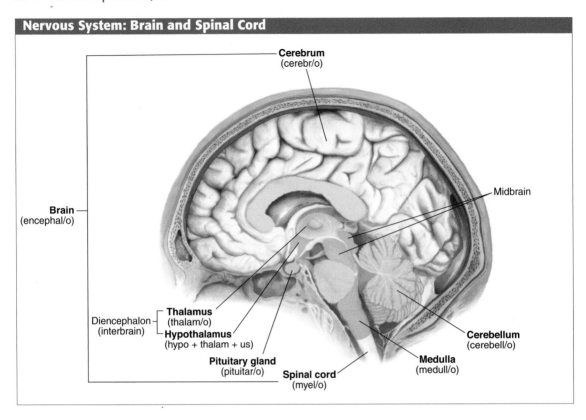

In the table below, CFs are listed alphabetically and other word parts are defined as needed. Review the medical word and study the elements that make up the term. Then complete the meaning of the medical words in the right-hand column. The first one is completed for you. You may also refer to *Appendix A: Glossary of Medical Word Elements* to complete this exercise.

Combining Form	Meaning	Medical Word	Meaning
cerebr/o	cerebrum	**cerebr/o**/spin/al (sĕr-ĕ-brō-SPĪ-năl) *spin:* spine *-al:* pertaining to	*Pertaining to the brain and spine or spinal cord*
encephal/o	brain	**encephal/**itis (ĕn-sĕf-ă-LĪ-tĭs) *-itis:* inflammation	
gli/o	glue; neuroglial tissue	**gli/**oma (glī-Ō-mă) *-oma:* tumor	

Combining Form	Meaning	Medical Word	Meaning
mening/o	meninges (membranes covering brain and spinal cord)	**mening/o**/cele (mĕn-ĬN-gō-sēl) *-cele:* hernia, swelling	
meningi/o		**meningi/**oma (mĕn-ĭn-jē-Ō-mă) *-oma:* tumor	
myel/o	bone marrow; spinal cord	**myel/**algia (mī-ĕl-ĂL-jē-ă) *-algia:* pain	
neur/o	nerve	**neur/o**/lysis (nū-RŎL-ĭs-ĭs) *-lysis:* separation; destruction; loosening	

Suffixes and Prefixes

In the table below, suffixes and prefixes are listed alphabetically and other word parts are defined as needed. Review the medical word and study the elements that make up the term. Then complete the meaning of the medical words in the right-hand column. You may also refer to *Appendix A: Glossary of Medical Word Elements* to complete this exercise.

Word Element	Meaning	Medical Word	Meaning
Suffixes			
-lepsy	seizure	epi/**lepsy** (ĔP-ĭ-lĕp-sē) *epi-:* above, upon	
-phasia	speech	a/**phasia** (ă-FĀ-zē-ă) *a-:* without, not	
Prefixes			
dys-	bad, painful, difficult	**dys/**phasia (dĭs-FĀ-zē-ă) -speech	
hemi-	one half	**hemi/**paresis (hĕm-ē-păr-Ē-sĭs) *-paresis:* partial paralysis	

(Continued)

Word Element	Meaning	Medical Word	Meaning
Prefixes			
para-	near; beside; beyond	**para**/plegia (păr-ă-PLĒ-jē-ă) *-plegia:* paralysis	
quadri-	four	**quadri**/plegia (kwŏd-rĭ-PLĒ-jē-ă) *-plegia:* paralysis Get a closer look at quadriplegia, see page 273 and page 274.	

 Competency Verification: Check your answers in Appendix B, Answer Key, page 376. If you are not satisfied with your level of comprehension, review the terms in the table and retake the review.

 Listen and Learn, the audio CD-ROM included in this book, will help you master pronunciation of selected medical words. Use it to practice pronunciations of the medical terms in the above "Word Building" tables and for instructions to complete the *Listen and Learn* exercise.

 Flash-Card Activity. Enhance your study and reinforcement of this chapter's word elements with the power of the DavisPlus flash-card activity. Do so by visiting *http://davisplus.fadavis.com/ gylys-express.* We recommend you complete the flash-card activity before continuing with the next section.

Medical Terminology Word Building

In this section, combine the word parts you have learned to construct medical terms related to the nervous system.

Use *neur/o* (nerve) to build words that mean:

1. tumor composed of nervous (tissue) _____

2. separation or destruction of a nerve _____

Use *encephal/o* (brain) to build words that mean:

3. inflammation of the brain _____

4. tumor composed of brain (tissue) _____

5. herniation or protrusion of brain (tissue) _____

Use *myel/o* (bone marrow; spinal cord) to build words that mean:

6. pain in the spinal cord _____

7. herniation of the spinal cord _____

Use *cerebr/o* (cerebrum) to build a word that means:

8. pertaining to the cerebrum and spinal cord _____

Use the suffix *-phasia* to build words that mean:

9. without or lacking speech _____

10. difficult speech _____

> **Competency Verification:** Check your answers in Appendix B, Answer Key, on page 377. Review material that you did not answer correctly.
>
> **Correct Answers** _____ × 10 = _____ %

Additional Medical Vocabulary

The following tables list additional terms related to the nervous system. Recognizing and learning these terms will help you understand the connection between common signs, symptoms, and diseases and their diagnoses. Included are medical and surgical procedures as well as pharmacological agents used to treat diseases.

Signs, Symptoms, and Diseases

dementia dĭ-MĔN-shē-ă	Progressive, irreversible deterioration of mental function marked by memory impairment and, commonly, deficits in reasoning, judgement, abstract thought, comprehension, learning, task execution, and use of language
Alzheimer disease ĂLTS-hī-mĕr	Chronic, organic brain syndrome characterized by death of neurons in the cerebral cortex and their replacement by microscopic "plaques," which results in dementia that progresses to complete loss of mental, emotional, and physical functioning and personality changes
epilepsy ĔP-ĭ-lĕp-sē	Disorder that results from the generation of electrical signals inside the brain, causing recurring seizures in which some people simply stare blankly for a few seconds during a seizure, while others have extreme convulsions

Huntington chorea HŬN-tĭng-tŭn kō-RĒ-ă	Inherited, degenerative disease of the CNS with symptoms developing in middle age as nerve cells in the brain waste away, resulting in uncontrolled bizarre movements, emotional disturbances, and mental deterioration

hydrocephalus
hī-drō-SĔF-ă-lŭs
hydro: water
cephal: head
  -us: condition,
    structure
	Condition caused by an accumulation of fluid within the ventricles of the brain that causes pressure builds up, distending the ventricles in the brain and compressing brain tissue, and which, if left untreated, causes a grossly enlarged head and mental retardation

multiple sclerosis (MS) MŬL-tĭ-pl sklĕ-RŌ-sĭs *scler:* hardening; sclera (white of eye) *-osis:* abnormal condition; increase (used primarily with blood cells)	Progressive degenerative disease of the CNS characterized by inflammation, hardening, and loss of myelin throughout the spinal cord and brain, which produces weakness and other muscle symptoms

neuroblastoma
nū-rō-blăs-TŌ-mă
neur/o: nerve
  blast: embryonic cell
  -oma: tumor
	Malignant tumor composed mainly of cells resembling neuroblasts that occurs most commonly in infants and children

neurosis nū-RŌ-sĭs *neur/o:* nerve *-osis:* abnormal condition; increase (used primarily with blood cells)	Nonpsychotic mental illness that triggers feelings of distress and anxiety and impairs normal behavior

palsy PAWL-zē	Partial or complete loss of motor function; also called *paralysis*
Bell	Facial paralysis on one side of the face due to inflammation of a facial nerve
cerebral sĕ-RĒ-brăl *cerebr:* cerebrum *-al:* pertaining to	Bilateral, symmetrical, nonprogressive motor dysfunction and partial paralysis, which is usually caused by damage to the cerebrum during gestation or birth trauma but can also be hereditary
paralysis pă-RĂL-ĭ-sĭs	Loss of muscle function, loss of sensation, or both as a result of spinal cord injury Get a closer look at spinal cord injuries on page 273 and 274.
Parkinson disease	Progressive neurological disorder caused by a neurotransmitter deficiency (dopamine) that affects the portion of the brain responsible for controlling movement and results in hand tremors, uncontrollable head nodding, shuffling gait, and difficulty talking, swallowing, or completing simple tasks

poliomyelitis
pō-lē-ō-mī-ĕl-Ī-tĭs
poli/o: gray; gray matter
   (of brain or spinal
   cord)
myel: bone marrow;
   spinal cord
  -itis: inflammation
	Inflammation of the gray matter of the spinal cord caused by a virus, commonly resulting in spinal and muscle deformity and paralysis

psychosis sī-KŌ-sĭs	Mental disorder marked by loss of contact with reality; often with delusions and hallucinations
sciatica sī-ĂT-ĭ-kă	Severe pain in the leg along the course of the sciatic nerve, which travels from the hip to the foot (See Figure 11-1.)

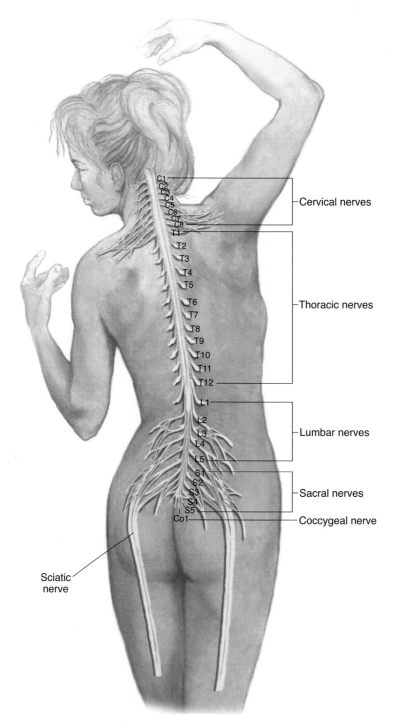

C1
C2
C3
C4
C5
C6
C7
C8

Cervical nerves

T1
T2
T3
T4
T5
T6
T7
T8
T9
T10
T11
T12

Thoracic nerves

L1
L2
L3
L4
L5

Lumbar nerves

S1
S2
S3
S4
S5

Sacral nerves

Co1

Coccygeal nerve

Sciatic
nerve

Figure 11–1. Spinal nerves.

shingles SHĬNG-lz	Eruption of acute, inflammatory, herpetic vesicles caused by herpes zoster virus on the trunk of the body along a peripheral nerve
spina bifida SPĪ-nă BĬF-ĭ-dă	Congenital neural tube defect characterized by incomplete closure of the spinal canal through which the spinal cord and meninges may or may not protrude (See Figure 11-2.)
spina bifida occulta SPĪ-nă BĬF-ĭ-dă ŏ-KŬL-tă	Most common and least severe form of spina bifida without protrusion of the spinal cord or meninges
spina bifida cystica SPĪ-nă BĬF-ĭ-dă SĬS-tĭk-ă	More severe type of spina bifida that involves protrusion of the meninges (meningocele), spinal cord (myelocele), or both (meningomyelocele)
stroke strōk	Brain tissue damage caused by a disorder within the blood vessels that is usually due to the formation of a clot or a ruptured blood vessel; also called *cerebrovascular accident* (CVA)
transient ischemic attack (TIA) TRĂN-zhĕnt ĭs-KĒ-mĭk *ischem:* to hold back, block *-ic:* pertaining to	Interruption in blood supply to the brain that does not cause permanent brain damage but may be an indication of a higher risk of a more serious and debilitating condition (stroke); also called *ministroke*

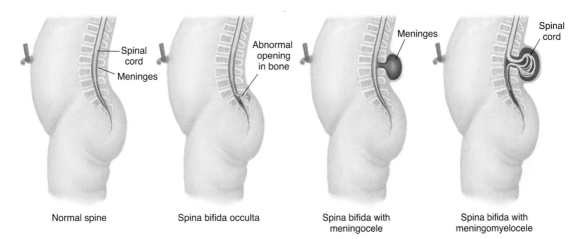

Normal spine   Spina bifida occulta   Spina bifida with meningocele   Spina bifida with meningomyelocele

Figure 11–2. Spina bifida.

Diagnostic Procedures

cerebrospinal fluid (CSF) analysis sĕr-ĕ-brō-SPĪ-năl *cerebr/o:* cerebrum *spin:* spine *-al:* pertaining to	Laboratory test used to examine a sample of CSF fluid obtained from a lumbar puncture which is analyzed for presence of blood, bacteria, malignant cells, as well as for the amount of protein and glucose present
lumbar puncture (LP) LŬM-băr *lumb:* loins (lower back) *-ar:* pertaining to	Insertion of a needle into the subarachnoid space of the spinal column to withdraw a sample of CSF used for biochemical, microbiological, and cytological laboratory analysis; also called *spinal tap* or *spinal puncture* (See Figure 11-3.)

Medical and Surgical Procedures

craniotomy krā-nē-ŎT-ō-mē *crani/o:* cranium (skull) *-tomy:* incision	Surgical procedure that creates an opening in the skull to gain access to the brain during neurosurgical procedures

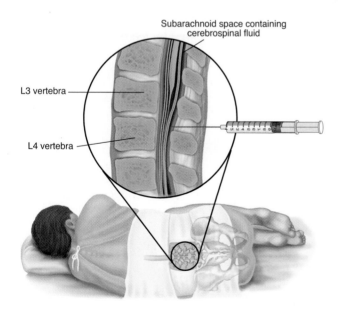

Figure 11–3. Lumbar puncture.

thalamotomy thăl-ă-MŎT-ō-mē *thalam/o:* thalamus *-tomy:* incision	Partial destruction of the thalamus to treat psychosis or intractable pain

Pharmacology

anesthetics
ăn-ĕs-THĔT-ĭks
  general
  local
	Produce partial or complete loss of sensation with or without loss of consciousness
	      Produce complete loss of feeling with loss of consciousness
	      Produce loss of feeling and affect a local area only

anticonvulsants ăn-tĭ-kŏn-VŬL-sănts	Prevent or control seizures

antiparkinsonian agents ăn-tĭ-păr-kĭn-SŌN-ē-ăn	Reduce the signs and symptoms associated with Parkinson disease

Pronunciation Help	Long Sound	ā in rāte	ē in rēbirth	ī in īsle	ō in ōver	ū in ūnite
	Short Sound	ă in ălone	ĕ in ĕver	ĭ in ĭt	ŏ in nŏt	ŭ in cŭt

Closer Look

Take a closer look at these nervous system disorders to enhance your understanding of the medical terminology associated with them.

Spinal Cord Injuries

Vertebral fractures and dislocations are severe injuries to the spinal cord that result in impairment of spinal cord function below the level of the injury. Spinal cord injuries are commonly the result of **trauma** caused by motor vehicle accidents, falls, diving in shallow water, or accidents associated with contact sports. Such trauma may cause varying degrees of paralysis. These injuries are seen most commonly in the male adolescent and young adult population. The loss of motor function may be confined to the lower extremities (**paraplegia**) or may be present in all four extremities (**quadriplegia**), accompanied by increased muscular tension and hyperactive reflexes (**spastic**) or by loss of reflexes and tone (**flaccid**).

(Continued)

Closer Look–cont'd

Paraplegia is paralysis of the lower portion of the body and both legs. It results in loss of sensory and motor control below the level of injury. **Quadriplegia** is paralysis of all four extremities and, usually, the trunk. It generally results in loss of motor and sensory function below the level of injury. Paralysis includes the trunk, legs, and pelvic organs with partial or total paralysis in the upper extremities. The higher the trauma, the more debilitating the motor and sensory impairments will be. The illustration below shows spinal cord injuries and their extent of paralysis.

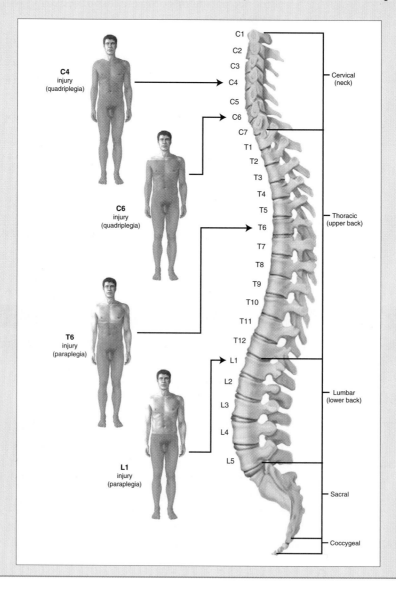

Additional Medical Vocabulary Recall

Match the medical term(s) below with the definitions in the numbered list.

Alzheimer disease   craniotomy   neuroblastoma   shingles
anesthetics   dementia   paralysis   spina bifida
anticonvulsants   epilepsy   Parkinson disease   stroke
antiparkinsonian   hydrocephalus   poliomyelitis   thalamotomy
Bell palsy   LP   sciatica   TIA

1. _____ is facial paralysis due to inflammation of a facial nerve.

2. _____ refers to brain tissue damage due to formation of a clot or a ruptured blood vessel; also called CVA.

3. _____ is a central nervous system disorder characterized by recurrent seizures.

4. _____ is a partial destruction of the thalamus to treat psychosis or intractable pain.

5. _____ involves insertion of a needle into the subarachnoid space to withdraw a sample of CSF for laboratory analysis.

6. _____ is a temporary interruption of blood supply to the brain without permanent brain damage.

7. _____ is a progressive degenerative neurological disorder that causes tremors, uncontrollable head nodding, and a shuffling gait.

8. _____ refers to inflammation of the gray matter caused by a virus.

9. _____ refers to severe pain in the leg along the course of the sciatic nerve.

10. _____ is a congenital defect characterized by incomplete closure of the spinal canal through which the spinal cord and meninges may or may not protrude.

11. _____ is a cranial enlargement caused by accumulation of fluid within the ventricles of the brain.

12. _____ is a malignant tumor, composed principally of cells resembling neuroblasts, that occurs mainly in infants and children.

13. _____ results in memory loss, mental deterioration, and decline in social skills and physical functioning.

14. _____ are used to prevent or control seizure activity.

15. _____ is a general term that refers to cognitive deficit, including memory impairment.

16. _____ refers to eruption of acute, inflammatory, herpetic vesicles on the trunk of the body along a peripheral nerve.

17. _____ produce partial or complete loss of sensation with our without loss of consciousness.

18. _____ agents reduce symptoms, such as tremors, in Parkinson disease.

19. _____ is the creation of an opening in the skull to gain access to the brain during neurosurgical procedures.

20. _____ is a loss of muscle function, sensation, or both resulting from spinal cord injury.

 Competency Verification: Check your answers in Appendix B, Answer Key, on page 377. Review material that you did not answer correctly.

Correct Answers _____ × 5 = _____ %

Pronunciation and Spelling

Use the following list to practice correct pronunciation and spelling of medical terms. First practice the pronunciation aloud. Then, write the correct spelling of the term. The first word is completed for you.

Pronunciation	Spelling
1. ĂLTS-hī-měr	*Alzheimer*
2. sĕr-ĕ-brō-VĂS-kū-lăr	
3. krā-nē-ŎT-ō-mē	
4. ĔP-ĭ-lĕp-sē	
5. LŬM-băr	
6. PAWL-zē	
7. pō-lē-ō-mī-ĕl-Ī-tĭs	
8. pă-RĂL-ĭ-sĭs	
9. păr-ă-PLĒ-jē-ă	
10. nū-rō-blăs-TŌ-mă	
11. kwŏd-rĭ-PLĒ-jē-ă	
12. SPĪ-nă BĬF-ĭ-dă ŏ-KŬL-tă	
13. sī-ĂT-ĭ-kă	
14. SĒ-zhūr	
15. SHĬNG-lz	

Competency Verification: Check your answers in Appendix B, Answer Key, on page 377. Review material that you did not answer correctly.

Correct Answers: _____ × 6.67 = _____ %

Abbreviations

The table below introduces abbreviations associated with the nervous system.

Abbreviation	Meaning	Abbreviation	Meaning
C1, C2, and so on	first cervical vertebra, second cervical vertebra, and so on	L1, L2, and so on	first lumbar vertebra, second lumbar vertebra, and so on
CNS	central nervous system	LP	lumbar puncture
CSF	cerebrospinal fluid	MS	mitral stenosis; musculoskeletal; multiple sclerosis; mental status; magnesium sulfate
CO	coccygeal nerves	S1, S2	first sacral vertebra, second sacral vertebra, and so on
CVA	cerebrovascular accident; costovertebral angle	T1-T12	first thoracic vertebra, second thoracic vertebra, and so on
CVD	cerebrovascular disease	TIA	transient ischemic attack
EEG	electrocardiogram; electroencephalography		

Chart Notes

Chart notes make up part of the medical record and are used in various types of health care facilities. The chart notes below were dictated by the patient's physician and reflect common clinical events using medical terminology to document the patient's care. By studying and completing the terminology and chart notes sections below you will learn and understand terms associated with the medical specialty of neurology.

Terminology

The following terms are linked to chart notes in the medical specialty of neurology. Practice pronouncing each term aloud and then use a medical dictionary such as *Taber's Cyclopedic Medical Dictionary, Appendix A: Glossary of Medical Word Elements* on page 337, or other resources to define each term.

Term	Meaning
adenocarcinoma ăd-ĕ-nō-kăr-sĭn-Ō-mă	
anorexia ăn-ō-RĔK-sē-ă	
aphasia ă-FĀ-zē-ă	
biliary BĬL-ē-ār-ē	
cardiovascular kăr-dē-ō-VĂS-kū-lăr	
cholecystojejunostomy kō-lē-sĭs-tō-jĕ-jū-NŎS-tō-mē	
deglutition dē-gloo-TĬSH-ŭn	
diplopia dĭp-LŌ-pē-ă	
jaundice JAWN-dĭs	
jejunojejunostomy jĕ-jū-nō-jĕ-jū-NŎS-tō-mē	
metastasis mĕ-TĂS-tă-sis	
pruritus proo-RĪ-tŭs	
stroke strōk	
vertigo VĔR-tĭ-gō	

Visit *http://davisplus.fadavis.com/gylys-express* for the terminology pronunciation exercise associated with this chart note.

Stroke

Read the chart note below aloud. Underline any term you have trouble pronouncing and any terms that you cannot define. If needed, refer to the Terminology section above for correct pronunciations and meanings of terms.

Patient is a moderately obese white woman who was admitted to Riverside Hospital because of a sudden episode of stroke. She recalls an episode of vertigo 3 days ago. Patient is being nursed at home by her daughter because of terminal adenocarcinoma of the head of the pancreas with metastasis to the liver, which was diagnosed in December. Patient fell to the floor with paralysis of the right arm and right leg and aphasia. She has not noticed any difficulty with deglutition. Apparently with the onset of the stroke, she also experienced diplopia. She denies any difficulty with her cardiovascular system in the past. Patient was in the hospital 5 years ago because of generalized biliary-type disease with jaundice, pruritus, weight loss, and anorexia. Subsequently, she was seen in consultation, and cholecystojejunostomy and jejunojejunostomy were performed.

Diagnosis:
1. Stroke, probably secondary to metastatic lesion of the brain or cerebrovascular disease.
2. Evidence of the previously described deterioration secondary to carcinoma of the pancreas with metastases to the liver.

Chart Note Analysis

From the chart note above, select the medical word that means

1. loss of appetite: _____

2. the act of swallowing: _____

3. double vision: _____

4. condition of yellowness of the skin and the mucous membranes: _____

5. a sensation of moving around in space: _____

6. a loss of sensation and voluntary movement: _____

7. a malignant tumor of a glandular organ: _____

8. creation of an opening between the gallbladder and the jejunum: _____

9. pertaining to bile: _____

10. spread of cancer (to the liver): _____

11. inability to communicate through speech: _____

12. itchy skin sensation that prompts a person to rub or scratch: _____

Competency Verification: Check your answers in Appendix B, Answer Key, on page 377.
Review material that you did not answer correctly.

Correct Answers: _____ × **8.4** = _____ %

Demonstrate What You Know!

To evaluate your understanding of how medical terms you have studied in this and previous
chapters are used in a clinical environment, complete the numbered sentences by selecting
an appropriate term from the list below.

aphasia	homeostasis	paresis
CNS	meningitis	PNS
cognition	meningomyelocele	quadriplegia
diplopia	myelalgia	TIAs
flaccid	neurosurgeon	vertigo

1. The baby born with spina bifida cystica is diagnosed with a herniation of the meninges and spinal
   cord, also known as _____.

2. A paralysis of four limbs is charted as _____.

3. CSF analysis indicates a patient is suffering from an infection of the meninges called _____.

4. Partial paralysis is charted as _____.

5. _____ refers to the ability to think and reason.

6. The brain and spinal cord make up the _____.

7. A patient complains of a strange sensation of moving around in space. This condition is diagnosed
   as _____.

8. The peripheral nerves are part of the _____.

9. The term used to describe pain in the spinal cord is _____.

10. A relative equilibrium in the internal environment of the body is known
    as _____.

11. The aging process results in a loss of reflexes and body tone, a condition called _____.

12. The physician who specializes in neurosurgery is a _____.

13. A patient has a history of mini-strokes, or _____, that preceded her stroke.

14. _____ is an absence of language function that may be the result of an injury to the cerebral cortex.

15. With the onset of stroke, a patient experiences double vision, or _____.

Competency Verification: Check your answers in Appendix B, Answer Key, on page 377. Review material that you did not answer correctly.

Correct Answers: _____ × **6.67 =** _____ **%**

Multimedia Review. If you are not satisfied with your retention level of the nervous system chapter, visit *http://davisplus.fadavis.com/gylys-express* and complete the website activities linked to this chapter. It is your choice whether or not you want to take advantage of these reinforcement exercises before continuing with the next chapter.

Musculoskeletal System

MULTIMEDIA STUDY TOOLS.
To enrich your medical terminology skills, look for this multimedia icon throughout the text. It will help alert you to when it is best to use the various multimedia resources available with this textbook to enhance your studies.

Objectives

Upon completion of this chapter, you will be able to:

- Describe types of medical treatment provided by orthopedists and chiropractors.
- Name the primary structures of the musculoskeletal system and discuss their functions.
- Identify combining forms, suffixes, and prefixes associated with the musculoskeletal system.
- Recognize, pronounce, build, and spell medical terms and abbreviations associated with the musculoskeletal system.
- Demonstrate your knowledge of this chapter by successfully completing the activities in this chapter.

Vocabulary Preview

Terms	Meanings
arthritis ăr-THRĪ-tĭs *arthr:* joint *-itis:* inflammation	Inflammation of a joint, usually accompanied by pain, swelling, and stiffness
arthroplasty ĂR-thrō-plăs-tē *arthr:* joint *-plasty:* surgical repair	Surgery to reshape, reconstruct, or replace a diseased or damaged joint
articulate ăr-TĬK-ū-lāt	Site of contact between two bones; also called a *joint*
contraction kŏn-TRĂK-shŭn	Shortening or tightening of a muscle
musculoskeletal mŭs-kū-lō-SKĔL-ĕ-tăl *muscul/o:* muscle *skelet:* skeleton *-al:* pertaining to	Pertaining to muscles and the skeleton
radiography rā-dē-OG-ră-fē *radi/o:* radiation, x-ray; radius (lower arm bone on thumb side) *-graphy:* process of recording	Production of captured shadow images on photographic film through the action of ionizing radiation passing through the body from an external source
synovial fluid sĭn-Ō-vē-ăl	Lubricating fluid of the joint secreted by the synovial membrane in the joint

Pronunciation Help	Long Sound	ā in rāte	ē in rēbirth	ī in īsle	ō in ōver	ū in ūnite
	Short Sound	ă in ălone	ĕ in ĕver	ĭ in ĭt	ŏ in nŏt	ŭ in cŭt

Orthopedics and Chiropractic

The **musculoskeletal** system is associated with the medical specialties of orthopedics and chiropractic medicine.

Orthopedics

Orthopedics is the branch of medicine concerned with prevention, diagnosis, care, and treatment of musculoskeletal disorders. These disorders include injury to or disease of the body's bones, joints, ligaments, muscles, and tendons. **Orthopedists** employ medical, physical, and surgical methods, such as hip **arthroplasty,** to restore function that is lost as a result of injury or disease to the musculoskeletal system. They also coordinate their treatments with other health care providers, such as physical therapists, occupational therapists, and sports medicine physicians. In addition to the orthopedist who treats bone and joint diseases, the **rheumatologist** (also a medical doctor) specializes in treatment of **arthritis** and other diseases of joints, muscles, and bones.

Chiropractic

Another health care provider who treats musculoskeletal disorders is the **chiropractor.** Unlike orthopedists, chiropractors are not physicians. They do not employ drugs or surgery, the primary basis of treatment used by medical physicians. **Chiropractic medicine** is a system of therapy based on the theory that disease is caused by pressure on nerves. Even so, chiropractors do employ the use of **radiography** to diagnose pathological disorders and determine the most effective type of treatment. In most instances, chiropractic treatment involves physical manipulation of the spinal column.

Musculoskeletal System Quick Study

The musculoskeletal system includes muscles, bones, joints, and related structures, such as the tendons and connective tissue. These structures function to support and move body parts and organs.

Muscles perform four primary functions: producing body movements, stabilizing body positions, storing and moving substances within the body, and generating heat. Through **contraction,** muscles cause and help maintain body posture. Less apparent motions provided by muscles include the passage and elimination of food through the digestive system, propulsion of blood through the arteries, and contraction of the bladder to eliminate urine. In addition, muscles function in body movements in several different ways to allow a range of motion for the contraction and relaxation of muscle fibers.

The main function of bones is to form a skeleton that supports and protects the body. It also serves as a storage area for mineral salts, especially calcium and phosphorus. Joints are the places where two bones **articulate. Synovial fluid** lubricates the joints to minimize friction upon motion. Because bones cannot move without the help of muscles, contraction must be provided by muscular tissue. (See *Anterior View of the Sheleton,* page 286.)

 An extensive anatomy and physiology review is included in *TermPlus,* the powerful, interactive CD-ROM program.

Medical Word Building

Building medical words using word elements related to the musculoskeletal system will enhance your understanding of those terms and reinforce your ability to use terms correctly.

Combining Forms

Begin your study of musculoskeletal terminology by reviewing the structures of the musculoskeletal system and their associated combining forms (CFs), which are illustrated in the figure *Anterior View of the Skeleton* on the next page.

Anterior View of the Skeleton

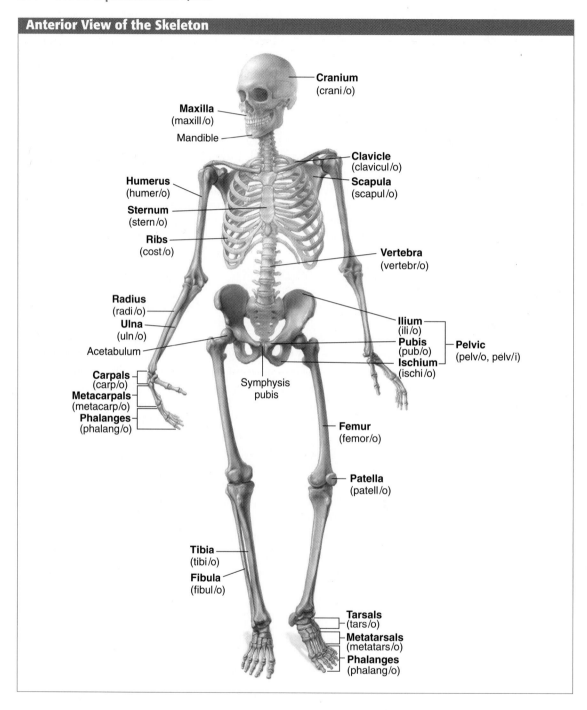

Cranium
(crani/o)

Maxilla
(maxill/o)

Mandible

Clavicle
(clavicul/o)

Scapula
(scapul/o)

Humerus
(humer/o)

Sternum
(stern/o)

Ribs
(cost/o)

Vertebra
(vertebr/o)

Radius
(radi/o)

Ulna
(uln/o)

Acetabulum

Ilium
(ili/o)

Pubis
(pub/o)

Ischium
(ischi/o)

Pelvic
(pelv/o, pelv/i)

Carpals
(carp/o)

Metacarpals
(metacarp/o)

Phalanges
(phalang/o)

Symphysis
pubis

Femur
(femor/o)

Patella
(patell/o)

Tibia
(tibi/o)

Fibula
(fibul/o)

Tarsals
(tars/o)

Metatarsals
(metatars/o)

Phalanges
(phalang/o)

In the table below, CFs are listed alphabetically and other word parts are defined as needed. Review the medical word and study the elements that make up the term. Then complete the meaning of the medical words in the right-hand column. The first one is completed for you. You may also refer to *Appendix A: Glossary of Medical Word Elements* to complete this exercise.

Combining Form	Meaning	Medical Word	Meaning
Muscles and Related Structures			
fasci/o	band, fascia (fibrous membrane supporting and separating muscles)	**fasci/o**/plasty (FĂSH-ē-ō-plăs-tē) *-plasty:* surgical repair	*surgical repair of fascia*
fibr/o	fiber, fibrous tissue	**fibr/**oma (fĭ-BRŌ-mă) *-oma:* tumor	
leiomy/o	smooth muscle (visceral)	**leiomy/**oma (lī-ō-mī-Ō-mă) *-oma:* tumor	
lumb/o	loins (lower back)	**lumb/o**/cost/al (lŭm-bō-KŎS-tăl) *cost:* ribs *-al:* pertaining to	
muscul/o	muscle	**muscul/**ar (MŬS-kū-lăr) *-ar:* pertaining to	
my/o		**my/o**/rrhexis (mī-or-ĔK-sĭs) *-rrhexis:* rupture	
ten/o	tendon	**ten/o**/tomy (tĕn-ŎT-ō-mē) *-tomy:* incision	
tend/o		**tend/o**/plasty (TĔN-dō-plăs-tē) *-plasty:* surgical repair	
tendin/o		**tendin/**itis (tĕn-dĭn-Ī-tĭs) *-itis:* inflammation	

(Continued)

Combining Form	Meaning	Medical Word	Meaning
Bones of the Upper Extremities			
carp/o	carpus (wrist bones)	**carp/o**/ptosis (kăr-pŏp-TŌ-sĭs) *-ptosis:* prolapse, downward displacement	
cervic/o	neck; cervix uteri (neck of uterus)	**cervic**/al (SĔR-vĭ-kăl) *-al:* pertaining to	
cost/o	ribs	sub/**cost**/al (sŭb-KŎS-tăl) *sub-:* under, below *-al:* pertaining to	
crani/o	cranium (skull)	**crani/o**/tomy (krā-nē-ŎT-ō-mē) *-tomy:* incision	
humer/o	humerus (upper arm bone)	**humer**/al (HŪ-mĕr-ăl) *-al:* pertaining to	
metacarp/o	metacarpus (hand bones)	**metacarp**/ectomy (mĕt-ă-kăr-PĔK-tō-mē) *-ectomy:* excision, removal	
phalang/o	phalanges (bones of fingers and toes)	**phalang**/itis (făl-ăn-JĪ-tĭs) *-itis:* inflammation	
spondyl/o*	vertebra (backbone)	**spondyl**/itis (spŏn-dĭl-Ī-tĭs) *-itis:* inflammation	
vertebr/o*		**vertebr**/al (VĔR-tĕ-brăl) *-al:* pertaining to	
stern/o	sternum (breastbone)	**stern/o**/cost/al (stĕr-nō-KŎS-tăl) *cost:* ribs *-al:* pertaining to	

*The CF spondyl/o is used to form words about the condition of the structure; the CF vertebr/o is used to form words that describe the structure.

Combining Form	Meaning	Medical Word	Meaning
Bones of the Lower Extremities			
calcane/o	calcaneum (heel bone)	**calcane/o**/dynia (kăl-kăn-ē-ō-DĬN-ē-ă) *-dynia:* pain	
femor/o	femur (thigh bone)	**femor/**al (FĔM-or-ăl) *-al:* pertaining to	
fibul/o	fibula (smaller, outer bone of lower leg)	**fibul/**ar (FĬB-ū-lăr) *-ar:* pertaining to	
patell/o	patella (kneecap)	**patell/**ectomy (păt-ĕ-LĔK-tō-mē) *-ectomy:* excision, removal	
pelv/i**	pelvis	**pelv/i**/metry (pĕl-VĬM-ĕ-trē) *-metry:* act of measuring	
pelv/o		**pelv/**is (PĔL-vĭs) *-is:* noun ending	
radi/o	radiation, x-ray; radius (lower arm bone, thumb side)	**radi/o**/graph (RĀ-dē-ō-grăf) *-graph:* instrument for recording	
tibi/o	tibia (larger bone of lower leg)	**tibi/**al (TĬB-ē-ăl) *-al:* pertaining to	
Other Related Structures			
ankyl/o	stiffness; bent, crooked	**ankyl/**osis (ăng-kĭ-LŌ-sĭs) *-osis:* abnormal condition; increase (used primarily with blood cells)	
arthr/o	joint	**arthr/o**/desis (ăr-thrō-DĒ-sĭs) *-desis:* binding, fixation (of a bone or joint)	

**The i *in* pelv/i/metry *is an exception to the rule of using the connecting vowel* o.

(Continued)

Combining Form	Meaning	Medical Word	Meaning
Other Related Structures			
chondr/o	cartilage	**cost/o**/chondr/itis (kŏs-tō-kŏn-DRĪ-tĭs) *cost/o:* ribs −*itis:* inflammation	
lamin/o	lamina (part of vertebral arch)	**lamin**/ectomy (lăm-ĭ-NĔK-tŏ-mē) −*ectomy:* excision, removal	
myel/o	bone marrow; spinal cord	**myel/o**/cele (MĪ-ĕ-lō-sēl) −*cele:* hernia, swelling	
orth/o	straight	**orth/o**/ped/ics (or-thō-PĒ-dĭks) *ped:* foot; child −*ics:* pertaining to	
oste/o	bone	**oste/o**/porosis (ŏs-tē-ō-por-Ō-sĭs) −*porosis:* porous	

Suffixes and Prefixes

In the table below, suffixes and prefixes are listed alphabetically and other word parts are defined as needed. Review the medical word and study the elements that make up the term. Then complete the meaning of the medical words in the right-hand column. You may also refer to *Appendix A: Glossary of Medical Word Elements* to complete this exercise.

Word Element	Meaning	Medical Word	Meaning
Suffixes			
-clasia	to break; surgical fracture	arthr/o/**clasia** (ăr-thrō-KLĀ-zē-ă) *arthr/o:* joint	
-clast	to break	oste/o/**clast** (ŎS-tē-ō-klăst) *oste/o:* bone	
-plegia	paralysis	hemi/**plegia** (hĕm-ē-PLĒ-jē-ă) *hemi−:* half	

Word Element	Meaning	Medical Word	Meaning
Suffixes			
-sarcoma	malignant tumor of connective tissue	my/o/**sarcoma** (mī-ō-sar-KŌ-mă) *my/o:* muscle	
Prefixes			
dia-	through, across	**dia**/physis (dī-ĂF-ĭ-sĭs) *-physis:* growth	
peri-	around	**peri**/oste/um (pĕr-ē-ŎS-tē-ŭm) *oste:* bone *um:* structure, thing	

 Competency Verification: Check your answers in Appendix B, Answer Key, page 378. If you are not satisfied with your level of comprehension, review the terms in the table and retake the review.

 Listen and Learn, the audio CD-ROM included in this book, will help you master pronunciation of selected medical words. Use it to practice pronunciations of the medical terms in the above "Word Building" tables and for instructions to complete the *Listen and Learn* exercise.

 Flash-Card Activity. Enhance your study and reinforcement of this chapter's word elements with the power of the DavisPlus flash-card activity. Do so by visiting *http://davisplus.fadavis.com/gylys-express.* We recommend you complete the flash-card activity before continuing with the next section.

Medical Terminology Word Building

In this section, combine the word parts you have learned to construct medical terms related to the musculoskeletal system.

Use *oste/o* (bone) to build words that mean:

1. bone cells _____

2. pain in bones _____

3. disease of bones and joints _____

4. beginning or formation of bones _____

Use *cervic/o* (neck) to build words that mean:

5. pertaining to the neck _____

6. pertaining to the neck and arm _____

7. pertaining to the neck and face _____

Use *myel/o* (bone marrow; spinal cord) to build words that mean:

8. tumor of bone marrow _____

9. sarcoma of bone marrow (cells) _____

10. radiography of the spinal cord _____

11. abnormal softening of the spinal cord _____

Use *stern/o* (sternum) to build words that mean:

12. pertaining to above the sternum _____

13. resembling the breastbone _____

Use *arthr/o* (joint) or *chondr/o* (cartilage) to build words that mean:

14. embryonic cell that forms cartilage _____

15. inflammation of a joint _____

16. inflammation of bones and joints _____

Use *pelv/i* (pelvis) to build a word that means:

17. instrument for measuring the pelvis _____

Use *my/o* (muscle) to build words that mean:

18. twitching of a muscle _____

19. any disease of muscle _____

20. rupture of a muscle _____

Competency Verification: Check your answers in Appendix B, Answer Key, on page 380. Review material that you did not answer correctly.

Correct Answers _____ × **5 =** _____ %

Additional Medical Vocabulary

The following tables list additional terms related to the musculoskeletal system. Recognizing and learning these terms will help you understand the connection between common signs, symptoms, and diseases and their diagnoses. Included are medical and surgical procedures as well as pharmacological agents used to treat diseases.

Signs, Symptoms, and Diseases
Muscles

muscular dystrophy (MD) MŬS-kū-lăr DĬS-trō-fē *muscul:* muscle *-ar:* pertaining to *dys-:* bad; painful; difficult *-trophy:* development, nourishment	Group of hereditary diseases characterized by progressive degeneration of the muscles, leading to increasing weakness and debilitation, including Duchenne dystrophy (most common form)
myasthenia gravis (MG) mī-ăs-THĒ-nē-ă GRĂV-ĭs	Autoimmune neuromuscular disorder characterized by progressive fatigue and severe muscle weakness, particularly evident with facial muscles and ptosis of the eyelids
rotator cuff injury	Injury to the capsule of the shoulder joint, which is reinforced by muscles and tendons; also called *musculotendinous rotator cuff injury*
sprain	Trauma to a joint that causes injury to the surrounding ligament, accompanied by pain and disability, such as an eversion sprain that occurs when the foot is twisted outward
strain	Trauma to a muscle from overuse or excessive forcible stretch
talipes equinovarus TĂL-ĭ-pēz ē-kwī-nō-VĀR-ŭs	Congenital deformity of the foot; also called *clubfoot* (See Figure 12-1.)
tendinitis tĕn-dĭn-Ī-tĭs	Inflammation of a tendon, usually caused by injury or overuse; also called *tendonitis*
torticollis tōr-tĭ-KŎL-ĭs	Spasmodic contraction of the neck muscles, causing stiffness and twisting of the neck; also called *wryneck*

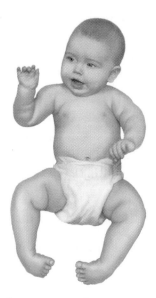

Figure 12–1. Talipes.

Bones and Joints

arthritis
ăr-THRĪ-tĭs
arthr: joint
-itis: inflammation

Inflammation of a joint usually accompanied by pain, swelling and, commonly, changes in structure

    gouty
    GOWT-ē

Arthritis caused by excessive uric acid in the body; also called *gout*

    osteoarthritis
    ŏs-tē-ō-ăr-THRĪ-tĭs
oste/o: bone
arthr: joint
-itis: inflammation

Progressive, degenerative joint disease characterized by bone spurs (osteophytes) and destruction of articular cartilage

rheumatoid arthritis (RA)
ROO-mă-toyd
ăr-THRĪ-tĭs

Chronic, systemic inflammatory disease affecting the synovial membranes of multiple joints, eventually resulting in crippling deformities and immobility

 Get a closer look at rheumatoid arthritis on page 302.

carpal tunnel syndrome (CTS) KĂR-păl TŬN-ĕl SĬN-drōm	Pain or numbness resulting from compression of the median nerve within the carpal tunnel (wrist canal through which the flexor tendons and median nerve pass)
contracture kŏn-TRĂK-chŭr	Fibrosis of connective tissue in the skin, fascia, muscle, or joint capsule that prevents normal mobility of the related tissue or joint
crepitation krĕp-ĭ-TĀ-shŭn	Grating sound made by movement of bone ends rubbing together, indicating a fracture or joint destruction
Ewing sarcoma Ū-ĭng săr-KŌ-mă	Malignant tumor that develops from bone marrow, usually in long bones or the pelvis, and most commonly in adolescent boys
fracture FRĂK-chŭr	Any break in a bone Get a closer look at bone fractures on pages 300 and 301.
herniated disk HĔR-nē-āt-ĕd	Herniation or rupture of the nucleus pulposus (center gelatinous material within an intervetebral disk) between two vertebrae; also called *prolapsed disk* (See Figure 12-2.)

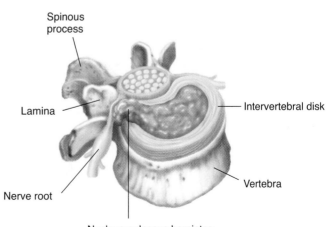

Figure 12–2. Herniated disk.

osteoporosis
ŏs-tē-ō-pōr-Ō-sĭs
  oste/o: bone
  -porosis: porous
	Decrease in bone density with an increase in porosity, causing bones to become brittle and increasing the risk of fractures

Paget disease PĂ-jĕt	Skeletal disease affecting elderly people that causes chronic inflammation of bones, resulting in thickening and softening of bones and bowing of long bones; also called *osteitis deformans*
rickets RĬK-ĕts	Form of osteomalacia in children caused by vitamin D deficiency; also called *rachitis*
sequestrum sē-KWĔS-trŭm	Fragment of a necrosed bone that has become separated from surrounding tissue

Spine

kyphosis
kī-FŌ-sĭs
  kyph: humpback
  -osis: abnormal condition; increase (used primarily with blood cells)
	Increased curvature of the thoracic region of the vertebral column, leading to a humpback posture; also called *hunchback* (See Figure 12-3.)

lordosis
lōr-DŌ-sĭs
  lord: curve, swayback
  -osis: abnormal condition; increase (used primarily with blood cells)
	Forward curvature of the lumbar region of the vertebral column, leading to a swayback posture (Figure 12-3.)

scoliosis
skō-lē-Ō-sĭs
  scoli: crooked, bent
  -osis: abnormal
       condition; increase
       (used primarily
       with blood cells)
	Abnormal sideward curvature of the spine to the left or right that eventually causes back pain, disk disease, or arthritis (Figure 12-3.)

spondylitis
spŏn-dĭl-Ī-tĭs
  ankylosing spondylitis
  ăng-kĭ-LŌS-ĭng
  spŏn-dĭl-Ī-tĭs
  spondyl: vertebra
       (backbone)
  -itis: inflammation
	Inflammation of one or more vertebrae
	
	Chronic inflammatory disease of unknown origin that first affects the spine and is characterized by fusion and loss of mobility of two or more vertebrae; also called *rheumatoid spondylitis*

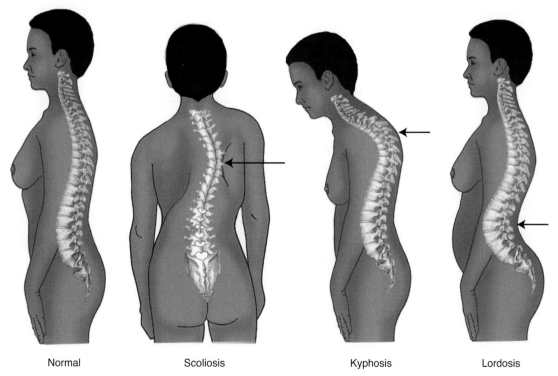

Normal   Scoliosis   Kyphosis   Lordosis

Figure 12–3. Spinal curvatures.

spondylolisthesis spŏn-dĭ-lō-lĭs-THĒ-sĭs *spondyl/o:* vertebra (backbone) *-listhesis:* slipping	Partial forward dislocation of one vertebra over the one below it, most commonly the fifth lumbar vertebra over the first sacral vertebra; also called *spinal cord compression*
subluxation sŭb-lŭk-SĀ-shŭn	Partial or incomplete dislocation of a bone from its normal location within a joint, causing loss of function of the joint; also called *partial dislocation*

Diagnostic Procedures

arthrocentesis ăr-thrō-sĕn-TĒ-sĭs *arthr/o:* joint *-centesis:* surgical puncture	Puncture of a joint space with a needle to obtain samples of synovial fluid for diagnostic purposes, instill medications, or remove accumulated fluid from joints to relieve pain
arthroscopy ăr-THRŌ S-kō-pē *arthr/o:* joint *-scopy:* visual examination	Visual examination of the interior of a joint and its structures using a thin, flexible, fiberoptic scope called an *arthroscope,* which contains a miniature camera and projects images on a monitor to guide instruments during procedures (See Figure 12-4.)

Medical and Surgical Procedures

arthroplasty ĂR-thrō-plăs-tē *arthr/o:* joint *-plasty:* surgical repair	Surgical reconstruction or replacement of a painful, degenerated joint to restore mobility in rheumatoid arthritis or osteoarthritis or to correct a congenital deformity
total hip arthroplasty	Replacement of the femoral head and acetabulum with prostheses that are fastened into the bone; also called *total hip replacement* (THR) (See Figure 12-5.)
sequestrectomy sē-kwĕs-TRĔK-tō-mē *sequestr:* separation *-ectomy:* excision, removal	Excision of a sequestrum (segment of necrosed bone)

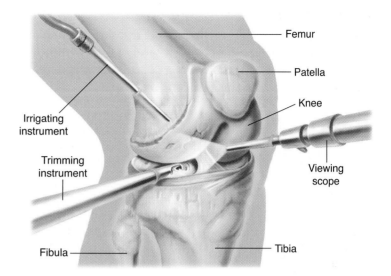

Figure 12–4. Arthroscopy.

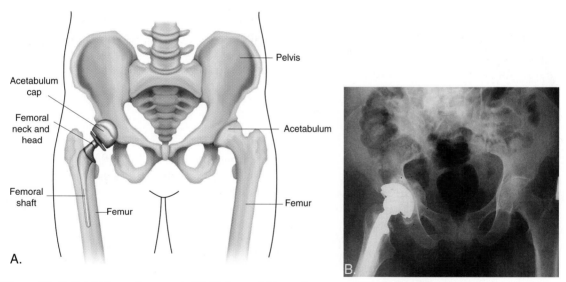

Figure 12–5. Total hip replacement. (A) Right total hip replacement. (B) Radiograph showing total hip replacement of arthritic hip. (From McKinnis: *Fundamentals of Musculoskeletal Imaging,* ed 2. FA Davis, Philadelphia, 2005, p 314, with permission.)

Pharmacology

bone reabsorption inhibitors	Reduce the reabsorption of bones in treatment of weak and fragile bones as seen in osteoporosis and Paget disease
gold salts	Treat rheumatoid arthritis by inhibiting activity within the immune system by preventing further disease progression
muscle relaxants	Relieve muscle spasms, pain, and stiffness
nonsteroidal anti-inflammatory drugs (NSAIDs) nŏn-STĒR-oyd-ăl ăn-tē-ĭn-FLĂM-ă-tō-rē	Relieve mild to moderate pain and reduce inflammation in treatment of musculoskeletal conditions, such as sprains and strains, and inflammatory disorders, including rheumatoid arthritis, osteoarthritis, bursitis, gout, and tendinitis

Pronunciation Help	Long Sound	ā in rāte	ē in rēbirth	ī in īsle	ō in ōver	ū in ūnite
	Short Sound	ă in ălone	ĕ in ĕver	ĭ in ĭt	ŏ in nŏt	ŭ in cŭt

Closer Look

Take a closer look at these musculoskeletal conditions to enhance your understanding of the medical terminology associated with them.

Bone Fractures

A **fracture** is a break or crack in a bone. Fractures occur when bones are broken as a result of an injury, an accident, or a disease process. They are classified according to the way in which the bone breaks and whether or not the skin is pierced with a bony fragment. A fracture that is caused by a disease process, such as **osteoporosis** or bone cancer, is known as a *pathologic fracture*. The illustration on the next page identifies and describes some common types of fractures. Specific methods of treatment for fractures depend on the type of fracture sustained, its location, and any related injuries. X-rays help confirm and determine the severity of the fracture.

Closer Look—cont'd

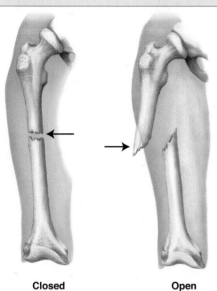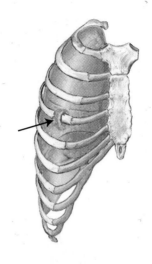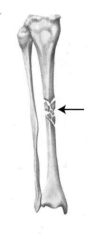

Closed
Bone is broken but
no open wound in skin

Open
Bone breaks
through skin

Complicated
Extensive soft tissue
injury such as a
broken rib piercing the lung above

Comminuted
Bone is crushed
into several pieces

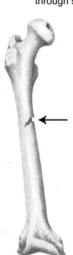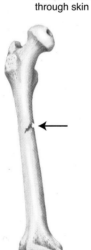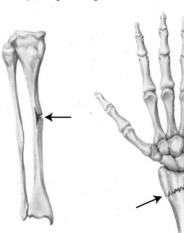

Impacted
Broken ends of a bone
are forced into one another

Incomplete
Line of fracture
does not include
the whole bone

Greenstick
Bone is broken only
on one side, commonly occurs
most in
children because
growing bones
are soft

Colles fracture
Distal radius is
broken by falling
onto an outstretched
hand

(Continued)

Closer Look–cont'd

Rheumatoid Arthritis

Rheumatoid arthritis (RA) is a chronic, systemic inflammatory disease that primarily attacks peripheral joints and surrounding muscles, tendons, ligaments, and blood vessels. Spontaneous remissions and unpredictable exacerbations mark the course of this potentially crippling disease. RA is an **autoimmune disease** in which a reaction against one's own joint tissues, especially synovial fluid, occurs. As RA develops, there is congestion and edema of the synovial membrane and joint, causing formation of a thick layer of granulation tissue. This tissue invades cartilage, destroying the joint and bone. Eventually, a fibrous immobility of joints **(ankylosis)** occurs, causing immobility and visible deformities, as seen in the illustration below. The disease is three times more common in women than men. RA usually requires lifelong treatment and, occasionally, surgery. The prognosis worsens with the development of nodules, **vasculitis,** and the presence of **rheumatoid factor** (substance detected in blood test of patients with rheumatoid arthritis).

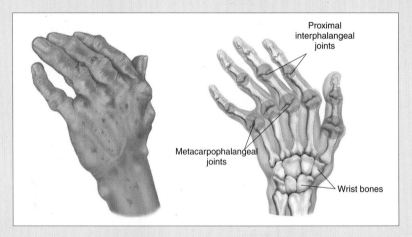

Treatment consists of physical therapy, heat applications, and such drugs as aspirin, nonsteroidal anti-inflammatory drugs (NSAIDs), and **corticosteroids** to reduce pain and inflammation. Other therapeutic drugs include disease-modifying antirheumatic drugs (DMARDs), such as gold salts.

Additional Medical Vocabulary Recall

Match the medical term(s) below with the definitions in the numbered list.

arthroplasty	gout	myasthenia gravis	sequestrum
contracture	herniated disk	osteoporosis	sprain
crepitation	kyphosis	Paget disease	strain
CTS	lordosis	RA	tendinitis
Ewing sarcoma	muscular dystrophy	scoliosis	torticollis

1. _____ means decrease in bone density and an increase in porosity, causing the risk of fractures.

2. _____ means inflammation of a tendon.

3. _____ refers to trauma to a joint, causing injury to the surrounding ligament.

4. _____ refers to muscular trauma that results from overuse or excessive, forcible stretch.

5. _____ means hunchback or humpback.

6. _____ is a malignant tumor that develops from bone marrow, usually in long bones or the pelvis, and occurs most commonly in adolescent boys.

7. _____ means wryneck.

8. _____ is a disease characterized by excessive uric acid in the blood and around the joints.

9. _____ is a disease characterized by inflammatory changes in joints and related structures that result in crippling deformities.

10. _____ is a skeletal disease of the elderly with chronic inflammation of bones, resulting in thickening and softening of bones and bowing of long bones and is also called *osteitis deformans*.

11. _____ is a fragment of necrosed bone that has become separated from surrounding tissue.

12. _____ means repair or replacement of a joint.

13. _____ is a grating sound made by the ends of bone rubbing together.

14. _____ is a neuromuscular disorder characterized by muscular weakness and progressive fatigue.

15. _____ means forward curvature of the lumbar spine; also called *swayback*.

16. _____ refers to a group of hereditary diseases characterized by gradual atrophy and weakness of muscle; the most common form is called *Duchenne*.

17. _____ is connective tissue fibrosis that prevents normal mobility of the related tissue or joint.

18. _____ is abnormal sideward curvature of the spine to the left or right.

19. _____ refers to rupture of the nucleus pulposus between two vertebrae.

20. _____ is pain or numbness resulting from compression of the median nerve within the carpal tunnel.

Competency Verification: Check your answers in Appendix B, Answer Key, page 380. Review material that you did not answer correctly.

Correct Answers _____ × 5 = _____ × %

Pronunciation and Spelling

Use the following list to practice correct pronunciation and spelling of medical terms. First practice the pronunciation aloud. Then, write the correct spelling of the term. The first word is completed for you.

Pronunciation	Spelling
1. ăb-DŬK-shŭn	*abduction*
2. ăr-thrō-KLĀ-zē-ă	
3. DOR-sĭ-flĕk-shŭn	
4. făl-ăn-JĪ-tĭs	
5. FĂSH-ē-ō-plăs-tē	
6. gowt	
7. krĕp-ĭ-TĀ-shŭn	
8. lī-ō-mī-Ō-mă	
9. mī-ō-săr-KŌ-mă	
10. mī-ăs-THĒ-nē-ă GRĂV-ĭs	
11. or-thō-PĒ-dĭks	
12. ŏs-tē-ō-ăr-THRŎP-ă-thē	
13. ŎS-tē-ō-klăst	
14. PĂJ-ĕt dĭ-ZĒZ	
15. pĕl-VĬM-ĕ-trē	

Pronunciation	Spelling
16. ROO-mă-toyd ăr-THRĪ-tĭs	
17. sē-kwĕs-TRĔK-tō-mē	
18. spŏn-dĭl-ō-mă-LĀ-shē-ă	
19. stĕr-nō-KŎS-tăl	
20. tōr-tĭ-KŎL-ĭs	

Competency Verification: Check your answers in Appendix B, Answer Key, on page380. Review material that you did not answer correctly.

Correct Answers: _____ × 5 = _____ %

Abbreviations

The table below introduces abbreviations associated with the musculoskeletal system.

Abbreviation	Meaning	Abbreviation	Meaning
BK	below the knee	L1, L2, to L5	first lumbar vertebra, second lumbar vertebra, and so on
C1, C2, to C7	first cervical vertebra, second cervical vertebra, and so on	MG	myasthenia gravis
CT	computed tomography	NSAIDs	nonsteroidal anti-inflammatory drugs
CTS	carpal tunnel syndrome	ORTH, Ortho	orthopedics
DMARDs	Disease-modifying antirheumatic drugs	RA	rheumatoid arthritis
Fx	fracture	S1, S2, to S5	first sacral vertebra, second sacral vertebra, and so on
HNP	herniated nucleus pulposus (herniated disk)	T1, T2, to T12	first thoracic vertebra, second thoracic vertebra, and so on
IM	intramuscular	THR	total hip replacement

Chart Notes

Chart notes make up part of the medical record and are used in various types of health care facilities. The chart notes that follow were dictated by the patient's physician, and reflect common clinical events using medical terminology to document the patient's care. By studying and completing the terminology and chart notes sections below you will learn and understand terms associated with the medical specialty of orthopedics.

Terminology

The following terms are linked to chart notes in the medical specialty of orthopedics. Practice pronouncing each term aloud and then use a medical dictionary such as *Taber's Cyclopedic Medical Dictionary, Appendix A: Glossary of Medical Word Elements* on page 337, or other resources to define each term.

Term	Meaning
anteroposterior ăn-tĕr-ō-pŏs-TĒ-rē-ŏr	
bilateral bī-LĂT-ĕr-ăl	
degenerative dĕ-JĔN-ĕr-ă-tĭv	
hypertrophic hī-pĕr-TRŌF-ĭk	
intervertebral ĭn-tĕr-VĔRT-ĕ-brăl	
L5	
laminectomies lăm-ĭ-NĔK-tŏ-mēz	
lateral views LĂT-ĕr-ăl	
lipping LĬP-ĭng	
lumbar LŬM-băr	
lumbosacral lŭm-bō-SĀ-krăl	

Term	Meaning
S1	
sacroiliac sā-krō-ĬL-ē-ăk	
sacrum SĀ-krŭm	

 Visit *http://davisplus.fadavis.com/gylys-express* for the terminology pronunciation exercise associated with this chart note.

Degenerative Intervertebral Disk Disease

Read the chart note below aloud. Underline any term you have trouble pronouncing and any terms that you cannot define. If needed, refer to the Terminology section above for correct pronunciations and meanings of terms.

Anteroposterior and lateral views of the lumbar spine and an AP view of the sacrum show a placement of L5 on S1. The L5-S1 intervertebral disk space contains a slight shadow of decreased density. There is now slight narrowing of the L3-4 and L4-5 spaces. Bilateral laminectomies appear to have been done at L5-S1. Slight hypertrophic lipping of the upper margin of the body of L4. The sacroiliac joint spaces are well preserved. Lateral view of the lumbosacral spine taken with the spine in flexion and extension demonstrates slight motion at all of the lumbar and lumbosacral levels.

Impression:
1. Degenerative, inververtebral disk disease at L5-S1, now also accompanied by slight narrowing of the L3-4 and L5-4 disk spaces.
2. Slight motion at all of the lumbar and lumbosacral levels.

Chart Note Analysis

From the chart note above, select the medical word that means:

1. Pertaining to the sacrum and ilium _____

2. Designates the third and fourth lumbar vertebrae _____

3. Bending motion of a limb _____

4. Directional term indicating *from the front to the back* _____

5. Pertaining to two sides _____

6. Pertaining to an increase in the size of an organ or structure _____

7. Pertaining to the lumbar vertebra and the sacrum _____

8. Pertaining to one side _____

9. Extending motion of a limb _____

10. Pertaining to between vertebrae _____

Competency Verification: Check your answers in Appendix B, Answer Key, on page 380. Review material that you did not answer correctly.

Correct Answers: _____ × 10 = _____ %

Demonstrate What You Know!

To evaluate your understanding of how medical terms you have studied in this and previous chapters are used in a clinical environment, complete the numbered sentences by selecting an appropriate term from the list below.

ankylosis	degenerative	NSAIDs
arthrocentesis	gouty	rheumatologist
articulate	greenstick	rickets
calcaneodynia	laminectomy	subluxation
carpoptosis	muscles	talipes

1. _____ is a congenital deformity of the foot.

2. The surgical puncture of a joint is known as _____.

3. Partial or incomplete dislocation of a bone is known as a _____.

4. Immobility of joints is known as _____.

5. An elderly patient suffers from arthritis. Her primary physician referred her to a specialist called a(n) _____.

6. A patient fell on her hand, resulting in a downward displacement of her wrist, a condition known as

   _____.

7. A joint is a place where two or more bones connect, or _____,
   to allow motion between the parts.

8. _____ is a form of osteomalacia in children caused by vitamin D deficiency.

9. _____ are responsible for movement, maintaining posture, and the
   propulsion of substances through the body.

10. _____ refers to an impairment of a body structure.

11. A laboratory result with findings of excessive uric acid probably indicates _____
    arthritis.

12. The surgical procedure to excise part of the vertebrae is known as a _____.

13. _____ fractures usually occur in children because their growing bones are
    soft and tend to splinter rather than break completely.

14. _____ relieve pain and reduce inflammation in the treatment of
    musculoskeletal disorders.

15. A person with a symptom of heel pain would be suffering from _____.

Competency Verification: Check your answers in Appendix B, Answer Key, page 380.
Review material that you did not answer correctly.

Correct Answers: _____ × 6.67 = _____ %

Multimedia Review: If you are not satisfied with your retention level of the musculoskeletal
chapter, visit *http://davisplus.fadavis.com/gylys-express* to complete the website activities linked
to this chapter. It is your choice whether or not you want to take advantage of these reinforcement
exercises before continuing with the next chapter.

Special Senses: Eyes and Ears

MULTIMEDIA STUDY TOOLS.
To enrich your medical terminology skills, look for this
multimedia icon throughout the text. It will help alert
you to when it is best to use the various multimedia
resources available with this textbook to enhance your
studies.

Objectives

*Upon completion of this chapter, you will be
able to:*

- Describe types of medical treatment provided by
  ophthalmologists and otolaryngologists.
- Name the primary structures of the eyes and
  ears and discuss their functions.
- Identify combining forms, suffixes, and prefixes
  associated with the eyes and the ears.
- Recognize, pronounce, build, and spell
  pathological, diagnostic, and therapeutic terms,
  and abbreviations associated with the eyes
  and ears.
- Demonstrate your knowledge of this chapter
  by successfully completing the activities in this
  chapter.

Vocabulary Preview

Term	Meaning
cataract KĂT-ă-răkt	Opacity of the lens of the eye, usually occurring as a result of aging, trauma, metabolic disease, or the adverse effect of certain medications or chemicals
cornea transplantation KOR-nē-ă	Procedure in which a damaged cornea is replaced by the cornea from the eye of a human cadaver; also known as *keratoplasty*
glaucoma glaw-KŌ-mă *glauc:* gray *-oma:* tumor	Eye disease in which increased eyeball pressure causes gradual loss of sight
ocular ŎK-ū-lăr *ocul:* eye *-ar:* pertaining to	Pertaining to the eye or sense of sight
radial keratotomy kĕr-ă-TŎT-ō-mē *kerat/o:* horny tissue; hard; cornea *-tomy:* incision	Surgery to correct myopia, or *nearsightedness,* by changing the shape of the cornea (transparent part of the eye that covers the iris and pupil)
sleep apnea ăp-NĒ-ă *a-:* without, not *-pnea:* breathing	Condition in which breathing stops for more than ten seconds during sleep

Pronunciation Help	Long Sound	ā in rāte	ē in rēbirth	ī in īsle	ō in ōver	ū in ūnite
	Short Sound	ă in ălone	ĕ in ĕver	ĭ in ĭt	ŏ in nŏt	ŭ in cŭt

Ophthalmology and Otolaryngology

The medical specialty of **ophthalmology** is associated with the eyes, the organs of sight. The medical specialty of **otolaryngology** is associated with the ears, the organs of hearing.

Ophthalmology

Ophthalmology is the branch of medicine concerned with diagnosis and treatment of eye disorders. The medical specialist in ophthalmology is called an *ophthalmologist.* Although ophthalmologists specialize in treatment of the eyes only, it is important for them to be aware of other abnormalities that an eye examination may reveal. For example, the examination may reveal the first signs of a systemic illness, such as diabetes, even though it is taking place in another part of the body.

The ophthalmologist also prescribes corrective lenses and performs corrective eye surgeries. These include, but are not limited to **cornea transplantation,** cataract removal, repair of **ocular** muscle dysfunction, **glaucoma,** treatment, lens removal, and **radial keratotomy.**

Two other health care practitioners, the **optometrist** and **optician,** specialize in providing corrective lenses for the eyes. They are not medical doctors, but are licensed to examine and test the eyes and treat visual defects by prescribing corrective lenses. The optician also specializes in filling prescriptions for corrective lenses.

Otolaryngology

Otolaryngology is the oldest medical specialty in the United States. Fifty years ago, otolaryngology was practiced along with ophthalmology. During that time, the medical practice consisted mainly of removing tonsils and adenoids and irrigating (cleansing a canal by flushing it with water or other fluids) the sinuses and ear canals.

Today, otolaryngology is greatly expanded to include medical and surgical management of patients with disorders of the ear, nose, and throat (ENT) and related structures of the head and neck. Thus, specialists in this practice are commonly called *ENT physicians,* or *otolaryngologists.* ENT physicians commonly treat disorders related to the sinuses, including allergies and disorders of the sense of smell. Their diagnostic techniques are used to detect the causes of such symptoms as hoarseness, hearing and breathing difficulty, and swelling around the head or neck. ENT physicians also treat sleep disorders, most commonly **sleep apnea.** Various types of procedures, including but not limited to surgery, may be performed to treat sleep apnea or snoring disorders.

Eyes and Ears Quick Study

The major senses of the body are sight, hearing, smell, taste, and touch. These sensations are identified by specific body organs. Senses of smell and taste have been discussed in previous chapters. This chapter focuses on the eyes and ears, which include the senses of sight and hearing.

Eyes

The eyes and their accessory structures are receptor organs that provide vision. It is one of the most important sense organs of the body. As such, the eyes provide most of the information about what we see, but also what we learn from printed material. Similar to other sensory organs, the eyes are constructed to detect stimuli in the environment and to transmit those observations to the brain for visual interpretation. (See *Eye Structures,* page 314.)

Ears

The ears and their accessory structures are receptor organs that enable us to hear and maintain balance. Each ear consists of three divisions: the external, middle, and inner ear. The external and middle ears conduct sound waves through the ear. The inner ear contains auditory structures that receive sound waves and transmit them to the brain for interpretation. The inner ear also contains specialized receptors that maintain balance and equilibrium in response to fluctuations in body position and motion. (See *Ear Structures,* page 315.)

 An extensive anatomy and physiology review is included in *TermPlus,* the powerful, interactive CD-ROM program.

Medical Word Building

Building medical words using word elements related to the special senses of sight and hearing will enhance your understanding of those terms and reinforce your ability to use terms correctly.

Combining forms

Begin your study of terminology related to the special senses by reviewing the organs of the eyes and ears and their associated combining forms (CFs), which are illustrated in the figures *Eye Structures* below and *Ear Structures* on the next page.

Eye Structures

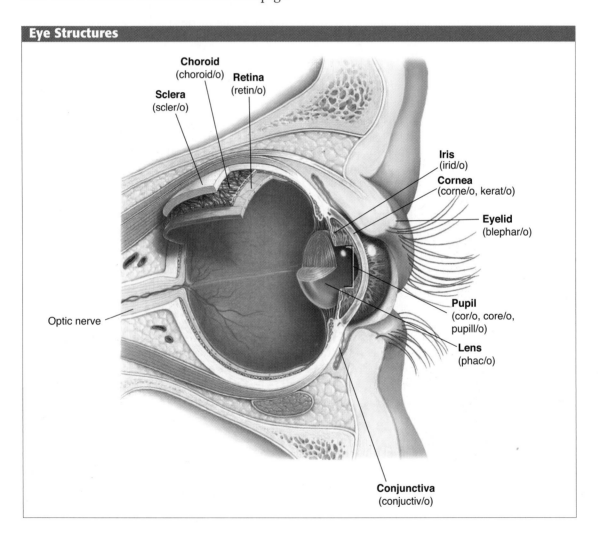

Choroid
(choroid/o)

Sclera
(scler/o)

Retina
(retin/o)

Iris
(irid/o)

Cornea
(corne/o, kerat/o)

Eyelid
(blephar/o)

Optic nerve

Pupil
(cor/o, core/o, pupill/o)

Lens
(phac/o)

Conjunctiva
(conjuctiv/o)

Ear Structures

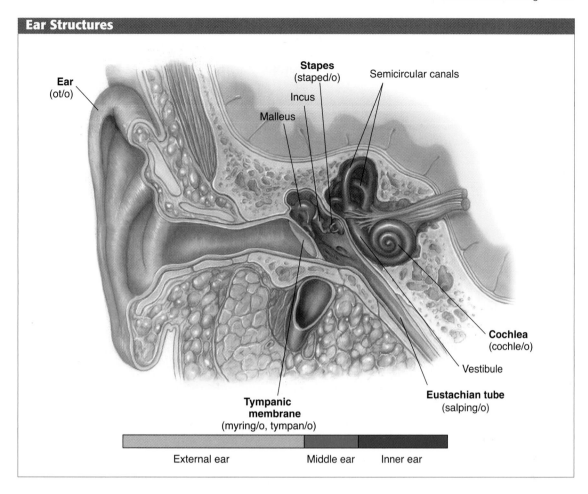

Ear
(ot/o)

Stapes
(staped/o)

Incus

Malleus

Semicircular canals

Cochlea
(cochle/o)

Vestibule

Eustachian tube
(salping/o)

Tympanic membrane
(myring/o, tympan/o)

External ear   Middle ear   Inner ear

In the table below, CFs are listed alphabetically and other word parts are defined as needed. Review the medical word and study the elements that make up the term. Then complete the meaning of the medical words in the right-hand column. The first one is completed for you. You may also refer to *Appendix A: Glossary of Medical Word Elements* to complete this exercise.

Combining Form	Meaning	Medical Word	Meaning
Eye			
blephar/o	eyelid	**blephar/o**/spasm (BLĔF-ă-rō-spăzm) *-spasm:* involuntary contraction, twitching	*Involuntary contraction of the eyelid*

(Continued)

Combining Form	Meaning	Medical Word	Meaning
Eye			
choroid/o	choroid	**choroid/o**/pathy (kō-roy-DŎP-ă-thē) -*pathy:* disease	
conjunctiv/o	conjuctiva	**conjunctiv**/itis (kŏn-jŭnk-tĭ-VĪ-tĭs) -*itis:* inflammation	
corne/o	cornea	**corne**/itis (kor-nē-Ī-tĭs) -*itis:* inflammation	
cor/o	pupil	aniso/**cor**/ia (ăn-ī-sō-KŌ-rē-ă) *aniso:* unequal, dissimilar -*ia:* condition	
core/o		**core/o**/meter (kō-rē-ŎM-ĕ-tĕr) -*meter:* instrument for measuring	
pupill/o		**pupill**/ary (PŪ-pĭ-lĕr-ē) -*ary:* pertaining to	
dacry/o	tear; lacrimal apparatus (duct, sac, or gland)	**dacry/o**/rrhea (dăk-rē-ō-RĒ-ă) -*rrhea:* discharge, flow	
lacrim/o		**lacrim**/ation (lăk-rĭ-MĀ-shŭn) -*ation:* process (of)	
dipl/o	double	**dipl**/opia (dĭp-LŌ-pē-ă) -*opia:* vision	
irid/o	iris	**irid/o**/plegia (ĭr-ĭd-ō-PLĒ-jē-ă) -*plegia:* paralysis	
kerat/o	horny tissue; hard; cornea	**kerat/o**/plasty (KĔR-ă-tō-plăs-tē) -*plasty:* surgical repair	

Combining Form	Meaning	Medical Word	Meaning
Eye			
ocul/o	eye	intra/**ocul**/ar (ĭn-tră-ŎK-ū-lăr) *intra-:* in, within *-ar:* pertaining to	
ophthalm/o		**ophthalm/o**/scope (ŏf-THĂL-mō-skōp) *-scope:* instrument for examining	
opt/o	eye, vision	**opt**/ic (ŎP-tĭk) *-ic:* pertaining to	
retin/o	retina	**retin/o**/pathy (rĕt-ĭn-ŎP-ă-thē) *-pathy:* disease	
Ear			
acous/o	hearing	**acous**/tic (ă-KOOS-tik) *-tic:* pertaining to	
audi/o		**audi/o**/meter (aw-dē-ŎM-ĕ-tĕr) *-meter:* instrument for measuring	
audit/o		**audit**/ory (AW-dĭ-tō-rē) *-ory:* pertaining to	
myring/o	tympanic membrane (eardrum)	**myring/o**/tomy (mĭr-ĭn-GŎT-ō-mē) *-tomy:* incision	
tympan/o		**tympan/o**/plasty (tĭm-păn-ō-PLĂS-tē) *-plasty:* surgical repair	
ot/o	ear	**ot/o**/rrhea (ō-tō-RĒ-ă) *-rrhea:* discharge, flow	
salping/o	tube (usually fallopian or eustachian [auditory] tubes)	**salping/o**/pharyng/eal (săl-pĭng-gō-fă-RĬN-jē-ăl) *pharyng:* pharynx (throat) *-eal:* pertaining to	

Suffixes and prefixes

In the table below, suffixes and prefixes are listed alphabetically and other word parts are defined as needed. Review the medical word and study the elements that make up the term. Then complete the meaning of the medical words in the right-hand column. You may also refer to *Appendix A: Glossary of Medical Word Elements* to complete this exercise.

Word Element	Meaning	Medical Words	Meaning
Suffixes			
-acusis	hearing	an/**acusis** (ăn-ă-KŪ-sĭs) *an-:* without, not	
-cusis		presby/**cusis** (prĕz-bĭ-KŪ-sĭs) *presby:* old age	
-opia	vision	ambly/**opia** (ăm-blē-Ō-pē-ă) *ambly:* dull, dim	
-opsia		heter/**opsia** (hĕt-ĕr-ŎP-sē-ă) *heter-:* different	
-ptosis	prolapse, downward displacement	blephar/o/**ptosis** (blĕf-ă-rō-TŌ-sĭs) *blephar/o:* eyelid	
Prefixes			
exo-	outside, outward	**exo**/tropia (ĕks-ō-TRŌ-pē-ă) *-tropia:* turning	
hyper-	excessive, above normal	**hyper**/opia (hī-pĕr-Ō-pē-ă) *-opia:* vision	

 Competency Verification: Check your answers in Appendix B, Answer Key, page 380. If you are not satisfied with your level of comprehension, review the terms in the table and retake the review.

 Listen and Learn, the audio CD-ROM included in this book, will help you master pronunciation of selected medical words. Use it·to practice pronunciations of the medical terms in the above "Word Building" tables and for instructions to complete the *Listen and Learn* exercise.

 Flash-Card Activity. Enhance your study and reinforcement of this chapter's word elements with the power of the DavisPlus flash-card activity. Do so by visiting *http://davisplus.fadavis.com/gylys-express.* We recommend you complete the flash-card activity before continuing with the next section.

Medical Terminology Word Building

In this section, combine the word parts you have learned to construct medical terms related to the eyes and the ears.

Use *ophthalm/o* (eye) to build words that mean:

1. paralysis of the eye _____

2. study of the eye _____

Use *pupill/o* (pupil) to build a word that means:

3. examination of the pupil _____

Use *kerat/o* (cornea) to build words that mean:

4. softening of the cornea _____

5. instrument for measuring the cornea _____

Use *scler/o* (sclera) to build words that mean:

6. inflammation of the sclera _____

7. softening of the sclera _____

Use *irid/o* (iris) to build words that mean:

8. paralysis of the iris _____

9. herniation of the iris _____

Use *retin/o* (retina) to build words that mean:

10. disease of the retina _____

11. inflammation of the retina _____

Use *blephar/o* (eyelid) to build words that mean:

12. paralysis of the eyelid _____

13. prolapse of the eyelid _____

14. surgical repair of the eyelid _____

Use *ot/o* (ear) to build a word that means:

15. flow of pus from the ear _____

Use *audi/o* (hearing) to build a word that means:

16. instrument for measuring hearing _____

Use *myring/o* (tympanic membrane [eardrum]) to build words that mean:

17. instrument for cutting the eardrum _____

18. surgical repair of the tympanic membrane _____

Use *salping/o* (tube, usually fallopian or eustachian [auditory] tubes) to build words that means:

19. inflammation of the eustachian tube _____

20. pertaining to the eustachian tube and throat _____

 Competency Verification: Check your answers in Appendix B, Answer Key, page 382. Review material that you did not answer correctly.

Correct Answers: _____ × 5 = _____ %

Additional Medical Vocabulary

The following tables list additional terms related to the eyes and ears. Recognizing and learning these terms will help you understand the connection between common signs, symptoms, and diseases and their diagnoses. Included are medical and surgical procedures as well as pharmacological agents used to treat diseases.

Signs, Symptoms, and Diseases

Eye

achromatopsia ă-krō-mă-TŎP-sē-ă 　　*a-:* without, not 　*chromat:* color 　　*-opsia:* vision	Congenital deficiency in color perception that is more common in men; also called *color blindness*
astigmatism ă-STĬG-mă-tĭzm 　　*a-:* without, not 　*stigmat:* point, mark 　　*-ism:* condition	Refractive disorder in which excessive curvature of the cornea or lens causes light to be scattered over the retina, rather than focused on a single point, resulting in a distorted image (See Figure 13-1.)
cataract KĂT-ă-răkt	Degenerative disease due mainly to the aging process in which the lens of the eye becomes progressively cloudy, causing decreased vision (See Figure 13-2.)

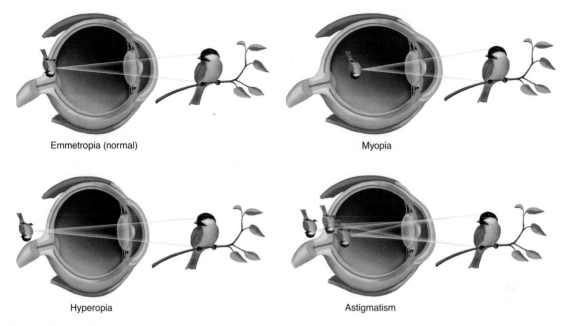

Emmetropia (normal)

Myopia

Hyperopia

Astigmatism

Figure 13–1. Refraction of the eye.

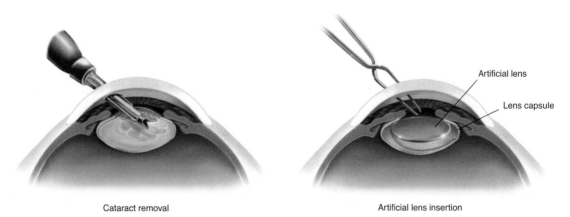

Cataract removal

Artificial lens insertion

Artificial lens

Lens capsule

Figure 13–2. Phacoemulsification.

conjunctivitis kŏn-jŭnk-tĭ-VĪ-tĭs *conjunctiv:* conjunctiva *-itis:* inflammation	Inflammation of the conjunctiva that can be caused by bacteria, allergy, irritation, or a foreign body; also called *pinkeye*
diabetic retinopathy dī-ă-BĔT-ĭk rĕt-ĭn-ŎP-ă-thē *retin/o:* retina *-pathy:* disease	Retinal damage marked by aneurysmal dilation and bleeding of blood vessels or the formation of new blood vessels causing visual changes in diabetic patients
hordeolum hor-DĒ-ō-lŭm	Small, purulent, inflammatory infection of a sebaceous gland of the eyelid; also called *sty* (See Figure 13-3.)
macular degeneration MĂK-ū-lăr	Breakdown of the tissues in the macula, resulting in loss of central vision (See Figure 13-4.)
photophobia fō-tō-FŌ-bē-ă *phot/o:* light *-phobia:* fear	Unusual intolerance and sensitivity to light that occurs in such disorders as meningitis, eye inflammation, measles, and rubella
retinal detachment RĔT-ĭ-năl *retin:* retina *-al:* pertaining to	Separation of the retina from the choroid, which disrupts vision and results in blindness if not repaired

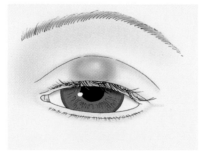

Figure 13–3. Hordeolum (sty).

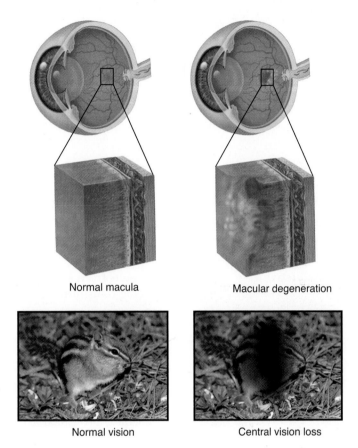

Normal macula

Macular degeneration

Normal vision

Central vision loss

Figure 13–4. Macular degeneration.

strabismus stră-BĬZ-mŭs	Muscular eye disorder in which the eyes turn from the normal position so that they deviate in different directions (See Figure 13-5.).
esotropia ĕs-ō-TRŌ-pē-ă *eso-:* inward *-tropia:* turning	Strabismus in which there is deviation of the visual axis of one eye toward that of the other eye, resulting in diplopia; also called *cross-eye* or *convergent strabismus* (See Figure 13-5A.)
exotropia ĕks-ō-TRŌ-pē-ă *exo-:* outside, outward *-tropia:* turning	Strabismus in which there is deviation of the visual axis of one eye away from that of the other, resulting in diplopia; also called *wall-eye* or *divergent strabismus* (See Figure 13-5B.)

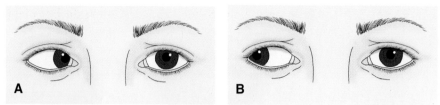

Figure 13–5. Types of strabismus. (A) Esotropia (affected eye turns inward). (B) Exotropia (affected eye turns outward).

Ear

hearing loss	Loss of the sense or perception of sound
anacusis ăn-ă-KŪ-sĭs *an-:* without, not *-acusis:* hearing	Total deafness (complete hearing loss)
conductive	Results from any condition that prevents sound waves from being transmitted to the auditory receptors
presbycusis prĕz-bĭ-KŪ-sĭs *presby:* old age *-cusis:* hearing	Impairment of hearing that results from the aging process
sensorineural sĕn-sō-rē-NŪ-răl	Inability of nerve stimuli to be delivered to the brain from the inner ear due to damage to the auditory (acoustic) nerve or cochlea; also called *nerve deafness*
Ménière disease mĕn-ē-ĀR	Rare disorder characterized by progressive deafness, vertigo, and tinnitus, possibly due to swelling of membranous structures within the labyrinth
otitis media (OM) ō-TĪ-tĭs MĒ-dē-ă *ot:* ear *-itis:* inflammation *med:* middle *-ia:* condition	Inflammation of the middle ear, which is commonly the result of an upper respiratory infection (URI) and may be treated with tympanostomy tube insertion Get a closer look at tympanostomy tube insertion on page 330.

otosclerosis
ō-tō-sklĕ-RŌ-sĭs
 	
  ot/o: ear
  scler: hardening; sclera
    (white of eye)
  -osis: abnormal condition; increase
    (used primarily
    with blood cells)
	Progressive deafness due to ossification in the bony labyrinth of the inner ear

tinnitus tĭn-Ī-tĭs	Ringing or tinkling noise heard constantly or intermittently in one or both ears, even in a quiet environment, that usually results from damage to inner ear structures associated with hearing
vertigo VĔR-tĭ-gō	Sensation of moving around in space or a feeling of spinning or dizziness that usually results from inner ear structure damage associated with balance and equilibrium

Diagnostic Procedures

Eye

tonometry
tōn-ŎM-ĕ-trē
 	
  ton/o: tension
  -metry: act of measuring
	Screening test to detect glaucoma that measures intraocular pressure and to determine if its elevated (See Figure 13-6.)

visual acuity test ă-KŪ-ĭ-tē	Standard eye examination to determine the smallest letters a person can read on a Snellen chart, or E chart, at a distance of 20 feet

Ear

audiometry
ăw-dē- ŎM-ĕ-trē
 	
  audi/o: hearing
  -metry: act of measuring
	Test that measures hearing acuity at various sound frequencies

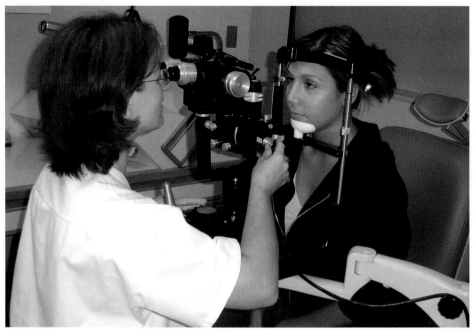

Figure 13–6. Tonometry.

otoscopy
ō-TŎS-kŏ-pē
   ot/o: ear
   -scopy: visual
       examination
	Visual examination of the external auditory canal and the tympanic membrane using an otoscope

tuning fork test
 	
  Rinne
  RĬN-nē,
  Weber
  WĔB-ĕr
	Hearing tests that use a tuning fork (instrument that produces a constant pitch when struck) that is struck and then placed against or near the bones on the side of the head to assess nerve and bone conduction of sound
	     Evaluates bone conduction of sound in one ear at a time
	
	     Evaluates bone conduction of sound in both ears at the same time

Medical and Surgical Procedures

Eye

cataract surgery KĂT-ă-răkt	Excision of a lens affected by a cataract

phacoemulsification
  FĂK-ō-ē-mŭl-sĭ-fĭ-
  kā-shŭn
	Excision of the lens by ultrasonic vibrations that break the lens into tiny particles, which are suctioned out of the eye; also called *small incision cataract surgery* (SICS) (See Figure 13-2.)

iridectomy
ĭr-ĭ-DĔK-tŏ-mē
  irid: iris
  -ectomy: excision,
      removal
	Excision of a portion of the iris used to relieve intraocular pressure in patients with glaucoma

laser iridotomy
ĭr-ĭ-DŎT-ō-mē
  irid/o: iris
  -tomy: incision
	Laser surgery that creates an opening on the rim of the iris to allow aqueous humor to flow between the anterior and posterior chambers to relieve IOP that occurs as a result of glaucoma and is replacing iridectomy because it is a safer procedure

laser photocoagulation fō-tō-kō-ăg-ū-LĀ-shŭn	Use of a laser beam to seal leaking or hemorrhaging retinal blood vessels used in treatment of diabetic retinopathy.

Ear

cochlear implant
KŎK-lē-ăr
  cochle: cochlea
  -ar: pertaining to
	Electronic transmitter surgically implanted into the cochlea of a deaf person to restore hearing

myringoplasty
mĭr-ĬN-gō-plăst-ē
  myring/o: tympanic
      membrane
      (eardrum)
  -plasty: surgical repair
	Surgical repair of a perforated eardrum with a tissue graft to correct hearing loss; also called *tympanoplasty*

myringotomy mĭr-ĭn-GŎT-ō-mē *myring/o:* tympanic membrane (eardrum) *-tomy:* incision	Incision of the tympanic membrane (eardrum) to relieve pressure and drain fluid from the middle ear or to insert tympanostomy tubes in the eardrum via surgery Get a closer look at tympanostomy tube insertion on page 330.

Pharmacology

antiglaucoma drugs ăn-tĭ-glaw-KŌ-mă	Reduce intraocular pressure by lowering the amount of aqueous humor in the eyeball, reducing its production, or increasing its outflow
miotics mī-ŎT-ĭks	Cause the pupil to constrict
mydriatics mĭd-rē-ĂT-ĭks	Cause the pupil to dilate and prepare the eye for an internal examination
vertigo and motion sickness drugs VĔR-tĭ-gō	Decrease sensitivity of the inner ear to motion and prevent nerve impulses from the inner ear from reaching the vomiting center of the brain
wax emulsifiers ē-MŬL-sĭ-fĭ-ĕrs	Loosen and help remove impacted cerumen (ear wax)

Pronunciation Help	Long Sound	ā in rāte	ē in rēbirth	ī in īsle	ō in ōver	ū in ūnite
	Short Sound	ă in ălone	ĕ in ĕver	ĭ in ĭt	ŏ in nŏt	ŭ in cŭt

 Closer Look

Take a closer look at these eye and ear procedures to enhance your understanding of the medical terminology associated with them.

Glaucoma

Glaucoma is a condition in which the aqueous humor fails to drain properly and accumulates in the anterior chamber of the eye, causing elevated **intraocular pressure (IOP)**. The IOP leads to degeneration and atrophy of the retina and optic nerve. There are two forms of glaucoma: open-angle and

Closer Look—cont'd

closed-angle. **Open-angle glaucoma** is the most common form. It results from degenerative changes that cause congestion and reduce flow of aqueous humor through the canal of Schlemm. This type of glaucoma is painless but destroys peripheral vision, causing tunnel vision. Closed-angle glaucoma is a medical emergency. This type of glaucoma is caused by an anatomically narrow angle between the iris and the cornea, which prevents outflow of aqueous humor from the eye into the lymphatic system, causing a sudden increase in IOP. Symptoms include severe pain, blurred vision, and photophobia. Glaucoma eventually leads to vision loss and, commonly, blindness. Treatment for glaucoma includes eyedrops **(miotics)** that cause the pupils to constrict, permitting aqueous humor to escape from the eye, thereby relieving pressure. If miotics are ineffective, surgery may be necessary. The illustration below shows the normal flow of aqueous humor (yellow arrows) and an abnormal flow of aqueous humor (red arrow), causing destruction of the optic nerve.

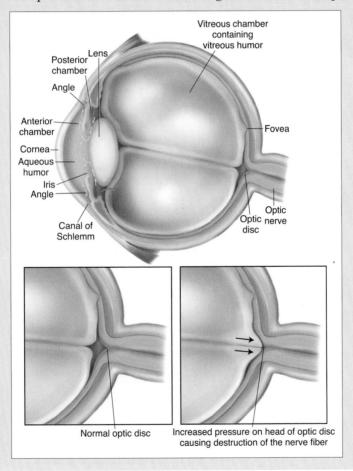

Tympanostomy Tube Insertion

Tympanostomy tubes, also known as *ear tubes* or *pressure-equalizing (PE) tubes*, are plastic cylinders surgically inserted into the eardrum to drain fluid and equalize pressure between the middle and outer ear. PE tubes are most commonly used in children who have recurrent ear infections that do not respond to antibiotics, or when fluid remains behind the eardrum. Tympanostomy tube insertion is an outpatient surgery performed by an otolaryngologist while the child is under general anesthesia. As seen in the illustration below, a small opening is made in the eardrum (tympanostomy, or **myringotomy**) followed by tube insertion. The tube decreases the feeling of pressure in the ears, reduces pain, and allows air to enter the middle ear and fluid to flow out of the middle ear and into the ear canal. Postsurgical recovery is usually rapid with little pain or other symptoms. Tubes normally remain in the ears for 6 to 12 months. They commonly fall out on their own or they may require surgical removal.

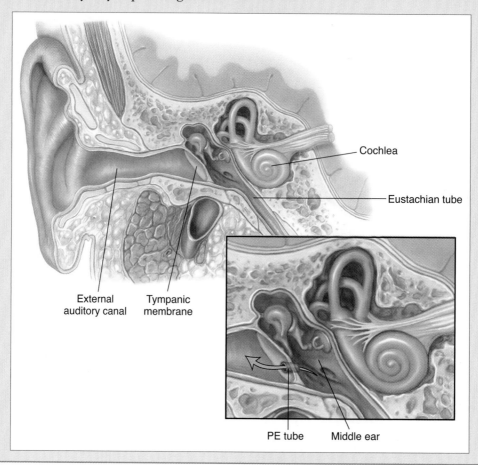

Additional Medical Vocabulary Recall

Match the medical term(s) below with the definitions in the numbered list.

achromatopsia	glaucoma	otitis media	Rinne
anacusis	hordeolum	otosclerosis	strabismus
astigmatism	iridectomy	photophobia	tinnitus
cataract	Ménière disease	presbycusis	tonometry
conjunctivitis	myringoplasty	retinal detachment	vertigo

1. _____ means ringing in the ears.

2. _____ is progressive deafness due to ossification in the bony labyrinth of the inner ear.

3. _____ means color blindness.

4. _____ is a rare disorder characterized by progressive deafness, vertigo, and tinnitus.

5. _____ is a muscular eye disorder in which the eyes deviate in different directions.

6. _____ means total deafness.

7. _____ refers to middle ear infection that is most commonly seen in young children.

8. _____ refers to pinkeye.

9. _____ means intolerance or unusual sensitivity to light.

10. _____ is hearing loss due to old age.

11. _____ refers to increased intraocular pressure caused by failure of the aqueous humor to drain.

12. _____ refers to a feeling of spinning or dizziness.

13. _____ refers to separation of the retina from the choroid.

14. _____ is another term for sty.

15. _____ is a refractive disorder in which light scatters over the retina rather than focuses on a single point, resulting in a distorted image.

16. _____ is a surgical repair of the eardrum.

17. _____ measures intraocular pressure and is used to diagnose glaucoma.

18. _____ refers to excision of a portion of the iris.

19. _____ is a hearing test performed with a vibrating tuning fork.

20. _____ refers to opacity (cloudiness) of the lens due to protein deposits.

Competency Verification: Check your answers in Appendix B, Answer Key, on page 382. Review material that you did not answer correctly.

Correct Answers: _____ × **5** = _____ **%**

Pronunciation and Spelling

Use the following list to practice correct pronunciation and spelling of medical terms. Practice the pronunciation aloud and then write the correct spelling of the term. The first word is completed for you.

Pronunciation	Spelling
1. a-KOOS-tĭk nū-RŌ-mă	*acoustic neuroma*
2. ă-krō-mă-TŎP-sē-ă	
3. ă-STĬG-mă-tĭzm	
4. AW-dĭ-tō-rē	
5. blĕf-ă-rō-TŌ-sĭs	
6. dăk-rē-ō-RĒ-ă	
7. ĕks-ō-TRŌ-pē-ă	
8. FĂK-ō-ē-mŭl-sĭ-fĭ-kā-shŭn	
9. glaw-KŌ-mă	
10. hor-DĒ-ō-lŭm	
11. ĭr-ĭd-ō-PLĒ-jē-ă	
12. kŏn-jŭnk-tĭ-VĪ-tĭs	
13. mĕn-ē-ĀR	
14. ŏf-THĂL-mō-skōp	
15. prĕz-bĭ-KŪ-sĭs	
16. săl-pĭng-gō-fă-RĬN-jē-ăl	
17. stră-BĬZ-mŭs	
18. tĭm-păn-ō-PLĂS-tē	
19. tĭn-Ī-tĭs	
20. VĔR-tĭ-gō	

Competency Verification: Check your answers in Appendix B, Answer Key, on page 382. Review material that you did not answer correctly.

Correct Answers: _____ × 5 = _____ %

Abbreviations

The table below introduces abbreviations associated with the eyes and the ears.

Abbreviation	Meaning	Abbreviation	Meaning
ARMD	age-related macular degeneration	O.D.	Doctor of Optometry
Ast	astigmatism	OD	right eye
ENT	ear, nose, and throat	OM	otitis media
EOM	extraocular movement	OS	left eye
IOP	intraocular pressure	OU	both eyes
Myop	myopia	ST	esotropia

Chart Notes

Chart notes make up part of the medical record and are used in various types of health care facilities. The chart notes that follow were dictated by the patient's physician and reflect common clinical events using medical terminology to document the patient's care. By studying and completing the terminology and chart notes sections below, you will learn and understand terms associated with the medical specialty of otolaryngology.

Terminology

The following terms are linked to chart notes in the specialty of otolaryngology. First, practice pronouncing each term aloud. Then use a medical dictionary such as *Taber's Cyclopedic Medical Dictionary, Appendix A: Glossary of Medical Word Elements* on page 337, or other resources to define each term.

Term	Meaning
cholesteatoma kō-lē-stē-ă-TŌ-mă	
ENT	

(Continued)

Term	Meaning
general anesthesia ăn-ĕs-THĒ-zē-ă	
mucoserous mū-kō-SĒR-ŭs	
otitis media ō-TĪ-tĭs MĒ-dē-ă	
postoperatively pōst-ŎP-ĕr-ă-tĭv-lē	
tympanoplasty tĭm-păn-ō-PLĂS-tē	

 Visit *http://davisplus.fadavis.com/gylys-express* for the terminology pronunciation exercise associated with this chart note.

Cholesteatoma

Read the chart note below aloud. Underline any term you have trouble pronouncing and any terms that you cannot define. If needed, refer to the Terminology section above for correct pronunciations and meanings of terms.

> This 30-year-old white female was seen by the ENT specialist for a diagnosis of mucoserous otitis media on the right. Patient was admitted to City Hospital and developed cholesteatoma. A tube was inserted for the chronic adhesive otitis media with secondary cholesteatoma. Patient progressed favorably postoperatively, but the cholesteatoma continues to enlarge in size. Presently she is in the hospital for a right tympanoplasty under general anesthetic.

Chart Note Analysis

From the chart note above, select the medical word that means:

1. of long duration _____

2. composed of mucus and serum _____

3. surgical repair of the eardrum _____

4. inflammation of the inner ear _____

5. abbreviation that refers to *ear, nose, and throat* _____

6. cystlike sac filled with cholesterol and epithelial cells _____

7. agent that causes loss of sensation to the entire body and results in a loss of consciousness

_____

8. term denoting the name of a disease a person has or is believed to have _____

9. causing two surfaces to unite _____

10. following a surgical procedure _____

Competency Verification: Check your answers in Appendix B, Answer Key, on page 382. Review material that you did not answer correctly.

Correct Answers _____ × **10 =** _____ %

Demonstrate What You Know!

To evaluate your understanding of how medical terms you have studied in this and previous chapters are used in a clinical environment, complete the numbered sentences by selecting an appropriate term from the list below.

blepharoplasty	diagnosis	heteropsia
blepharoptosis	esotropia	mydriatics
cholesteatoma	exotropia	ophthalmoplegia
		tympanitis

1. When a person suffers a stroke and is unable to move his eyes, the condition is called _____.

2. A deviation of one eye toward the other eye is a type of strabismus called _____.

3. An eyetuck, also called a(n) _____, is a cosmetic procedure to remove wrinkles from the eyelid.

4. Agents that dilate the pupil to prepare the eye for an internal examination are called _____.

5. A patient is diagnosed with an inequality of vision. The diagnosis was charted as _____.

6. A deviation of one eye away from the other eye is a type of strabismus called _____; also known as *wall-eye*.

7. If a stroke results in facial paralysis, the patient may experience drooping eyelids. This condition would be charted as _____.

8. _____ is a term denoting the disease a person has or is believed to have.

9. The medical term for a cystlike sac filled with cholesterol is _____.

10. The diagnosis for a patient with inflammation of an eardrum is _____.

Competency Verification: Check your answers in Appendix B, Answer Key, on page 382. Review material that you did not answer correctly.

Correct Answers: _____ × 10 = _____ %

Multimedia Review: If you are not satisfied with your retention level of the special senses chapter, visit *http://davisplusfadavis.com/gylys-express* and complete the website activities linked to this chapter. It is your choice whether or not you want to take advantage of these reinforcement exercises.

Glossary of Medical Word Elements

Medical Word Element	Meaning	Medical Word Element	Meaning
A		alveol/o	alveolus; air sac
a-	without, not	ambly/o	dull, dim
ab-	from, away from	amni/o	amnion (amniotic sac)
abdomin/o	abdomen	an-	without, not
abort/o	to miscarry	an/o	anus
-ac	pertaining to	ana-	against; up; back
acid/o	acid	andr/o	male
acous/o	hearing	aneurysm/o	widened blood vessel
acr/o	extremity	angi/o	vessel (usually blood or
acromi/o	acromion		lymph)
	(projection of	aniso-	unequal, dissimilar
	scapula)	ankyl/o	stiffness; bent, crooked
-acusis	hearing	ante-	before, in front of
-ad	toward	anter/o	anterior, front
ad-	toward	anthrac/o	coal, coal dust
aden/o	gland	anti-	against
adenoid/o	adenoids	aort/o	aorta
adip/o	fat	append/o	appendix
adren/o	adrenal glands	appendic/o	appendix
adrenal/o	adrenal glands	aque/o	water
aer/o	air	-ar	pertaining to
af-	toward	-arche	beginning
agglutin/o	clumping, gluing	arteri/o	artery
-al	pertaining to	arteriol/o	arteriole (small artery)
albin/o	white	arthr/o	joint
albumin/o	albumin (protein)	-ary	pertaining to
-algesia	pain	-asthenia	weakness, debility
-algia	pain	astr/o	star
allo-	other		

(Continued)

Medical Word Element	Meaning	Medical Word Element	Meaning
-ate	having the form of, possessing	carcin/o	cancer
atel/o	incomplete; imperfect	cardi/o	heart
		-cardia	heart condition
		carp/o	carpus (wrist bones)
ather/o	fatty plaque	caud/o	tail
-ation	process (of)	cauter/o	heat, burn
atri/o	atrium	cec/o	cecum
audi/o	hearing	-cele	hernia, swelling
audit/o	hearing	-centesis	surgical puncture
aur/o	ear	cephal/o	head
auricul/o	ear	-ceps	head
auto-	self, own	-ception	conceiving
azot/o	nitrogenous compounds	cerebell/o	cerebellum
		cerebr/o	cerebrum
		cervic/o	neck; cervix uteri (neck of uterus)
B			
bacteri/o	bacteria (singular, *bacterium*)	chalic/o	limestone
		cheil/o	lip
balan/o	glans penis	chem/o	chemical; drug
bas/o	base (alkaline, opposite of acid)	chlor/o	green
		chol/e	bile, gall
bi-	two	cholangi/o	bile vessel
bi/o	life	cholecyst/o	gallbladder
bil/i	bile, gall	choledoch/o	bile duct
-blast	embryonic cell	chondr/o	cartilage
blast/o	embryonic cell	chori/o	chorion
blephar/o	eyelid	choroid/o	choroid
brachi/o	arm	chrom/o	color
brachy-	short	chromat/o	color
brady-	slow	-cide	killing
bronch/o	bronchus (plural, *bronchi*)	cine-	movement
		circum-	around
bronchi/o	bronchus (plural, *bronchi*)	cirrh/o	yellow
		-cision	a cutting
bronchiol/o	bronchiole	-clasia	to break; surgical fracture
bucc/o	cheek	-clasis	to break; surgical fracture
		-clast	to break
C		clavicul/o	clavicle (collar bone)
calc/o	calcium	-cleisis	closure
calcane/o	calcaneum (heel bone)	-clysis	irrigation, washing
		coccyg/o	coccyx (tail bone)
-capnia	carbon dioxide (CO_2)		

Medical Word Element	Meaning	Medical Word Element	Meaning
cochle/o	cochlea	-derma	skin
col/o	colon	dermat/o	skin
colon/o	colon	-desis	binding, fixation (of a bone or joint)
colp/o	vagina		
condyl/o	condyle	di-	double
coni/o	dust	dia-	through, across
conjunctiv/o	conjunctiva	dipl-	double
-continence	to hold back	dipl/o	double
contra-	against, opposite	diplo-	double
cor/o	pupil	dips/o	thirst
core/o	pupil	-dipsia	thirst
corne/o	cornea	dist/o	far, farthest
coron/o	heart	dors/o	back (of body)
corp/o	body	duct/o	to lead; carry
corpor/o	body	-duction	act of leading, bringing, conducting
cortic/o	cortex		
cost/o	ribs	duoden/o	duodenum (first part of small intestine)
crani/o	cranium (skull)		
crin/o	secrete	dur/o	dura mater; hard
-crine	secrete	-dynia	pain
cruci/o	cross	dys-	bad; painful; difficult
cry/o	cold		
crypt/o	hidden	**E**	
-cusia	hearing	-eal	pertaining to
-cusis	hearing	ec-	out, out from
cutane/o	skin	echo-	a repeated sound
cyan/o	blue	-ectasis	dilation, expansion
cycl/o	ciliary body of eye; circular; cycle	ecto-	outside, outward
		-ectomy	excision, removal
-cyesis	pregnancy	-edema	swelling
cyst/o	bladder	ef-	away from
cyt/o	cell	electr/o	electricity
-cyte	cell	-ema	state of; condition
		embol/o	embolus (plug)
D		-emesis	vomiting
dacry/o	tear; lacrimal apparatus (duct, sac, or gland)	-emia	blood condition
		emphys/o	to inflate
		en-	in, within
dacryocyst/o	lacrimal sac	encephal/o	brain
dactyl/o	fingers; toes	end-	in, within
de-	cessation	endo-	in, within
dent/o	teeth	enter/o	intestine (usually small intestine)
derm/o	skin		

(Continued)

Medical Word Element	Meaning	Medical Word Element	Meaning
epi-	above, upon	-genesis	forming, producing, origin
epididym/o	epididymis		
epiglott/o	epiglottis	genit/o	genitalia
episi/o	vulva	gest/o	pregnancy
erot/o	sexual desire	gingiv/o	gum(s)
erythem/o	red	glauc/o	gray
erythemat/o	red	gli/o	glue; neuroglial tissue
erythr/o	red	-glia	glue; neuroglial tissue
eschar/o	scab	-globin	protein
-esis	condition	glomerul/o	glomerulus
eso-	inward	gloss/o	tongue
esophag/o	esophagus	glott/o	glottis
esthes/o	feeling	gluc/o	sugar, sweetness
-esthesia	feeling	glucos/o	sugar, sweetness
eti/o	cause	glyc/o	sugar, sweetness
eu-	good, normal	glycos/o	sugar, sweetness
ex-	out, out from	gnos/o	knowing
exo-	outside, outward	-gnosis	knowing
extra-	outside	gon/o	seed (ovum or spermatozoon)
F		gonad/o	gonads, sex glands
faci/o	face	-grade	to go
fasci/o	band, fascia (fibrous membrane supporting and separating muscles)	-graft	transplantation
		-gram	record, writing
		granul/o	granule
		-graph	instrument for recording
		-graphy	process of recording
femor/o	femur (thigh bone)	-gravida	pregnant woman
-ferent	to carry	gyn/o	woman, female
fibr/o	fiber, fibrous tissue	gynec/o	woman, female
fibul/o	fibula (smaller bone of lower leg)	**H**	
fluor/o	luminous, fluorescence	hem/o	blood
		hemangi/o	blood vessel
G		hemat/o	blood
galact/o	milk	hemi-	one half
gangli/o	ganglion (knot or knotlike mass)	hepat/o	liver
		hetero-	different
gastr/o	stomach	hidr/o	sweat
-gen	forming, producing, origin	hirsut/o	hairy
		hist/o	tissue
gen/o	forming, producing, origin	histi/o	tissue
		home/o	same, alike
		homeo-	same, alike

Medical Word Element	Meaning	Medical Word Element	Meaning
homo-	same	infer/o	lower, below
humer/o	humerus (upper arm bone)	infra-	below, under
		inguin/o	groin
hydr/o	water	insulin/o	insulin
hyp-	under, below, deficient	inter-	between
		intra-	in, within
hyp/o	under, below, deficient	-ion	the act of
		-ior	pertaining to
hyper-	excessive, above normal	irid/o	iris
		-is	noun ending
hypn/o	sleep	isch/o	to hold back, block
hypo-	under, below, deficient	ischi/o	ischium (lower portion of hip bone)
hyster/o	uterus (womb)	-ism	condition
		iso-	same, equal
I		-ist	specialist
-ia	condition	-isy	state of; condition
-iac	pertaining to	-itic	pertaining to
-iasis	abnormal condition (produced by something specified)	-itis	inflammation
		-ive	pertaining to
		-ization	process (of)
iatr/o	physician; medicine; treatment	**J**	
		jaund/o	yellow
-iatry	medicine; treatment	jejun/o	jejunum (second part of small intestine)
-ic	pertaining to		
-ical	pertaining to		
-ice	noun ending	**K**	
ichthy/o	dry, scaly	kal/i	potassium (an electrolyte)
-ician	specialist	kary/o	nucleus
-icle	small, minute	kerat/o	horny tissue; hard; cornea
-icterus	jaundice	ket/o	ketone bodies (acids and acetones)
idi/o	unknown, peculiar		
-ile	pertaining to	keton/o	ketone bodies (acids and acetones)
ile/o	ileum (third part of small intestine)		
		kinesi/o	movement
ili/o	ilium (lateral, flaring portion of hip bone)	-kinesia	movement
		kinet/o	movement
		klept/o	to steal
im-	not	kyph/o	humpback
immun/o	immune, immunity, safe		
		L	
in-	in; not	labi/o	lip
-ine	pertaining to	labyrinth/o	labyrinth (inner ear)

(Continued)

Medical Word Element	Meaning	Medical Word Element	Meaning
lacrim/o	tear; lacrimal apparatus (duct, sac, or gland)	-mania	state of mental disorder, frenzy
		mast/o	breast
lact/o	milk	mastoid/o	mastoid process
-lalia	speech, babble	maxill/o	maxilla (upper jaw bone)
lamin/o	lamina (part of vertebral arch)	meat/o	opening, meatus
		medi-	middle
lapar/o	abdomen	medi/o	middle
laryng/o	larynx (voice box)	mediastin/o	mediastinum
later/o	side, to one side	medull/o	medulla
lei/o	smooth	mega-	enlargement
leiomy/o	smooth muscle (visceral)	megal/o	enlargement
		-megaly	enlargement
-lepsy	seizure	melan/o	black
lept/o	thin, slender	men/o	menses, menstruation
leuk/o	white	mening/o	meninges (membranes covering brain and spinal cord)
lingu/o	tongue		
lip/o	fat		
lipid/o	fat	meningi/o	meninges (membranes covering brain and spinal cord)
-listhesis	slipping		
-lith	stone, calculus		
lith/o	stone, calculus	ment/o	mind
lob/o	lobe	meso-	middle
log/o	study of	meta-	change, beyond
-logist	specialist in the study of	metacarp/o	metacarpus (hand bones)
		metatars/o	metatarsus (foot bones)
-logy	study of	-meter	instrument for measuring
lord/o	curve, swayback	metr/o	uterus (womb); measure
-lucent	to shine; clear	metri/o	uterus (womb)
lumb/o	loins (lower back)	-metry	act of measuring
lymph/o	lymph	mi/o	smaller, less
lymphaden/o	lymph gland (node)	micr/o	small
lymphangi/o	lymph vessel	micro-	small
-lysis	separation; destruction; loosening	mono-	one
		morph/o	form, shape, structure
		muc/o	mucus
		multi-	many, much
M		muscul/o	muscle
macro-	large	mut/a	genetic change
mal-	bad	my/o	muscle
-malacia	softening	myc/o	fungus (plural, *fungi*)
mamm/o	breast	mydr/o	widen, enlarge

Medical Word Element	Meaning	Medical Word Element	Meaning
myel/o	bone marrow; spinal cord	optic/o	eye, vision
		or/o	mouth
myos/o	muscle	orch/o	testis (plural, *testes*)
myring/o	tympanic membrane (eardrum)	orchi/o	testis (plural, *testes*)
		orchid/o	testis (plural, *testes*)
myx/o	mucus	-orexia	appetite
		orth/o	straight
N		-ory	pertaining to
narc/o	stupor; numbness; sleep	-ose	pertaining to; sugar
		-osis	abnormal condition; increase (used primarily with blood cells)
nas/o	nose		
nat/o	birth		
natr/o	sodium (an electrolyte)	-osmia	smell
		oste/o	bone
necr/o	death, necrosis	ot/o	ear
neo-	new	-ous	pertaining to
nephr/o	kidney	ovari/o	ovary
neur/o	nerve	ox/i	oxygen
neutr/o	neutral; neither	ox/o	oxygen
nid/o	nest	-oxia	oxygen
noct/o	night		
nucle/o	nucleus	**P**	
nulli-	none	pan-	all
nyctal/o	night	pancreat/o	pancreas
		para-	near, beside; beyond
O		-para	to bear (offspring)
obstetr/o	midwife	parathyroid/o	parathyroid glands
ocul/o	eye	-paresis	partial paralysis
odont/o	teeth	patell/o	patella (kneecap)
-oid	resembling	path/o	disease
-ole	small, minute	-pathy	disease
olig/o	scanty	pector/o	chest
-oma	tumor	ped/i	foot; child
omphal/o	navel (umbilicus)	ped/o	foot; child
onc/o	tumor	pedicul/o	lice
onych/o	nail	pelv/i	pelvis
oophor/o	ovary	pelv/o	pelvis
-opaque	obscure	pen/o	penis
ophthalm/o	eye	-penia	decrease, deficiency
-opia	vision	-pepsia	digestion
-opsia	vision	per-	through
-opsy	view of	peri-	around
opt/o	eye, vision		

(Continued)

Medical Word Element	Meaning	Medical Word Element	Meaning
perine/o	perineum (area between scrotum [or vulva in the female] and anus)	pneum/o	air; lung
		pneumon/o	air; lung
		pod/o	foot
		-poiesis	formation, production
		poli/o	gray; gray matter (of brain or spinal cord)
peritone/o	peritoneum		
-pexy	fixation (of an organ)	poly-	many, much
		polyp/o	small growth
phac/o	lens	-porosis	porous
phag/o	swallowing, eating	post-	after, behind
-phage	swallowing, eating	poster/o	back (of body), behind, posterior
-phagia	swallowing, eating		
phalang/o	phalanges (bones of fingers and toes)	-potence	power
		-prandial	meal
pharmaceutic/o	drug, medicine	pre-	before, in front of
pharyng/o	pharynx (throat)	presby/o	old age
-phasia	speech	primi-	first
-phil	attraction for	pro-	before, in front of
phil/o	attraction for	proct/o	anus, rectum
-philia	attraction for	prostat/o	prostate gland
phleb/o	vein	proxim/o	near, nearest
-phobia	fear	pseudo-	false
-phonia	voice	psych/o	mind
-phoresis	carrying, transmission	-ptosis	prolapse, downward displacement
-phoria	feeling (mental state)	ptyal/o	saliva
		-ptysis	spitting
phot/o	light	pub/o	pelvis bone (anterior part of pelvic bone)
phren/o	diaphragm; mind		
-phylaxis	protection	pulmon/o	lung
-physis	growth	pupill/o	pupil
pil/o	hair	py/o	pus
pituitar/o	pituitary gland	pyel/o	renal pelvis
-plakia	plaque	pylor/o	pylorus
plas/o	formation, growth	pyr/o	fire
-plasia	formation, growth		
-plasm	formation, growth	**Q, R**	
-plasty	surgical repair	quadri-	four
-plegia	paralysis	rachi/o	spine
pleur/o	pleura	radi/o	radiation, x-ray; radius (lower arm bone on thumb side)
-plexy	stroke		
-pnea	breathing		

Medical Word Element	Meaning	Medical Word Element	Meaning
radicul/o	nerve root	-scopy	visual examination
rect/o	rectum	scot/o	darkness
ren/o	kidney	seb/o	sebum, sebaceous
reticul/o	net, mesh	semi-	one half
retin/o	retina	semin/i	semen; seed
retro-	backward, behind	semin/o	semen; seed
rhabd/o	rod-shaped (striated)	sept/o	septum
rhabdomy/o	rod-shaped (striated) muscle	sequestr/o	separation
		ser/o	serum
rhin/o	nose	sial/o	saliva, salivary gland
rhytid/o	wrinkle	sider/o	iron
roentgen/o	x-rays	sigmoid/o	sigmoid colon
-rrhage	bursting forth (of)	sin/o	sinus, cavity
-rrhagia	bursting forth (of)	sinus/o	sinus, cavity
-rrhaphy	suture	-sis	state of; condition
-rrhea	discharge, flow	somat/o	body
-rrhexis	rupture	somn/o	sleep
-rrhythm/o	rhythm	son/o	sound
rube/o	red	-spadias	slit, fissure
		-spasm	involuntary contraction, twitching
S			
sacr/o	sacrum	sperm/i	spermatozoa, sperm cells
salping/o	tube (usually fallopian or eustachian [auditory] tubes)	sperm/o	spermatozoa, sperm cells
		spermat/o	spermatozoa, sperm cells
		sphygm/o	pulse
-salpinx	tube (usually fallopian or eustachian [auditory] tubes)	-sphyxia	pulse
		spin/o	spine
		spir/o	breathe
		splen/o	spleen
		spondyl/o	vertebra (backbone)
sarc/o	flesh (connective tissue)	squam/o	scale
		staped/o	stapes
-sarcoma	malignant tumor of connective tissue	-stasis	standing still
		steat/o	fat
scapul/o	scapula (shoulder blade)	sten/o	narrowing, stricture
		-stenosis	narrowing, stricture
-schisis	a splitting	stern/o	sternum (breast bone)
schiz/o	split	steth/o	chest
scler/o	hardening; sclera (white of eye)	sthen/o	strength
		stomat/o	mouth
scoli/o	crooked, bent	-stomy	forming an opening (mouth)
-scope	instrument for examining	sub-	under, below

(Continued)

Medical Word Element	Meaning	Medical Word Element	Meaning
sudor/o	sweat	-tome	instrument to cut
super-	upper, above	-tomy	incision
super/o	upper, above	ton/o	tension
supra-	above; excessive; superior	tonsill/o	tonsils
		tox/o	poison
sym-	union, together, joined	-toxic	poison
		toxic/o	poison
syn-	union, together, joined	trache/o	trachea (windpipe)
		trans-	across, through
synapt/o	synapsis, point of contact	tri-	three
		trich/o	hair
synov/o	synovial membrane; synovial fluid	-tripsy	crushing
		-trophy	development, nourishment
		-tropia	turning
T		-tropin	stimulate
tachy-	rapid	tubercul/o	a little swelling
tars/o	tarsals	tympan/o	tympanic membrane (eardrum)
tax/o	order, coordination		
-taxia	order, coordination		
ten/o	tendon	**U**	
tend/o	tendon	-ula	small, minute
tendin/o	tendon	-ule	small, minute
-tension	to stretch	uln/o	ulna (lower arm bone on opposite side of thumb)
test/o	testis (plural, *testes*)		
thalam/o	thalamus	ultra-	excess, beyond
thec/o	sheath (usually refers to meninges)	-um	structure, thing
		umbilic/o	umbilicus, navel
thel/o	nipple	ungu/o	nail
therapeut/o	treatment	uni-	one
-therapy	treatment	ur/o	urine, urinary tract
therm/o	heat	ureter/o	ureter
thorac/o	chest	urethr/o	urethra
-thorax	chest	-uria	urine
thromb/o	blood clot	urin/o	urine, urinary tract
thym/o	thymus gland	-us	condition; structure
thyr/o	thyroid gland	uter/o	uterus (womb)
thyroid/o	thyroid gland	uvul/o	uvula
tibi/o	tibia (larger bone of lower leg)		
		V	
-tic	pertaining to	vagin/o	vagina
-tocia	childbirth, labor	valv/o	valve
tom/o	to cut	varic/o	dilated vein

Medical Word Element	Meaning	Medical Word Element	Meaning
vas/o	vessel; vas deferens; duct	vest/o	clothes
		viscer/o	internal organs
vascul/o	vessel (usually blood or lymph)	vitr/o	vitreous body (of eye)
		vitre/o	glassy
ven/o	vein	vol/o	volume
ventr/o	belly, belly side	vulv/o	vulva
ventricul/o	ventricle (of heart or brain)	**W, X, Y, Z**	
venul/o	venule (small vein)	xanth/o	yellow
-version	turning	xen/o	foreign, strange
vertebr/o	vertebra (backbone)	xer/o	dry
vesic/o	bladder	xiph/o	sword
vesicul/o	seminal vesicle	-y	condition; process

Answer Key

CHAPTER 1

Introduction to Medical Terminology

Review Activity 1-1: Matching Word Elements

1. J	**3.** G	**5.** I	**7.** E	**9.** B
2. D	**4.** H	**6.** F	**8.** C	**10.** A

Review Activity 1-2: Understanding Medical Word Elements

1. root, combining form, suffix, and prefix
2. arthr

Identify the following statements as either true or false. If false, rewrite the statement correctly in the space provided.

3. False-A combining vowel is usually an "o."
4. False-A word root links a suffix that begins with a vowel.
5. True
6. True
7. False- Whenever a prefix stands alone it will be followed by a hyphen.
8. True

Underline the word root in each of following Combining forms.

9. <u>splen</u>/o	**12.** <u>neur</u>/o	**15.** <u>hydr</u>/o
10. <u>hyster</u>/o	**13.** <u>ot</u>/o	
11. <u>enter</u>/o	**14.** <u>dermat</u>/o	

Review Activity 1-3: Identifying Word Roots and Combining Forms

1. <u>nephr</u>itis	6. nephr (word root)
2. <u>arthr</u>odesis	7. <u>hepat/o</u>
3. <u>dermat</u>itis	8. arthr (word root)
4. <u>arthr</u>ocentesis	9. <u>oste/o</u>/arthr
5. <u>gastr</u>ectomy	10. <u>cholangi/o</u>

Review Activity 1-4: Defining Medical Words

1. *breast*	9. gastr/o
2. inflammation	10. -pathy
3. colon	11. mast/o
4. bone	12. -scope
5. after	13. appendix
6. joint	14. intestine (usually
7. disease	small intestine)
8. pre-	15. -centesis

Review Activity 1-5: Defining and Building Medical Words

Term	Definition
1. col/itis	inflammation (of) colon
2. gastr/o/scope	instrument for examining the stomach
3. hepat/itis	inflammation of the liver
4. pre/nat/al	pertaining to (the period) before birth
5. tonsill/ectomy	excision of the tonsils
6. tonsill/itis	inflammation of the tonsils

Write the number for the rule that applies to each listed term as well as a short summary of the rule.

Term	Rule	Summary of the Rule
7. append/ectomy	*1*	*A WR links a suffix that begins with a vowel.*
8. arthr/o/centesis	2	A CF links a suffix that begins with a consonant.
9. col/ectomy	1	A WR links a suffix that begins with a vowel.
10. colon/o/scope	2	A CF links a suffix that begins with a consonant.
11. gastr/itis	1	A WR links a suffix that begins with a vowel.
12. gastr/o/enter/o/ col/itis	3,1	A CF links multiple roots to each other. This rule holds true even if the next word root begins with a vowel. A WR links a suffix that begins with a vowel.
13. arthr/o/pathy	2	A CF links a suffix that begins with a consonant.
14. oste/o/arthr/itis	3,1	A CF links multiple roots to each other. This rule holds true even if the next word root begins with a vowel. A WR links a suffix that begins with a vowel.
15. oste/o/chondr/itis	3,1	A CF links multiple roots to each other. This rule holds true even if the next word root begins with a vowel. A WR links a suffix that begins with a vowel.

Review Activity 1-6: Understanding Pronunciations

1. macron	**3.** long	**5.** k	**7.** is	**9.** second
2. breve	**4.** short	**6.** n	**8.** eye	**10.** separate

Review Activity 1-7: Plural Suffixes

Singular	Plural	Rule
1. sarcoma	*sarcomata*	*Retain the* ma *and add* ta.
2. thrombus	thrombi	Drop *us* and add *i.*
3. appendix	appendices	Drop *ix* and add *ices.*
4. diverticulum	diverticula	Drop *um* and add *a.*
5. ovary	ovaries	Drop *y* and add *ies.*
6. diagnosis	diagnoses	Drop *is* and add *es.*
7. lumen	lumina	Drop *en* and add *ina.*
8. vertebra	vertebrae	Retain the *a* and add *e.*
9. thorax	thoraces	Drop the *x* and add *ces.*
10. spermatozoon	spermatozoa	Drop *on* and add *a.*

Review Activity 1-8: Common Suffixes

Surgical Suffixes

Term	Meaning
arthr/o/**centesis**	*Surgical puncture of a joint*
oste/o/**clasis**	surgical breaking or fracture of a bone to correct a deformity; also called *osteoclasia*
arthr/o/**desis**	binding or fixation of a joint
append/**ectomy**	excision or removal of the appendix
thromb/o/**lysis**	separation, destruction, or loosening of a blood clot
mast/o/**pexy**	surgical fixation of the breast(s)
rhin/o/**plasty**	surgical repair of the nose (to change shape or size)
my/o/**rrhaphy**	suture of a muscle

(Continued)

Term	Meaning
trache/o/**stomy**	forming an opening (mouth) into the trachea
oste/o/**tome**	instrument to cut bone
trache/o/**tomy**	incision of the trachea
lith/o/**tripsy**	crushing a stone or calculus

Diagnostic Suffixes

Term	Meaning
electr/o/cardi/o/**gram**	record of electrical activity of the heart
cardi/o/**graph**	instrument to record electrical activity of the heart
angi/o/**graphy**	process of recording images of blood vessels (recording images of blood vessels after injection of a contrast medium)
pelv/i/**meter**	instrument for measuring the pelvis
pelv/i/**metry**	act of measuring the pelvis
endo/**scope**	instrument for examining within (instrument for examining inside a hollow organ or cavity)
endo/**scopy**	visual examination within; visual examination of a cavity or canal using a specialized lighted instrument called an *endoscope*

Pathological Suffixes

Term	Meaning
neur/**algia** ot/o/**dynia**	pain in a nerve; pain along the path of a nerve pain in the ear (earache)
hepat/o/**cele**	hernia or swelling of the liver
bronchi/**ectasis**	dilation or expansion of a bronchus or bronchi
lymph/**edema**	swelling of lymph tissue (swelling and accumulation of tissue fluid)
hyper/**emesis**	excessive or above normal vomiting
an/**emia**	without blood (blood condition caused by iron deficiency or decrease in red blood cells)

Term	Meaning
chol/e/lith/**iasis**	presence or formation of gallstones (in the gallbladder or common bile duct)
gastr/**itis**	inflammation of the stomach
chol/e/**lith**	gallstone
chondr/o/**malacia**	softening of cartilage
cardi/o/**megaly**	enlargement of the heart
neur/**oma**	tumor composed of nerve cells
cyan/**osis**	abnormal condition of blueness (bluish discoloration of the skin and mucous membrane)
my/o/**pathy**	disease of muscle
erythr/o/**penia**	abnormal decrease or deficiency in red (blood cells)
hem/o/**phobia**	fear of blood
hemi/**plegia**	paralysis of one half (paralysis of one side of the body)
hem/o/**rrhage**	bursting forth of blood (loss of large amounts of blood within a short period, either externally or internally)
men/o/**rrhagia**	bursting forth of menses (profuse discharge of blood during menstruation)
dia/**rrhea**	discharge or flow through (frequent discharge or flow of fluid fecal matter from the bowel)
arteri/o/**rrhexis**	rupture of an artery
arteri/o/**stenosis**	narrowing or stricture of an artery
hepat/o/**toxic**	poisonous or toxic to the liver
dys/**trophy**	bad development or nourishment (abnormal condition caused by defective nutrition or metabolism)

Review Activity 1-9: Common Prefixes

Term	Meaning
a/mast/ia **an**/esthesia	without a breast without feeling (partial or complete loss of sensation with or without loss of consciousness)

(Continued)

Term	Meaning
circum/duction	act of leading around (movement of a part, such as an extremity, in a circular direction)
peri/odont/al	pertaining to around a tooth
dia/thermy	process of generating heat through (some part of the body)
trans/vagin/al	pertaining to through or across the vagina
dipl/opia	double vision
diplo/bacteri/al	pertaining to a paired bacteria
dys/phonia	difficulty in speaking
endo/crine	secrete within (gland that secretes hormones directly into the bloodstream)
intra/muscul/ar	pertaining to within the muscle
homo/graft	transplantation of same (transplantion of tissue between the same species)
homeo/plasia	formation or growth of new tissue similar to that already existing in a part
hypo/derm/ic	pertaining to under the skin (under or inserted under the skin, as in a hypodermic injection)
macro/cyte	abnormally large erythrocyte, such as those found in pernicious anemia
micro/scope	instrument for examining small (minute) objects
mono/therapy	one treatment
uni/nucle/ar	pertaining to one nucleus
post/nat/al	pertaining to (the period) after birth
pre/nat/al	pertaining to (the period) before birth
pro/gnosis	before knowing (prediction of the course and end of a disease and the estimated chance of recovery)
primi/gravida	woman pregnant for the first time
retro/version	turning backward (tipping backward of an organ, such as the uterus, from its normal position)
super/ior	pertaining to upper or above (toward the head or upper portion of a structure)

Chapter 2

Body Structure

Figure 2-2: Anatomical Position, Directional Terms, and Body Planes.

1. Median plane
2. Frontal plane
3. Horizontal plane

Figure 2-3A: Regions and Quadrants. (A) Four Quadrants of the Abdomen.

1. Right upper quadrant
2. Right lower quadrant
3. Left upper quadrant
4. Left lower quadrant

Combining Forms

Medical Word	Meaning
Body Regions	
abdomin/al	*pertaining to the abdomen*
caud/ad	toward the tail; in a posterior direction
cephal/ad	toward the head
cervic/al	pertaining to the neck of the body or the neck of the uterus
crani/al	pertaining to the cranium or skull
gastr/ic	pertaining to the stomach
ili/ac	pertaining to the ilium
inguin/al	pertaining to the groin
lumb/ar	pertaining to the loins or lower back
pelv/i/meter pelv/ic	instrument for measuring the pelvis pertaining to the pelvis
spin/al	pertaining to the spine or spinal column
thorac/ic	pertaining to the chest
umbilic/al	pertaining to the umbilicus or navel
Directional Terms	
anter/ior	pertaining to the front of the body, an organ, or a structure
dist/al	pertaining to a point farthest from the center, a medial line, or the trunk; opposite of proximal

(Continued)

Medical Word	Meaning
Directional Terms	
dors/al	pertaining to the back or posterior (of the body)
infer/ior	pertaining to below or lower; toward the tail
later/al	pertaining to the side
medi/al	pertaining to the middle
poster/ior	pertaining to back or posterior side (of the body)
proxim/al	nearest the point of attachment, center of the body, or point of reference
super/ior	pertaining to above or higher; toward the head
ventr/al	pertaining to the belly side or front (of the body)
Other CFs Related to Body Structure	
cyt/o/meter	instrument for counting and measuring cells
hist/o/lysis	separation, destruction, or disintegration of tissue
nucle/ar	pertaining to a nucleus
radi/o/graphy	process of recording an x-ray

Suffixes and Prefixes

Medical Words	Meaning
Suffixes	
medi/**ad**	toward the middle or center
coron/**al**	pertaining to the heart
cost/**algia** thorac/o/**dynia**	pain in the ribs pain in the chest
path/o/**gen** carcin/o/**genesis**	forming, producing, or origin of a disease forming, producing, or origin of cancer
hist/o/**logist**	specialist in study of tissues
eti/o/**logy**	study of the causes (of disease)

Medical Words	Meaning
Suffixes	
cyt/o/**lysis**	destruction, dissolution, or separation of a cell
therm/o/**meter**	instrument for measuring heat
hyper/**plasia**	excessive growth of tissue
hepat/o/**toxic**	pertaining to poison in the liver
Prefixes	
bi/later/al	pertaining to or affecting two sides
epi/gastr/ic	pertaining to above or on the stomach
infra/cost/al	pertaining to below or under the ribs
trans/vagin/al	pertaining to or across the vagina

Medical Terminology Word Building

1. caudad
2. caudal
3. thoracocentesis
4. thoracic
5. thoracoplasty
6. gastric
7. gastroplasty
8. pelvic
9. pelvimeter
10. abdominal
11. abdominoplasty
12. cranial
13. cranioplasty
14. medial
15. mediad
16. cytology
17. cytologist
18. cytolysis
19. histology
20. histologist

Additional Medical Vocabulary Recall

1. CT scan
2. fluoroscopy
3. US
4. MRI
5. PET
6. endoscope
7. inflammation
8. SPECT
9. tomography
10. radiopharmaceutical
11. endoscopy
12. nuclear scan
13. adhesion
14. radiography
15. sepsis

Pronunciation and Spelling

1. bilateral
2. adhesion
3. cervical
4. cranial
5. distal
6. endoscope
7. fluoroscopy
8. inflammation
9. lumbar
10. radiopharmaceutical
11. radiography
12. sepsis
13. sigmoidoscope
14. speculum
15. tomography

Demonstrate What You Know!

1. i
2. n
3. j
4. h
5. a
6. m
7. c
8. b
9. d
10. e
11. k
12. o
13. l
14. f
15. g

Chapter 3

Integumentary System
Combining Forms

Medical Word	Meaning
adip/o/cele **lip/o**/cyte **steat**/oma	*hernia containing fat or fatty tissue* cell containing fat or fatty tissue tumor composed of fat
sub/**cutane**/ous **dermat/o**/logist hypo/**derm**/ic	pertaining to beneath the skin specialist or physician who studies or treats skin disorders pertaining to under or inserted under the skin, as in a hypodermic injection
cyan/osis	abnormal condition of blue (skin)
erythem/a **erythemat**/ous **erythr/o**/cyte	redness of skin caused by capillary dilation pertaining to redness (of the skin) red blood cell
hidr/osis **sudor**/esis	abnormal condition of sweat condition of profuse sweating
ichthy/**osis**	abnormal condition of dry, scaly (skin)
kerat/osis	abnormal condition of a horny growth, or abnormal condition of the skin characterized by overgrowth and thickening of skin
melan/oma	black tumor (malignant tumor of melanocytes)
dermat/o/**myc**/osis	abnormal condition of a fungal infection of the skin
onych/o/malacia	abnormal softening of nails
pil/o/nid/al **trich/o**/pathy	pertaining to growth of hair in a cyst or other internal structure disease of the hair
scler/o/derma	hardening of the skin or chronic disease with abnormal hardening of the skin
seb/o/rrhea	discharge or flow of sebum (secreted by sebaceous glands)
squam/ous	pertaining to scales (scalelike)
therm/al	pertaining to heat, such as thermal burn caused by heat
xer/o/derma	dry skin or skin condition characterized by excessive roughness and dryness

Suffixes and Prefixes

Medical Words	Meaning
Suffixes	
leuk/o/**cyte**	white blood cell
py/o/**derma**	pyogenic infection of the skin
carcin/**oma**	cancerous tumor
dia/**phoresis**	carrying or transmitting across or condition of profuse sweating; also called *sudoresis* or *hyperhidrosis*
dermat/o/**plasty**	surgical repair of the skin
cry/o/**therapy**	treatment using cold as a destructive medium
Prefixes	
an/hidr/osis	abnormal condition of absence of sweat
epi/derm/oid	resembling or pertaining to the epidermis
homo/graft	transplantation of tissue from an individual of one species to an individual of the same species; also called *allograft*
hyper/hidr/osis	abnormal condition of excessive or profuse sweating; also called *diaphoresis* or *sudoresis*

Medical Terminology Word Building

1. adipoma, lipoma
2. adipocyte, lipocyte
3. ichthyosis
4. onychoma
5. onychopathy
6. onychomalacia
7. trichopathy
8. trichosis
9. xeroderma
10. xerosis
11. erythrocyte
12. leukocyte
13. melanocyte
14. anhidrosis
15. hyperhidrosis

Additional Medical Vocabulary Recall

1. verruca
2. vitiligo
3. tinea
4. pressure ulcer
5. eczema
6. autograft
7. biopsy
8. dermabrasion
9. hirsutism
10. cryosurgery
11. debridement
12. scabies
13. alopecia
14. comedo
15. metastasize

Pronunciation and Spelling

1. abrasion
2. abscess
3. acne
4. alopecia
5. biopsy
6. cryotherapy
7. diaphoresis
8. epidermoid
9. erythematous
10. furuncle
11. keloid
12. hematoma
13. hirsutism
14. lesions
15. onychomalacia
16. petechia
17. scabies
18. psoriasis
19. seborrhea
20. vitiligo

Chart Note Analysis

1. macule
2. intermittent
3. syncope
4. vulgaris
5. colitis
6. chronic
7. sclerosed
8. enteritis
9. pruritus
10. Bartholin glands
11. psoriasis
12. erythematous
13. sinusitis
14. papule
15. diaphoresis

Demonstrate What You Know!

1. dermis	**5.** xenograft	**9.** carcinoma	**13.** lipocyte
2. sudoriferous	**6.** epidermis	**10.** ichthyosis	**14.** psoriasis
3. onychopathy	**7.** dermatologist	**11.** onychomalacia	**15.** pyoderma
4. mycosis	**8.** sebaceous	**12.** antibiotic	

Chapter 4

Respiratory System
Combining Forms

Medical Word	Meaning
Upper Respiratory Tract	
adenoid/ectomy	*excision of the adenoids*
laryng/o/scope	instrument for examining the larynx
nas/al **rhin/o**/rrhea	pertaining to the nose discharge from the nose (runny nose), often the result of a cold or allergy
pharyng/o/spasm	twitching or involuntary contractions of the pharynx (throat)
tonsill/ectomy	excision of the tonsils
trache/o/tomy	incision of the trachea
Lower Respiratory Tract	
alveol/ar	pertaining to an alveolus (alveoli, plural)
bronch/o/scopy **bronchi**/ectasis	visual examination of the bronchus (or bronchi) through a bronchoscope expansion or dilation of a bronchus (or bronchi)
bronchiol/itis	inflammation of the bronchiole(s)
phren/algia	pain in the diaphragm
pleur/o/dynia	pain in the pleura
pneum/o/melan/osis **pneumon**/ia	abnormal condition of blackening of the lung tissue(caused by inhalation of coal dust or other black particles)abnormal condition of the lungs
pulmon/o/logist	physician or medical specialist who treats pulmonary diseases
thorac/o/pathy	disease of the thorax

Medical Word	Meaning
Other Related Combining Forms	
aer/o/phagia	swallowing air
cyan/osis	abnormal condition of blue (skin)
mastoid/itis	inflammation of one of the mastoid bones, usually an extension of a middle ear infection
muc/oid	resembling mucus
myc/osis	any diseease induced by a fungus
orth/o/**pnea**	(labored) breathing that improves when standing or sitting up
py/o/thorax	pus in the chest

Suffixes and Prefixes

Medical Word	Meaning
Suffixes	
chondr/**oma**	tumor composed of cartilage
rhin/o/**plasty**	surgical repair of the nose
laryng/o/**plegia**	paralysis of the larynx (voice box)
Prefixes	
a/pnea	not breathing
brady/pnea	slow breathing
dys/pnea	bad, painful, or difficult breathing
eu/pnea	normal, unlabored breathing
tachy/pnea	rapid breathing

Medical Terminology Word Building

1. rhinoplasty
2. rhinorrhea
3. laryngoplegia
4. laryngitis
5. bronchiectasis
6. bronchoscopy
7. pleurodynia *or* pleuralgia
8. pleuritis
9. cyanosis
10. dyspnea
11. bradypnea
12. tachypnea
13. eupnea
14. pyothorax
15. aerophagia

Additional Medical Vocabulary Recall

1. pleurisy
2. croup
3. hypoxemia
4. corticosteroids
5. CF
6. stridor
7. asthma
8. bronchodilators
9. pneumothorax
10. ABGs
11. epistaxis
12. anosmia
13. PFT
14. Mantoux
15. atelectasis

Pronunciation and Spelling

1. *acidosis*
2. aerophagia
3. anosmia
4. asphyxia
5. asthma
6. atelectasis
7. bradypnea
8. bronchiectasis
9. bronchodilators
10. bronchoscopy
11. emphysema
12. corticosteroids
13. coryza
14. crackle
15. dyspnea
16. hypoxemia
17. hypoxia
18. pertussis
19. pleurisy
20. rhonchi

Demonstrate What You Know!

1. tracheotomy
2. alveoli
3. laryngectomy
4. emphysema
5. laryngoscope
6. pharyngitis
7. bronchioles
8. apnea
9. rhonchi
10. O_2
11. pneumonia
12. phrenalgia
13. hypoxia
14. diaphragm
15. tachypnea

Chart Note Analysis

1. polypoid
2. meatus
3. biopsy
4. metastatic
5. polypectomy
6. snare
7. hemorrhage
8. anesthesia
9. cm
10. carcinoma

Chapter 5

Cardiovascular System

Combining Forms

Medical Word	Meaning
aneurysm/o/rrhaphy	suture (of the sac) of an aneurysm; suture of a widened blood vessel
arteri/o/scler/osis	hardening of an artery; disorder characterized by thickening, loss of elasticity, and calcification of arterial walls
ather/oma	tumor of fatty plaque; fatty degeneration or thickening of the larger arterial walls, as in atherosclerosis
atri/um	structure of the atrium (a cavity, such as the atrium of the heart)
cardi/o/megaly coron/ary	enlargement of the heart pertaining to the heart
phleb/itis ven/ous	inflammation of a vein pertaining to the veins or blood passing through them
thromb/o/lysis	destruction or breaking up of a thrombus (blood clot)
varic/ose	pertaining to a dilated vein

Medical Word	Meaning
vas/o/spasm	involuntary contraction or spasm of a blood vessel
vascul/ar	pertaining to or composed of blood vessels
inter/**ventricul**/ar	within a ventricle (of the heart)

Suffixes and Prefixes

Medical Word	Meaning
Suffixes	
tachy/**cardia**	rapid heart rate
electr/o/cardi/o/**gram**	record of electrical activity of the heart
electr/o/cardi/o/**graph**	instrument for recording electrical activity of the heart
angi/o/**graphy**	process of recording (radiography) the heart and blood vessels
aort/o/**stenosis**	narrowing of the aorta
Prefixes	
brady/cardi/ac	pertaining to a slow heart (rate)
endo/cardi/um	structure (serous membrane that lines the interior of the heart) within the heart
epi/cardi/um	structure (outermost layer of the heart) above the heart
peri/cardi/um	structure (fibrous sac) around the heart

Medical Terminology Word Building

1. atheroma
2. atherosclerosis
3. phlebitis
4. phlebothrombosis
5. venous
6. venospasm
7. cardiologist
8. electrocardiograph
9. cardiomegaly *or* megalocardia
10. angiopathy
11. angioma
12. aortostenosis
13. arteriostenosis
14. tachycardia
15. bradycardia

Additional Medical Vocabulary Recall

1. varicose veins
2. fibrillation
3. thrombolytics
4. embolus
5. HF
6. DVT
7. HTN
8. arrhythmia
9. statin
10. bruit
11. stroke
12. rheumatic heart disease
13. Holter monitor
14. Raynaud disease
15. endarterectomy

Pronunciation and Spelling

1. *aneurysm*
2. arrhythmia
3. atherosclerosis
4. bruit
5. cardiomegaly
6. diastole
7. electrocardiography
8. fibrillation
9. infarction
10. hypertension
11. ischemia
12. myocardial
13. tachycardia
14. thrombus
15. varicose

Demonstrate What You Know!

1. cardiologist
2. arteriole
3. angioplasty
4. statin
5. tricuspid
6. oxygen
7. arteriosclerosis
8. cardiomegaly
9. phlebitis
10. nitrate
11. ischemia
12. arteriostenosis
13. aneurysm
14. tachycardia
15. MI

Chart Note Analysis

1. apnea
2. postoperative
3. anxiety
4. thyroiditis
5. syncope
6. desiccated
7. fibrillation
8. malaise
9. sinus tachycardia
10. EKG
11. dyspnea
12. mg

Chapter 6

Blood, Lymphatic, and Immune Systems

Combining Forms

Medical Word	Meaning
Blood System	
agglutin/ation	*process by which particles are caused to adhere and form into clumps*
embol/ectomy	excision of an embolus. It may be done surgically or by use of enzymes that dissolve the clot
erythr/o/cyte	red bood cell
hem/o/phobia **hemat**/oma	fear of blood tumor composed of blood (usually clotted)
leuk/o/cyte	white blood cell
myel/o/gen/ic	pertaining to, producing, or originating in bone marrow
thromb/o/lysis	dissolution of a blood clot
ven/ous	pertaining to a vein

Medical Word	Meaning
Lymphatic and Immune Systems	
aden/o/pathy	disease of a gland
immun/o/gen	producing immunity or an immune response
lymph/o/poiesis	formation of lymphocytes or lymphoid tissue
lymphaden/itis	inflammation of a lymph gland
lymphangi/oma	tumor of a lymph vessel
phag/o/cyte	cell that ingests (and destroys microorganisms and other cell debris)
splen/o/megaly	enlargement of the spleen
thym/oma	tumor of the thymus gland

Suffixes and Prefixes

Medical Words	Meaning
Suffixes	
leuk/**emia**	white blood; hematological malignancies of bone marrow cells
macr/o/**phage**	eating or swallowing large (pathogens); monocyte that transforms into a phagocyte capable of ingesting pathogens
ana/**phylaxis**	against protection; exaggerated, life-threatening hypersensitivity (allergic) reaction to a previously encountered antigen
hem/o/**poiesis**	formation or production of blood
hem/o/**stasis**	standing still of blood
Prefixes	
micro/cyte	small (red) cell
mono/nucle/osis	abnormal increase of mononuclear (leukocytes in the blood)

Medical Terminology Word Building

1. hematoma
2. hematopoiesis
3. hematologist
4. thrombectomy
5. thromboid
6. thrombolysis
7. erythrocytes
8. leukocytes *or* leucocytes
9. phagocytes
10. lymphopoiesis
11. lymphocytes
12. lymphadenopathy
13. immunology
14. immunogen
15. agglutination
16. agglutinogen
17. splenomegaly
18. hepatosplenomegaly
19. myelogenic
20. anaphylaxis

Additional Medical Vocabulary Recall

1. anemia
2. mononucleosis
3. thrombolytics
4. SLE
5. lymphadenitis
6. HIV
7. lymphangiography
8. tissue typing
9. Hodgkin disease
10. AIDS
11. leukemia
12. ELISA
13. lymphedema
14. hemophilia
15. anticoagulants

Pronunciation and Spelling

1. adenopathy
2. agglutination
3. anaphylaxis
4. anticoagulant
5. erythrocyte
6. hematoma
7. hemostasis
8. immunogen
9. leukemia
10. lymphangiography
11. macrocyte
12. mononucleosis
13. phagocyte
14. splenomegaly
15. vaccination

Chart Note Analysis

1. dyspnea
2. antiretroviral therapy
3. chills, night sweats
4. Tylenol
5. hemoglobin
6. persistent
7. *Pneumocystis*
8. WNL
9. CD4
10. sputum

Demonstrate What You Know!

1. hematology
2. hemopoiesis
3. oncology
4. lymphocytes
5. phagocytes
6. aplastic
7. Hodgkin
8. HIV
9. pernicious
10. antigen
11. splenomegaly
12. lymphadenitis
13. immunodeficiency
14. pathogen
15. agglutination

Chapter 7

Digestive System
Combining Forms

Medical Word	Meaning
Oral Cavity	
dent/ist orth/**odont**/ist	*specialist in treatment of the teeth* dental specialist that prevents and corrects abnormally positioned or misaligned teeth
gingiv/itis	inflammation of gums
hypo/**gloss**/al sub/**lingu**/al	pertaining to under the tongue pertaining to under the tongue

Medical Word	Meaning
Oral Cavity	
or/al **stomat/o**/pathy	pertaining to the mouth disease of the mouth
ptyal/ism	condition of excessive salivation
sial/o/rrhea	excessive flow of saliva; also called *hypersalivation* or *ptyalism*
Esophagus, Pharynx, and Stomach	
esophag/o/scope	instrument for examining the esophagus
gastr/o/scopy	visual examination of the stomach
pharyng/o/tonsill/itis	inflammation of the pharynx (throat) and tonsils
pylor/o/tomy	incision of the pylorus (lower portion of the stomach)
Small Intestine	
duoden/o/scopy	visual examination of the duodenum (a type of endoscopic procedure)
enter/o/pathy	disease of the intestine (usually small); any intestinal disease
jejun/o/rrhaphy	suture of the jejunum
ile/o/stomy	surgical creation of an opening in the ileum (to drain urine or feces into an exterior pouch)
Large Intestine	
peri/**an**/al	pertaining to around the anus
append/ectomy	removal of the appendix
appendic/itis	inflammation of the appendix
col/o/stomy **colon/o**/scopy	creation of an opening between the colon and the abdominal wall visual examination of the colon using a long, flexible endoscope (a type of endoscopic procedure)
proct/o/logist	physician who specializes in treating disorders of the colon, rectum, and anus
rect/o/cele	herniation or protrusion of the rectum; also called *proctocele*
sigmoid/o/tomy	incision of sigmoid colon
Accessory Organs of Digestion	
cholangi/ole	small terminal portion of the bile duct
chol/e/lith	gallstone

(Continued)

Medical Word	Meaning
Accessory Organs of Digestion	
cholecyst/ectomy	removal of the gallbladder by laparoscopic or open surgery
choledoch/o/tomy	incision of the common bile duct
hepat/itis	inflammation of the liver
pancreat/o/lysis	destruction of the pancreas by pancreatic enzymes

Suffixes and Prefixes

Medical Words	Meaning
Suffixes	
gastr/**algia** gastr/o/**dynia**	pain in the stomach pain in the stomach
hyper/**emesis**	excessive vomiting
chol/e/lith/**iasis**	presence or formation of gallstones
hepat/o/**megaly**	enlargement of the liver
an/**orexia**	without appetite; loss of appetite
cirrh/**osis**	abnormal condition of yellowness
dys/**pepsia**	difficult or painful digestion; also called *indigestion*
dys/**phagia**	difficulty swallowing or eating
post/**prandial**	following or after a meal
dia/**rrhea**	frequent, watery bowel movements
Prefixes	
endo/scopy	visual examination within (an organ or cavity using an endoscope)
hemat/emesis	vomiting blood
hypo/gastr/ic	pertaining to below the stomach

Medical Terminology Word Building

1. esophagospasm
2. esophagostenosis
3. gastritis
4. gastrodynia *or* gastralgia
5. gastropathy
6. jejunectomy
7. ileitis
8. jejunoileal
9. enteritis
10. enteropathy
11. colorectal
12. coloptosis
13. proctostenosis *or* rectostenosis
14. proctocele *or* rectocele
15. proctoplegia *or* proctoparalysis
16. cholecystitis
17. cholelithiasis
18. hepatoma
19. hepatomegaly
20. pancreatitis

Additional Medical Vocabulary Recall

1. stool guaiac
2. nasogastric intubation
3. polyp
4. ascites
5. Crohn disease
6. lithotripsy
7. fistula
8. jaundice
9. barium enema
10. IBD
11. hematochezia
12. volvulus
13. cirrhosis
14. barium swallow
15. IBS

Pronunciation and Spelling

1. appendicitis
2. ascites
3. bilirubin
4. borborygmus
5. cholangiopancreatography
6. cholecystectomy
7. choledochoplasty
8. cholelithiasis
9. cirrhosis
10. colostomy
11. Crohn disease
12. duodenitis
13. enteropathy
14. esophagogastroduodenoscopy
15. gastroesophageal
16. glossectomy
17. hepatitis
18. ileorectal
19. jaundice
20. sigmoidotomy

Chart Note Analysis

1. postprandial
2. anorectal
3. angulation
4. polyp
5. diverticulum
6. dysphagia
7. enteritis
8. ileostomy
9. hematemesis
10. carcinoma

Demonstrate What You Know!

1. sublingually
2. orthodontist
3. gastroesophagitis
4. bariatric
5. sigmoidoscopy
6. hemorrhoids
7. pylorotomy
8. constipation
9. hematemesis
10. bile ducts
11. nausea
12. stool
13. stones
14. stomach
15. GERD

Chapter 8

Urinary System
Combining Forms

Medical Word	Meaning
cyst/o/scopy vesic/o/cele	*visual examination of the bladder* hernial protrusion of the urinary bladder; also called *cystocele*
glomerul/o/pathy	disease of the glomerulus
meat/us	opening or tunnel through any part of the body, such as the external opening of the urethra

(Continued)

Medical Word	Meaning
hydr/o/**nephr**/osis	abnormal condition of water in the kidney(s)
ren/al	pertaining to the kidney
pyel/o/plasty	surgical repair of the renal pelvis
ur/emia	excessive levels of urea and other nitrogenous waste products in the blood; also called *azotemia*
urin/ary	pertaining to urine or the urinary tract
ureter/o/stenosis	narrowing or stricture of a ureter
urethr/o/cele	hernia or swelling of the urethra

Suffixes and Prefixes

Medical Words	Meaning
Suffixes	
azot/**emia**	nitrogenous compounds in the blood
lith/**iasis**	abnormal condition of a stone or calculus
dia/**lysis**	process of removing toxic wastes from blood when kidneys are unable to do so
nephr/o/**pathy**	disease of the kidney(s)
nephr/o/**pexy**	surgical fixation of a kidney
nephr/o/**ptosis**	downward displacement or dropping of a kidney
lith/o/**tripsy**	crushing of a stone
olig/**uria**	diminished or scanty capacity to form and pass urine
Prefixes	
an/uria	without urine
poly/uria	excessive urination
supra/ren/al	pertaining to the area above the kidney

Medical Terminology Word Building

1. nephrolith
2. nephropathy
3. nephrohydrosis
   or hydroneprhosis
4. pyelectasis
   or pyelectasia
5. pyelopathy
6. ureterocele
7. ureteroplasty
8. cystitis
9. cystoscope
10. azoturia
11. azotemia
12. urethrostenosis
13. urethrotome
14. urography
15. uropathy

Additional Medical Vocabulary Recall

1. UA
2. Wilms tumor
3. azoturia
4. dysuria
5. diuresis
6. retrograde pyelography
7. hydronephrosis
8. interstitial nephritis
9. BUN
10. enuresis
11. catheterization
12. VCUG
13. uremia
14. renal hypertension
15. dialysis

Pronunciation and Spelling

1. azotemia
2. catheterization
3. cystoscopy
4. cystourethroscope
5. glomerulonephritis
6. incontinence
7. lithotripsy
8. nephrolithotomy
9. nephroptosis
10. nephrosclerosis
11. oliguria
12. polyuria
13. proteinuria
14. pyeloplasty
15. pyonephrosis
16. retrograde pyelography
17. ureterectasis
18. ureterostenosis
19. urethrocele
20. urologist

Chart Note Analysis

1. cystitis
2. nocturia
3. hematuria
4. cystoscopy
5. epigastric
6. urgency
7. appendectomy
8. cholelithiasis
9. cholecystitis
10. choledocholithiasis
11. polyuria
12. incontinence
13. choledocholithotomy
14. cholecystectomy
15. gallbladder

Demonstrate What You Know!

1. edema
2. diuretic
3. urinary
4. pyelopathy
5. intravenous
6. hematuria
7. pyuria
8. anuria
9. urologist
10. continence
11. nephromegaly
12. hernia
13. pus
14. lithotomy
15. nephrologist

Chapter 9

Reproductive System
Combining Forms

Medical Word	Meaning
Female Reproductive System	
amni/o/centesis	*surgical puncture of the amniotic sac (to remove fluid for laboratory analysis)*
cervic/itis	inflammation of cervix uteri
colp/o/scopy	examination of the vagina and cervix with an optical magnifying instrument
vagin/o/cele	herniation into the vagina; also called *colpocele*
galact/o/rrhea	discharge or flow of milk
lact/o/gen	(substance that stimulates) formation or production of milk
gynec/o/logist	physician specializing in treating disorders of the female reproductive system
hyster/ectomy	excision of the uterus
uter/o/vagin/al	pertaining to the uterus and vagina
mamm/o/gram	radiography of the breast
mast/o/pexy	surgical fixation of the breast(s)
men/o/rrhagia	bursting forth of menses; heavy menstrual bleeding
endo/**metr/**itis	inflammation of the endometrium
pre/**nat/**al	pertaining to (the period) before birth
oophor/oma	ovarian tumor
ovari/o/rrhexis	rupture of an ovary
perine/o/rrhaphy	suture of the perineum, which is performed to repair a laceration that occurs spontaneously or is made surgically during the delivery of the fetus
salping/ectomy	excision of a fallopian tube
vulv/o/pathy	disease of the vulva
episi/o/tomy	incision of the perineum, which is performed to enlarge the vaginal opening for delivery of a fetus

Medical Word	Meaning
Male Reproductive System	
andr/o/gen	substance producing or stimulating the development of male characteristics
balan/itis	inflammation of the glans penis
gonad/o/tropin	gonad-stimulating hormone that stimulates the function of the testes and ovaries
olig/o/sperm/ia	condition of scanty sperm cells
crypt/**orch**/ism	condition of a hidden testicle; failure of the testicles to descend into the scrotum
orchi/o/pexy	surgical fixation of one or both testes
orchid/ectomy	excision of one or both testes
test/algia	pain in one or both testes
prostat/itis	inflammation of the prostate gland
spermat/o/cide	agent that kills spermatozoa; also called *spermicide*
sperm/i/cide	agent that kills spermatozoa; also called *spermatocide*
a/**sperm**/ia	failure to form semen or ejaculate
varic/o/cele	dilated or enlarged vein of the spermatic cord
vas/ectomy	removal of all or part of the vas deferens
vesicul/itis	inflammation of the seminal vesicle

Suffixes and Prefixes

Medical Words	Meaning
Suffixes	
men/**arche**	initial menstrual period
pseudo/**cyesis**	false pregnancy; condition in which a woman believes she is pregnant when she is not
primi/**gravida**	woman during her first pregnancy
multi/**para**	woman who has delivered more than one viable infant
hemat/o/**salpinx**	blood in the fallopian tube
dys/**tocia**	painful, difficult childbirth
Prefix	
retro/version	tipping back of an organ

Medical Terminology Word Building

1. gynecopathy
2. gynecologist
3. cervicovaginitis
4. cervicectomy
5. colposcope
6. colposcopy
7. hysterrhexis
8. hysteropathy
9. metrorrhagia
10. metritis
11. salpingocele
12. salpingitis
13. salpingopexy
14. prostatomegaly
15. prostatodynia, prostatalgia
16. orchidopathy, orchiopathy
17. orchialgia, orchiodynia, orchidalgia
18. balanorrhea
19. balanitis
20. balanoplasty

Additional Medical Vocabulary Recall

1. cryptorchidism
2. PSA
3. sterility
4. anorchism
5. candidiasis
6. chlamydia
7. circumcision
8. cerclage
9. lumpectomy
10. endometriosis
11. mammography
12. gonorrhea
13. syphilis
14. TSS
15. trichomoniasis
16. D&C
17. phimosis
18. impotence
19. preeclampsia
20. fistula

Pronunciation and Spelling

1. cerclage
2. cervicitis
3. chlamydia
4. circumcision
5. epispadias
6. gonadotropin
7. gynecologist
8. hysterosalpingo-oophorectomy
9. mammography
10. oophoroma
11. orchiopexy
12. Papanicolaou
13. perineorrhaphy
14. phimosis
15. prostatitis
16. pseudocyesis
17. spermicide
18. syphilis
19. trichomoniasis
20. varicocele

Chart Note Analysis

1. metastases (*metastasis,* singular)
2. postmenopausal
3. lesion
4. neoplastic
5. Premarin
6. mastectomy
7. menstrual
8. laparoscopy
9. gravida 4
10. para 4

Demonstrate What You Know!

1. ovaries
2. galactorrhea
3. hysterectomy
4. obstetrics
5. colpocystocele
6. infertility
7. fallopian tube
8. dystocia
9. fertilization
10. cryptorchidism
11. spermicide
12. urologists
13. prostatitis
14. aspermia
15. sperm

Chapter 10

Endocrine System
Combining Forms

Medical Word	Meaning
aden/oma	*tumor composed of glandular tissue.*
adrenal/ectomy **adren**/al	excision or removal of one or both adrenal glands pertaining to the adrenal glands

Medical Word	Meaning
hypo/**calc**/emia	deficiency of calcium in the blood
gluc/o/genesis hyper/**glyc**/emia	forming or producing glucose (sugar) greater than normal amount of glucose in the blood
pancreat/itis	inflammation of the pancreas
parathyroid/ectomy	excision or removal of one or both parathyroid glands
hypo/**pituitar**/ism	condition of inadequate levels of pituitary hormone in the body
thym/oma	tumor of the thymus gland
thyr/o/megaly **thyroid**/ectomy	enlargement of the thyroid gland excision of the thyroid gland
toxic/o/logist	specialist in the study of poisons or toxins

Suffixes and Prefixes

Medical Word	Meaning
Suffixes	
endo/**crine**	to secrete internally or within
hirsut/**ism**	condition of excessive hair growth in unusual places, especially in women
thyr/o/**toxic**	pertaining to toxic activity of the thyroid gland
Prefixes	
hyper/thyroid/ism	excessive secretion of the thyroid gland
poly/dipsia	excessive thirst

Medical Terminology Word Building

1. hyperglycemia
2. hypoglycemia
3. glycogenesis
4. pancreatitis
5. pancreatolysis
6. pancreatopathy
7. thyroiditis
8. thyromegaly
9. parathyroidectomy
10. adrenalectomy

Additional Medical Vocabulary Recall

1. total calcium
2. type 1 diabetes
3. cretinism
4. exophthalmos
5. insulinoma
6. myxedema
7. TFT
8. Cushing syndrome
9. panhypopituitarism
10. HRT

Pronunciation and Spelling

1. adenoma
2. adrenalectomy
3. diabetes
4. exophthalmos
5. glucose
6. hypocalcemia
7. hyperglycemia
8. insulinoma
9. mellitus
10. myxedema
11. pancreatitis
12. peripheral
13. pituitarism
14. polydipsia
15. toxicologist

Demonstrate What You Know!

1. hypocalcemia
2. hypersecretion
3. insulin
4. aerobic
5. ulceration
6. hormones
7. RAIU
8. Graves
9. GTT
10. homeostasis
11. toxicologist
12. pancreas
13. hyperglycemia
14. FBG
15. thymoma

Chart Note Analysis

1. erythema
2. antibiotic
3. vascular
4. calcaneal
5. ulceration
6. peripheral diabetic neuropathy
7. malleolus
8. trophic
9. type 1 diabetes mellitus
10. anaerobic

Chapter 11

Nervous System
Combining Forms

Medical Word	Meaning
cerebr/o/spin/al	*pertaining to the brain and spine or spinal cord*
encephal/itis	inflammation of the brain
gli/oma	tumor composed of neuroglial tissue (supportive tissue of the nervous system)
mening/o/cele	herniation, or saclike protrusion of the meninges through the skull or vertebral column
meningi/oma	tumor composed of meninges
myel/algia	pain of the spinal cord or its membranes
neur/o/lysis	destruction of a nerve

Suffixes and Prefixes

Medical Word	Meaning
Suffixes	
epi/**lepsy**	seizure disorder
a/**phasia**	absence of speech
Prefixes	
dys/phagia	difficulty speaking or impairment in the production of speech
hemi/paresis	paralysis of one half of the body (right half or left half)
para/plegia	paralysis of both legs and the lower part of the body
quadri/plegia	paralysis of all four extremities

Medical Terminology Word Building

1. neuroma
2. neurolysis
3. encephalitis
4. encephaloma
5. encephalocele
6. myelalgia, myelodynia
7. myelocele
8. cerebrospinal
9. aphasia
10. dysphasia

Additional Medical Vocabulary Recall

1. Bell palsy
2. stroke
3. epilepsy
4. thalamotomy
5. LP
6. TIA
7. Parkinson disease
8. poliomyelitis
9. sciatica
10. spina bifida
11. hydrocephalus
12. neuroblastoma
13. Alzheimer disease
14. anticonvulsants
15. dementia
16. shingles
17. anesthetics
18. antiparksonian
19. craniotomy
20. paralysis

Pronunciation and Spelling

1. Alzheimer
2. cerebrovascular
3. craniotomy
4. epilepsy
5. lumbar
6. palsy
7. poliomyelitis
8. paralysis
9. paraplegia
10. neuroblastoma
11. quadriplegia
12. spina bifida occulta
13. sciatica
14. seizure
15. shingles

Chart Note Analysis

1. anorexia
2. deglutition
3. diplopia
4. jaundice
5. vertigo
6. paralysis
7. adenocarcinoma
8. cholecystojejunostomy
9. biliary
10. metastasis
11. aphasia
12. pruritus

Demonstrate What You Know!

1. meningomyelocele
2. quadriplegia
3. meningitis
4. paresis
5. cognition
6. CNS
7. vertigo
8. PNS
9. myelalgia
10. homeostasis
11. flaccid
12. neurosurgeon
13. TIAs
14. aphasia
15. diplopia

Chapter 12

Musculoskeletal System
Combining Forms

Medical Word	Meaning
Muscles and Related Structures	
fasci/o/plasty	*surgical repair of fascia*
fibr/oma	tumor of fibrous tissue
leiomy/oma	tumor of smooth muscle
lumb/o/cost/al	pertaining to the lumbar region and the ribs
muscul/ar **my/o**/rrhexis	pertaining to muscles rupture of a muscle
ten/o/tomy **tend/o**/plasty **tendin**/itis	incision of a tendon surgical repair of a tendon inflammation of a tendon, usually resulting from strain; also called *tendonitis*
Bones of the Upper Extremities	
carp/o/ptosis	downward displacement of the wrist; also called *dropped wrist*
cervic/al	pertaining to the neck
sub/**cost**/al	beneath the ribs
crani/o/tomy	incision through the cranium, usually to gain access to the brain during neurosurgical procedures
humer/al	pertaining to the humerus
metacarp/ectomy	excision or resection of one or more metacarpal bones
phalang/itis	inflammation of one or more phalanges
spondyl/itis **vertebr**/al	inflammation of any of the vertebrae, usually characterized by stiffness and pain pertaining to a vertebra or the vertebral column
stern/o/cost/al	pertaining to the sternum and ribs
Bones of the Lower Extremities	
calcane/o/dynia	painful condition of the heel
femor/al	pertaining to the femur
fibul/ar	pertaining to the fibula

Medical Word	Meaning
Bones of the Lower Extremities	
patell/ectomy	excision of the patella
pelv/i/metry	measurement of the pelvic dimensions or proportions
pelv/is	refers to the pelvis (hipbone)
radi/o/graph	x-ray image
tibi/al	pertaining to the tibia (shin bone)
Other Related Structures	
ankyl/osis	immobility of a joint
arthr/o/desis	surgical fixation of a joint
cost/o/chondr/itis	inflammation of cartilage of the anterior chest wall (ribs)
lamin/ectomy	excision of the lamina (bony arches of one or more vertebrae)
myel/o/cele	herniation of the spinal cord
orth/o/ped/ics	branch of medicine concerned with prevention and correction of musculoskeletal system disorders
oste/o/porosis	porous bone

Suffixes and Prefixes

Medical Word	Meaning
Suffixes	
arthr/o/**clasia**	surgical breaking of adhesions to improve mobility of a joint
oste/o/**clast**	cell that breaks down bone
hemi/**plegia**	paralysis of one side of the body
my/o/**sarcoma**	malignant tumor of muscle tissue
Prefixes	
dia/physis	shaft or middle region of a long bone
peri/oste/um	layer that covers the surface of a bone

Medical Terminology Word Building

1. osteocytes
2. ostealgia, osteodynia
3. osteoarthropathy
4. osteogenesis
5. cervical
6. cervicobrachial
7. cervicofacial
8. myeloma
9. myelosarcoma
10. myelography
11. myelomalacia
12. suprasternal
13. sternoid
14. chondroblast
15. arthritis
16. osteoarthritis
17. pelvimeter
18. myospasm
19. myopathy
20. myorrhexis

Additional Medical Vocabulary Recall

1. osteoporosis
2. tendinitis
3. sprain
4. strain
5. kyphosis
6. Ewing sarcoma
7. torticollis
8. gout
9. RA
10. Paget disease
11. sequestrum
12. arthroplasty
13. crepitation
14. myasthenia gravis
15. lordosis
16. muscular dystrophy
17. contracture
18. scoliosis
19. herniated disk
20. CTS

Pronunciation and Spelling

1. abduction
2. arthroclasia
3. dorsiflexion
4. phalangitis
5. fascioplasty
6. gout
7. crepitation
8. leiomyoma
9. myosarcoma
10. myasthenia gravis
11. orthopedics
12. osteoarthropathy
13. osteoclast
14. Paget disease
15. pelvimetry
16. rheumatoid arthritis
17. sequestrectomy
18. spondylomalacia
19. sternocostal
20. torticollis

Chart Note Analysis

1. sacroiliac
2. L3-4
3. flexion
4. anteroposterior
5. bilateral
6. hypertrophic
7. lumbosacral
8. lateral
9. extension
10. intervertebral

Demonstrate What You Know!

1. talipes
2. arthrocentesis
3. subluxation
4. ankylosis
5. rheumatologist
6. carpoptosis
7. articulate
8. rickets
9. muscles
10. degenerative
11. gouty
12. laminectomy
13. greenstick
14. NSAIDs
15. calcaneodynia

Chapter 13

Special Senses: Eyes and Ears
Combining Forms

Medical Word	Meaning
Eye	
blephar/o/spasm	*involuntary contraction of the eyelid*
choroid/o/pathy	disease of the choroid (layer between the retina and sclera)

Medical Word	Meaning
Eye	
conjunctiv/itis	inflammation of the conjunctiva; also called *pinkeye*
corne/itis	inflammation of the cornea; also called *keratitis*
aniso/**cor**/ia **core**/o/meter **pupill**/ary	inequality of pupil size instrument for measuring the pupil pertaining to the pupil
dacry/o/rrhea	excessive secretion of tears
lacrim/ation	secretion and discharge of tears
dipl/opia	two images of an object seen at the same time; also called *double vision*
irid/o/plegia	paralysis of the sphincter of the iris
kerat/o/plasty	surgical repair of the cornea; also called *corneal transplant*
intra/**ocul**/ar **ophthalm**/o/scope	pertaining to within the eyeball instrument for examining the eye
opt/ic	pertaining to the eye or vision
retin/o/pathy	disease of the retina
Ear	
acous/tic **audi**/o/meter **audit**/ory	pertaining to hearing instrument for measuring levels of hearing pertaining to sense of hearing
myring/o/tomy **tympan**/o/plasty	incision of the tympanic membrane surgical repair of the tympanic membrane
ot/o/rrhea	discharge from the ear
salping/o/pharyng/eal	pertaining to the eustachian tube and pharynx

Suffixes and Prefixes

Medical Word	Meaning
Suffixes	
an/**acusis** presby/**cusis**	without hearing; total deafness hearing loss associated with old age

(Continued)

Medical Word	Meaning
Suffixes	
ambly/**opia** heter/**opsia**	reduction or dimness of vision usually in one eye with no apparent pathological condition; also called *lazy eye* inequality of vision in the two eyes
blephar/o/**ptosis**	downward displacement or drooping of the upper eyelid
Prefixes	
exo/tropia	abnormal turning outward of one or both eyes; also called *divergent strabismus*
hyper/opia	excess (farsighted) vision

Medical Terminology Word Building

1. ophthalmoplegia, ophthalmoparalysis
2. ophthalmology
3. pupilloscopy
4. keratomalacia
5. keratometer
6. scleritis
7. scleromalacia
8. iridoplegia, iridoparalysis
9. iridocele
10. retinopathy
11. retinitis
12. blepharoplegia
13. blepharoptosis
14. blepharoplasty
15. otopyorrhea
16. audiometer
17. myringotome
18. myringoplasty
19. salpingitis
20. salpingopharyngeal

Additional Medical Vocabulary Recall

1. tinnitus
2. otosclerosis
3. achromatopsia
4. Ménière disease
5. strabismus
6. anacusis
7. otitis media
8. conjunctivitis
9. photophobia
10. presbycusis
11. glaucoma
12. vertigo
13. retinal detachment
14. hordeolum
15. astigmatism
16. myringoplasty
17. tonometry
18. iridectomy
19. Rinne
20. cataract

Pronunciation and Spelling

1. acoustic neuroma
2. achromatopsia
3. astigmatism
4. auditory
5. blepharoptosis
6. dacryorrhea
7. exotropia
8. phacoemulsification
9. glaucoma
10. hordeolum
11. iridoplegia
12. conjunctivitis
13. Ménière
14. ophthalmoscope
15. presbycusis
16. salpingopharyngeal
17. strabismus
18. tympanoplasty
19. tinnitus
20. vertigo

Chart Note Analysis

1. chronic
2. mucoserous
3. tympanoplasty
4. otitis media
5. ENT
6. cholesteatoma
7. general anesthetic
8. diagnosis
9. adhesive
10. postoperatively

Demonstrate What You Know!

1. ophthalmoplegia
2. esotropia
3. blepharoplasty
4. mydriatics
5. heteropsia
6. exotropia
7. blepharoptosis
8. diagnosis
9. cholesteatoma
10. tympanitis

Abbreviations and Symbols

Abbreviations

The table below lists common abbreviations used in health care and related fields along with their meanings.

Abbreviation	Meaning	Abbreviation	Meaning
A		AF	atrial fibrillation
A&P	anatomy and physiology; auscultation and percussion	AFB	acid-fast bacillus (TB organism)
A, B, AB, O	blood types in ABO blood group	AGN	acute glomerulonephritis
		AI	artificial insemination
AAA	abdominal aortic aneurysm	AICD	automatic implantable cardioverter defibrillator
AB, Ab, ab	antibody; abortion		
ABC	aspiration biopsy cytology	AIDS	acquired immune deficiency syndrome
ABG	arterial blood gas(es)		
a.c.*	before meals	AK	above the knee
ACL	anterior cruciate ligament	ALL	acute lymphocytic leukemia
ACTH	adrenocorticotropic hormone	ALS	amyotrophic lateral sclerosis (also called *Lou Gehrig disease*)
ad lib.	as desired		
AD*	right ear	ALT	alanine aminotransferase
ADH	antidiuretic hormone (vasopressin)	AM, a.m.	in the morning (before noon)
		AML	acute myelogenous leukemia
ADHD	attention-deficit hyperactivity disorder	ANA	antinuclear antibody (test)
		ANS	autonomic nervous system
ADLs	activities of daily living	ant	anterior
AE	above the elbow	AOM	acute otitis media
AED	automatic external defibrillator	AP	anteroposterior

(Continued)

Abbreviation	Meaning	Abbreviation	Meaning
ARDS	acute respiratory distress syndrome	CA	cancer; chronological age; cardiac arrest
ARF	acute renal failure	Ca	calcium; cancer
ARMD, AMD	age-related macular degeneration	CABG	coronary artery bypass graft
AS	aortic stenosis	CAD	coronary artery disease
AS*	left ear	CAH	chronic active hepatitis; congenital adrenal hyperplasia
ASD	atrial septal defect		
ASHD	arteriosclerotic heart disease	CAT	computed axial tomography
AST	angiotensin sensitivity test	Cath	catheterization; catheter
Ast	astigmatism	CBC	complete blood count
AU*	both ears	CC	cardiac catheterization; chief complaint
AV	atrioventricular; arteriovenous		
		cc*	cubic centimeters; same as milliliters (1/1,000 of a liter)
B		CCU	coronary care unit
Ba	barium	CDH	congenital dislocation of the hip
baso	basophil (type of white blood cell)		
BBB	bundle-branch block	CF	cystic fibrosis
BC	bone conduction	CHD	coronary heart disease
BCC	basal cell carcinoma	chemo	chemotherapy
BE	barium enema; below the elbow	CHF	congestive heart failure
		Chol	cholesterol
BG	blood glucose	CK	creatine kinase (cardiac enzyme); conductive keratoplasty
b.i.d.*	twice a day		
BK	below the knee		
BKA	below-knee amputation	CLL	chronic lymphocytic leukemia
BM	bowel movement		
BMI	body mass index	cm	centimeter (1/100 of a meter)
BMR	basal metabolic rate	CML	chronic myelogenous leukemia
BNO	bladder neck obstruction		
BP, B/P	blood pressure	CNS	central nervous system
BPH	benign prostatic hyperplasia; benign prostatic hypertrophy	c/o	complains of, complaints
		CO	cardiac output
BS	blood sugar	CO₂	carbon dioxide
BSE	breast self-examination	COPD	chronic obstructive pulmonary disease
BSO	bilateral salpingo-oophorectomy		
		CP	cerebral palsy
BUN	blood urea nitrogen	CPAP	continuous positive airway pressure
Bx, bx	biopsy		
		CPD	cephalopelvic disproportion
C		CPK	creatine phosphokinase (enzyme released into the bloodstream after a heart attack)
C1, C2, and so on	first cervical vertebra, second cervical vertebra, and so on		

Abbreviation	Meaning	Abbreviation	Meaning
CPR	cardiopulmonary resuscitation	D.P.M.	Doctor of Podiatric Medicine
CRF	chronic renal failure	DPT	diphtheria, pertussis, tetanus
CRRT	continuous renal replacement therapy	DRE	digital rectal examination
C&S	culture and sensitivity	DSA	digital subtraction angiography
CS, C-section	cesarean section	DUB	dysfunctional uterine bleeding
CSF	cerebrospinal fluid	DVT	deep vein thrombosis; deep venous thrombosis
CT	computed tomography		
CTS	carpal tunnel syndrome	Dx	diagnosis
CV	cardiovascular		
CVA	cerebrovascular accident; costovertebral angle	**E**	
		EBV	Epstein-Barr virus
CVD	cardiovascular disease	ECCE	extracapsular cataract extraction
CVS	chorionic villus sampling		
CWP	childbirth without pain	ECG, EKG	electrocardiogram; electrocardiography
CXR	chest x-ray, chest radiograph		
cysto	cystoscopy	ECHO	echocardiogram; echocardiography; echoencephalogram; echoencephalography
D			
D	diopter (lens strength)		
dc, DC, D/C*	discharge; discontinue	ED	erectile dysfunction; emergency department
D&C	dilatation (dilation) and curettage		
Decub.	decubitus (lying down)	EEG	electroencephalogram; electroencephalography
derm	dermatology		
DES	diffuse esophageal spasm; drug-eluting stent	EENT	eyes, ears, nose, and throat
		EF	ejection fraction
DEXA, DXA	dual energy x-ray absorptiometry	EGD	esophagogastroduodenoscopy
		ELT	endovenous laser ablation; endoluminal laser ablation
DI	diabetes insipidus; diagnostic imaging		
		Em	emmetropia
diff	differential count (white blood cells)	EMG	electromyography
		ENT	ears, nose, and throat
DJD	degenerative joint disease	EOM	extraocular movement
DKA	diabetic ketoacidosis	eos	eosinophil (type of white blood cell)
DM	diabetes mellitus		
DMARDs	disease modifying antirheumatic drugs	ERCP	endoscopic retrograde cholangiopancreatography
DNA	deoxyribonucleic acid	ESR	erythrocyte sedimentation rate
D.O., DO	Doctor of Osteopathy	ESRD	end-stage renal disease
DOE	dyspnea on exertion	ESWL	extracorporeal shock-wave lithotripsy
DPI	dry powder inhaler		
		ETT	exercise tolerance test

(Continued)

Abbreviation	Meaning	Abbreviation	Meaning
F		HCl	hydrochloric acid
FBS	fasting blood sugar	HCT, Hct	hematocrit
FECG, FEKG	fetal electrocardiogram	HCV	hepatitis C virus
FH	family history	HD	hemodialysis; hip disarticulation; hearing distance
FHR	fetal heart rate		
FHT	fetal heart tone	HDL	high-density lipoprotein
FS	frozen section	HDN	hemolytic disease of the newborn
FSH	follicle-stimulating hormone		
		HDV	hepatitis D virus
FTND	full-term normal delivery	HEV	hepatitis E virus
FVC	forced vital capacity	HF	heart failure
Fx	fracture	HIV	human immunodeficiency virus
G			
G	gravida (pregnant)	HMD	hyaline membrane disease
g, gm	gram	HNP	herniated nucleus pulposus (herniated disk)
GB	gallbladder		
GBS	gallbladder series (x-ray studies)	HP	hemipelvectomy
		HPV	human papillomavirus
GC	gonococcus (*Neisseria gonorrhoeae*)	HRT	hormone replacement therapy
G-CSF	granulocyte colony-stimulating factor	hs*	half strength
		h.s.*	at bedtime
GER	gastroesophageal reflux	HSG	hysterosalpingography
GERD	gastroesophageal reflux disease	HSV	herpes simplex virus
		HTN	hypertension
GH	growth hormone	Hx	history
GI	gastrointestinal		
GTT	glucose tolerance test	**I, J**	
GU	genitourinary	IAS	interatrial septum
GVHD	graft-versus-host disease	IBD	irritable bowel disease
GVHR	graft-versus-host reaction	IBS	irritable bowel syndrome
GYN	gynecology	ICD	implantable cardioverter-defibrillator
H		ICP	intracranial pressure
H_2O	water	ICU	intensive care unit
HAV	hepatitis A virus	I&D	incision and drainage; irrigation and debridement
Hb, Hgb, hgb	hemoglobin		
HBV	hepatitis B virus	ID	intradermal
HCG	human chorionic gonadotropin	IDDM	insulin-dependent diabetes mellitus
		Ig	immunoglobulin

Abbreviation	Meaning	Abbreviation	Meaning
IM	intramuscular; infectious mononucleosis	LDL	low-density lipoprotein
		LES	lower esophageal sphincter
IMP	impression (synonymous with diagnosis)	LFT	liver function test
		LH	luteinizing hormone
IOL	intraocular lens	LLQ	left lower quadrant
IOP	intraocular pressure	LMP	last menstrual period
IPPB	intermittent positive-pressure breathing	LOC	loss of consciousness
		LP	lumbar puncture
IRDS	infant respiratory distress syndrome	LPR	laryngopharyngeal reflux
		LS	lumbosacral spine
IT	inhalation therapy; intensive therapy	LSO	left salpingo-oophorectomy
		lt	left
IUD	intrauterine device	LUQ	left upper quadrant
IUGR	intrauterine growth rate; intrauterine growth retardation	LV	left ventricle
		lymphos	lymphocytes
IV	intravenous	**M**	
IVC	intravenous cholangiogram; intravenous cholangiography	MCH	mean cell hemoglobin (average amount of hemoglobin per red cell)
IVF	in vitro fertilization		
IVF-ET	in vitro fertilization and embryo transfer	MCHC	mean cell hemoglobin concentration (average concentration of hemoglobin per red cell)
IVP	intravenous pyelogram; intravenous pyelography		
		MCV	mean cell volume (average volume or size per red cell)
K		MDI	metered-dose inhaler
K	potassium (an electrolyte)	MEG	magnetoencephalography
KD	knee disarticulation	MG	myasthenia gravis
KUB	kidney, ureter, bladder	mg	milligram (1/1,000 of a gram)
		mg/dl, mg/dL	milligram per deciliter
L		MI	myocardial infarction
L	liter	mix astig	mixed astigmatism
L1, L2 (and so on)	first lumbar vertebra, second lumbar vertebra (and so on)	ml, mL	milliliter (1/1,000 of a liter)
LA	left atrium	mm	millimeter (1/1,000 of a meter)
LASIK	laser-assisted in situ keratomileusis	mm Hg	millimeters of mercury
LAT, lat	lateral	MR	mitral regurgitation
LBBB	left bundle-branch block	MRA	magnetic resonance angiogram; magnetic resonance angiography
LD	lactate dehydrogenase; lactic acid dehydrogenase (cardiac enzyme)		
		MRI	magnetic resonance imaging

(Continued)

Abbreviation	Meaning	Abbreviation	Meaning
MSH	melanocyte-stimulating hormone	**P**	
MUGA	multiple-gated acquisition (scan)	P	phosphorus; pulse
		PA	posteroanterior; pernicious anemia; pulmonary artery; physician assistant
MVP	mitral valve prolapse		
MVR	mitral valve replacement; massive vitreous retraction (blade); microvitreoretinal	PAC	premature atrial contraction
		Pap	Papanicolaou (test)
Myop	myopia (nearsightedness)	para 1, 2, 3 (and so on)	unipara, bipara, tripara (and so on) (number of viable births)
N		PAT	paroxysmal atrial tachycardia
Na	sodium (an electrolyte)	PBI	protein-bound iodine
NB	newborn	pc, p.c.*	after meals
NCV	nerve conduction velocity	PCL	posterior cruciate ligament
NG	nasogastric	PCNL	percutaneous nephrolithotomy
NIDDM	non–insulin-dependent diabetes mellitus	P_{CO_2}	partial pressure of carbon dioxide
NIHL	noise-induced hearing loss	PCP	*Pneumocystis* pneumonia; primary care physician; phen-cyclidine (hallucinogen)
NK	natural killer cell		
NMT	nebulized mist treatment		
NPO, n.p.o.*	nothing by mouth		
NSAID	nonsteroidal anti-inflammatory drug	PE	physical examination; pulmonary embolism; pressure-equalizing (tube)
NSR	normal sinus rhythm		
		PERRLA	pupils equal, round, and reactive to light and accommodation
O			
O₂	oxygen		
OB	obstetrics	PET	positron emission tomography
OCP	oral contraceptive pill		
OD	overdose	PFT	pulmonary function test
OD*	right eye	PGH	pituitary growth hormone
O.D.	Doctor of Optometry	pH	symbol for degree of acidity or alkalinity
OM	otitis media		
OP	outpatient; operative procedure	PID	pelvic inflammatory disease
		PIH	pregnancy-induced hypertension
OR	operating room		
ORTH, ortho	orthopedics	PKD	polycystic kidney disease
OS*	left eye	PMH	past medical history
os	opening; mouth	PMI	point of maximum impulse
OSA	obstructive sleep apnea	PMN, PMNL	polymorphonuclear leukocyte
OU*	both eyes	PMP	previous menstrual period

Abbreviation	Meaning	Abbreviation	Meaning
PMS	premenstrual syndrome	RDS	respiratory distress syndrome
PND	paroxysmal nocturnal dyspnea	RF	rheumatoid factor; radio frequency
PNS	peripheral nervous system	RGB	Roux-en-Y gastric bypass
p.o.*	by mouth	RIA	radioimmunoassay
Po$_2$	partial pressure of oxygen	RK	radial keratotomy
poly	polymorphonuclear leukocyte	RLQ	right lower quadrant
		R/O	rule out
post	posterior	ROM	range of motion
p.r.n.*	as required	RP	retrograde pyelogram; retrograde pyelography
PSA	prostate-specific antigen		
PT	prothrombin time; physical therapy	RSO	right salpingo-oophorectomy
		rt	right
pt	patient	RUQ	right upper quadrant
PTCA	percutaneous transluminal coronary angioplasty	RV	residual volume; right ventricle
PTH	parathyroid hormone (also called *parathormone*)		
		S	
PTHC	percutaneous transhepatic cholangeography	S1, S2 (and so on)	first sacral vertebra, second sacral vertebra (and so on)
PTT	partial thromboplastin time	SA, S-A	sinoatrial
PUD	peptic ulcer disease	Sao$_2$	arterial oxygen saturation
PVC	premature ventricular contraction	SCC	squamous cell carcinoma
		SD	shoulder disarticulation
		SIADH	syndrome of inappropriate antidiuretic hormone
Q			
q.2h.*	every 2 hours	SICS	small incision cataract surgery
qAM*	every morning		
q.d.*	every day	SIDS	sudden infant death syndrome
q.h.*	every hour		
q.i.d.*	four times a day	SLE	systemic lupus erythematosus; slit-lamp examination
q.o.d.*	every other day		
qPM*	every evening	SMAS	superficial musculoaponeurotic system (flap)
R		SNS	sympathetic nervous system
RA	right atrium; rheumatoid arthritis	SOB	shortness of breath
		sono	sonogram
RAI	radioactive iodine	sp. gr.	specific gravity
RAIU	radioactive iodine uptake	SPECT	single photon emission computed tomography
RBC, rbc	red blood cell		
RD	respiratory distress	ST	esotropia

(Continued)

Abbreviation	Meaning	Abbreviation	Meaning
stat., STAT	immediately	TVH-BSO	total vaginal hysterectomy–
STD	sexually transmitted disease		bilateral salpingo-
subcu, *	subcutaneous (injection)		oophorectomy
Sub-Q, *		Tx	treatment
subQ*			
Sx	symptom	**U**	
		UA	urinalysis
T		UC	uterine contractions
T1, T2	first thoracic vertebra, second	UGI	upper gastrointestinal
(and so on)	thoracic vertebra (and so on)	UGIS	upper gastrointestinal series
T_3	triiodothyronine (thyroid	U&L, U/L	upper and lower
	hormone)	ung	ointment
T_4	thyroxine (thyroid hormone)	UPP	uvulopalatopharyngoplasty
T&A	tonsillectomy and	URI	upper respiratory infection
	adenoidectomy	US	ultrasound; ultrasonography
TAH	total abdominal	UTI	urinary tract infection
	hysterectomy	UV	ultraviolet
TB	tuberculosis		
TFT	thyroid function test	**V**	
THA	total hip arthroplasty	VA	visual acuity
ther	therapy	VC	vital capacity
THR	total hip replacement	VCUG	voiding cystourethrography
TIA	transient ischemic attack	VD	venereal disease
TIBC	total iron–binding capacity	VF	visual field
t.i.d.*	three times a day	VSD	ventricular septal defect
TKA	total knee arthroplasty	VT	ventricular tachycardia
TKR	total knee replacement	VUR	vesicoureteral reflux
TPPV	trans pars plana vitrectomy		
TPR	temperature, pulse, and	**W**	
	respiration	WBC, wbc	white blood cell
TRAM	transverse rectus abdominis	WD	well-developed
	muscle	WN	well-nourished
TSE	testicular self-examination	WNL	within normal limits
TSH	thyroid-stimulating hor-		
	mone	**X, Y, Z**	
TSS	toxic shock syndrome	XP, XDP	xeroderma pigmentosum
TURP	transurethral resection of	XT	exotropia
	the prostate		
TVH	total vaginal hysterectomy		

*Although these abbreviations are currently found in medical records and clinical notes, they are easily misinterpreted. Thus, The Joint Commission (formerly JCAHO) requires their discontinuance. Instead, they recommend to write out their meanings. For a summary of these abbreviations, see the table below.

Summary of Discontinued Abbreviations

As noted above, the Joint Commission has recommended the discontinuance of certain abbreviations that are easily misinterpreted in medical records. The table below lists these abbreviations along with their meanings.

Abbreviation	Meaning
Medication and Therapy Time Schedule	
a.c.	before meals
b.i.d.	twice a day
hs	half strength
h.s.	at bedtime
NPO, n.p.o.	nothing by mouth
p.c.	after meals
p.o.	by mouth (orally)
p.r.n.	as required
qAM	every morning
q.d.	every day
q.h.	every hour
q.2h.	every 2 hours
q.i.d.	four times a day
q.o.d.	every other day
qPM	every evening
t.i.d.	three times a day
Other Related Abbreviations	
AD	right ear
AS	left ear
AU	both ears
cc	cubic centimeters; same as ml (1/1000 of a liter) *Use ml for milliliters or write out the meaning.*
dc, DC, D/C	discharge; discontinue
OD	right eye

(Continued)

Abbreviation	Meaning
Other Related Abbreviations	
OS	left eye
OU	both eyes
subcu, Sub-Q, subQ	subcutaneous (injection)
U	unit

Common Symbols

The table below lists some common symbols used in health care and related fields.

Symbol	Meaning	Symbol	Meaning
@	at	−	minus, negative
āā	of each	±	plus or minus; either positive or negative; indefinite
′	foot	∅	no
″	inch	#	number; following a number; pounds
c̄	with	÷	divided by
Δ	change; heat	/	divided by
p̄	after	×	multiplied by; magnification
pH	degree of acidity or alkalinity	=	equals
℞	prescription, treatment, therapy	≈	approximately equal
s̄	without	°	degree
→	to, in the direction of	%	percent
↑	increase(d), up	♀	female
↓	decrease(d), down	♂	male
+	plus, positive		

Drug Classifications

This section provides a quick reference of common drug categories. They include prescription and over-the-counter drugs that are used to treat symptoms, signs, and diseases of the various body systems.

Drug Classification	Description
alkylates	Treat certain types of malignancies *Alkylates break deoxyribonucleic acid (DNA) strands in the cancerous cell by substituting an alkyl group for a hydrogen molecule in the DNA.*
analgesics	Relieve minor to severe pain *Analgesics include nonprescription drugs, such as aspirin and other nonsteroidal anti-inflammatory agents, and those classified as controlled substances and available only by prescription.*
angiotensin-converting enzyme inhibitors	Lower blood pressure by inhibiting conversion of angiotensin I (an inactive enzyme) to angiotensin II (a potent vasoconstrictor)
androgens	Increase testosterone levels *Hyposecretion of testosterone may be due to surgical removal of testes, or decreased levels of luteinizing hormone (LH) from the anterior pituitary gland.*
anesthetics	Produce partial or complete loss of sensation, with or without loss of consciousness *General anesthetics act upon the brain to produce complete loss of feeling with loss of consciousness. Local anesthetics act upon nerves or nerve tracts to affect a local area only.*

(Continued)

Drug Classification	Description
antacids	Neutralize excess acid in the stomach and help relieve gastritis and ulcer pain *Antacids are also used to relieve indigestion and reflux esophagitis (heartburn).*
antianginals	Relieve angina pectoris by vasodilation
antianxiety drugs	Reduce anxiety and neurosis *Antianxiety drugs are classified as minor tranquilizers and anxiolytics.*
antiarrhythmics	Treat cardiac arrhythmias by stabilizing the electrical conduction of the heart
antibiotics	Inhibit growth of or destroy microorganisms *Antibiotics are used extensively in treatment of infectious diseases.*
anticoagulants	Prevent or delay blood coagulation *Anticoagulants prevent deep vein thrombosis (DVT) and postoperative clot formation and decrease the risk of stroke.*
anticonvulsants	Prevent or reduce the severity of epileptic or other convulsive seizures; also called *antiepileptics*
antidepressants	Regulate mood and reduce symptoms of depression by affecting the amount of neurotransmitters in the brain
antidiabetics	Stimulate the pancreas to produce more insulin and decrease peripheral resistance to insulin *Antidiabetics are taken orally to treat type 2 diabetes mellitus.*
antidiarrheals	Control loose stools and relieve diarrhea by absorbing excess water in the bowel or slowing peristalsis in the intestinal tract
antidiuretics	Reduce the production of urine
antiemetics	Prevent or suppress vomiting *Antiemetics are also used in the treatment of vertigo, motion sickness, and nausea.*
antifungals	Alter the cell wall of fungi or disrupt enzyme activity, resulting in cellular death
antihistamines	Counteract the effects of a histamine *Antihistamines inhibit allergic reactions of inflammation, redness, and itching, especially hay fever and other allergic disorders of the nasal passages.*

Drug Classification	Description
antihyperlipidemics	Lower lipid levels in the bloodstream *Antihyperlipidemics reduce the risk of heart attack by lowering lipid levels.*
antihypertensives	Lower blood pressure
anti-impotence	Treat erectile dysfunction (impotence) by increasing blood flow to the penis, resulting in an erection
anti-infectives, antibacterials, antifungals	Eliminate or inhibit bacterial or fungal infections *Anti-infectives, antibacterials, and antifungals can be administered either topically or systemically.*
anti-inflammatories	Relieve the swelling, tenderness, redness, and pain of inflammation *Anti-inflammatories may be classified as steroidal (corticosteroids) or nonsteroidal.*
corticosteroids (glucocorticoids)	Relieve inflammation and replace hormones for adrenal insufficiency (Addison disease) *Corticosteroids are widely used to suppress the immune system's inflammatory response to tissue damage, controlling allergic reactions, reducing the rejection process in tissue and organ transplantation, and treating some cancers.*
nonsteroidals (NSAIDs)	Relieve inflammation associated with arthritis and related disorders
antimetabolites	Interfere with the use of enzymes required for cell division *Antimetabolites block folic acid, a B vitamin required for synthesis of some amino acids in the DNA of cancerous cells.*
antimicrobials	Destroy or inhibit the growth of bacteria, fungi, and protozoa, depending on the particular drug, generally by interfering with the functions of their cell membrane or their reproductive cycle
antiparkinsonians	Control tremors and muscle rigidity associated with Parkinson disease by increasing dopamine levels in the brain
antipruritics	Prevent or relieve itching
antipsychotics	Treat psychosis, paranoia, and schizophrenia by altering chemicals in the brain, including the limbic system (group of brain structures), which controls emotions
antiseptics	Topically applied agent that destroys or inhibits the growth of bacteria, preventing infection in cuts, scratches, and surgical incisions
antispasmodics	Act on the autonomic nervous system to reduce spasms in the bladder or GI tract

(Continued)

Drug Classification	Description
antithyroids	Treat hyperthyroidism by impeding the formation of T_3 and T_4 hormone
antituberculars	Used in the treatment of tuberculosis *Several of these drugs are used in combination to produce effective treatment.*
antitussives	Relieve or suppress coughing by blocking the cough reflex in the medulla of the brain
antivirals	Prevent replication of viruses within host cells *Antivirals are used in treatment of HIV infection and AIDS.*
astringents	Shrink the blood vessels locally, dry up secretions from seeping lesions, and lessen skin sensitivity
beta-adrenergic blockers	Treat cardiac arrhythmias, angina pectoris, and hypertension and improve outcomes after myocardial infarction; also called *beta blockers* *Beta-adrenergic blocking agents block the effect of epinephrine on beta receptors, slowing the nerve pulses that pass through the heart, thereby causing a decrease in heart rate and contractility. Some beta-adrenergic blockers are also used to treat glaucoma.*
bone resorption inhibitors	Inhibit breakdown of bone *Bone resorption inhibitors are used to treat osteoporosis.*
bronchodilators	Stimulate bronchial muscles to relax, thereby expanding air passages and resulting in increased air flow to the lungs
calcium channel blockers	Selectively block movement of calcium (required for blood vessel contraction) into myocardial cells and arterial walls, causing heart rate and blood pressure to decrease *Calcium channel blockers are used to treat angina pectoris, arrhythmias, heart failure, and hypertension.*
chrysotherapy	Treat certain diseases with gold compounds; also called *gold therapy* *Chrysotherapy is used to treat rheumatoid arthritis.*

Drug Classification	Description
contraceptives	Prevent conception or ovulation; also called *birth control*
birth control patch	Delivers two synthetic hormones, progestin and estrogen, through a transdermal patch, impeding pregnancy by preventing the ovaries from releasing eggs (ovulation) and thickening the cervical mucus *The patch is applied directly to the skin (buttocks, abdomen, upper torso, or upper outer arm) and has an effectiveness rate of 95%.*
injectable	Delivers a synthetic drug similar to progesterone (medroxyprogesterone acetate) through an injection administered four times per year that prevents the ovaries from releasing eggs (ovulation) and thickens the cervical mucus *When used as directed, an injectable contraceptive (Depo-Provera) may prevent pregnancy more than 99% of the time.*
oral	Inhibits ovulation and pituitary secretion of luteinizing hormone (LH), causing changes in cervical mucus that render it unfavorable to penetration by sperm and altering the nature of the endometrium; also called *birth control pills* *Oral contraceptives (OCs) contain mixtures of estrogen and progestin in various levels of strength. When used as directed, oral contraceptives (OCs) are nearly 100% effective.*
cycloplegics	Paralyze the ciliary muscles, resulting in pupil dilation *Cycloplegics are used to dilate the pupils to facilitate certain eye examinations and surgical procedures.*
cytotoxics	Disrupt nucleic acid and protein synthesis, causing immunosuppression and cancer cell death *Cytotoxics are used to treat cancer and autoimmune diseases, such as inflammatory bowel disease and systemic vasculitis. They are also used to prevent rejection in transplant recipients.*
decongestants	Decrease congestion of mucous membranes of sinuses and nose *Decongestants are used for temporary relief of nasal congestion associated with the common cold, hay fever, other upper respiratory allergies, and sinusitis.*
diuretics	Act on the kidney to promote the excretion of sodium and water *Diuretics are used to treat edema and hypertension.*
emetics	Used to induce vomiting, especially in cases of poisoning
estrogen hormone	Used in estrogen replacement therapy (ERT) during menopause to correct estrogen deficiency and as chemotherapy for some types of cancer, including tumors of the prostate

(Continued)

Drug Classification	Description
expectorants	Liquefy respiratory secretions so that they are more easily dislodged during coughing episodes
fibrinolytics	Trigger the body to produce plasmin, an enzyme that dissolves clots *Fibrinolytics are used to treat acute pulmonary embolism and, occasionally, deep vein thrombosis.*
gonadotropins	Raise sperm count in infertility cases
growth hormone replacements	Increase skeletal growth in children and growth hormone deficiencies in adults
H$_2$ blockers	Block histamine-2 (H$_2$) receptors in the stomach to decrease the release of hydrochloric acid *H$_2$ blockers are used to treat peptic ulcers.*
hemostatics	Prevent or control bleeding *Hemostatics are used to treat blood disorders and certain bleeding problems associated with surgery.*
hypnotics	Depress the central nervous system (CNS) to induce or maintain sleep
inotropics, cardiotonics	Increase the efficiency of contractions of the heart muscle *Inotropics are used to treat cardiac arrhythmias and cardiac failure.*
insulins	Synthetic form of insulin hormone for diabetes administered by injection to lower the glucose (sugar) level in the blood
keratolytics	Destroy and soften the outer layer of skin so that it is sloughed off or shed. *Strong keratolytics are effective for removing warts and corns. Milder preparations are used to promote the shedding of scales and crusts in eczema, psoriasis, and seborrheic dermatitis. Weak keratolytics irritate inflamed skin, acting as tonics that speed up the healing process.*
laxatives (cathartic, purgative)	Induce bowel movements or loosen stool *When used in smaller doses, laxatives relieve constipation. When used in larger doses, they evacuate the entire gastrointestinal tract—for example, as preparation for surgery or intestinal radiologic examinations.*
miotics	Constrict the pupil of the eye *Miotics are used in the treatment of glaucoma.*
mucolytics	Liquefy sputum or reduce its viscosity so that it can be coughed up more easily

Drug Classification	Description
mydriatics	Dilate the pupil and paralyze the muscles of accommodation of the iris *Mydriatics are used to prepare the eye for internal examination and to treat inflammatory conditions of the iris.*
nitrates	Treat angina pectoris by dilating arteries and increasing blood flow to the myocardium
opiates	Relieve pain *Opiates contain opium or its derivative. They are commonly prescribed on a short-term basis due to their strong addictive property.*
parasiticides	Destroy systemic parasites, such as pinworm or tapeworm, in oral form or insect parasites, such as mites and lice, in topical form
potassium supplements	Increase the potassium level of the blood *Potassium can be administered orally or intravenously (IV) when dangerously low levels occur. It is used as a replacement for potassium loss due to diuretics.*
prostaglandins	Used to induce labor, terminate pregnancy, or treat erectile dysfunction, patent ductus arteriosis, or pulmonary hypertension
protectives	Function by covering, cooling, drying, or soothing inflamed skin *Protectives do not penetrate or soften the skin but form a long-lasting film that protects the skin from air, water, and clothing during the natural healing process.*
proton pump inhibitors	Block the final stage of hydrochloric acid production in the stomach *Proton pump inhibitors are used to treat peptic ulcers and gastroesophageal reflux disease (GERD).*
psychotropics	Alter chemical balance in the brain, causing changes in perception, mood, and behavior *Psychotropics are commonly employed in the management of psychiatric disorders.*
relaxants	Reduce tension, causing relaxation of muscles or bowel
salicylates	Relieve mild to moderate pain and reduce inflammation
sclerotherapy	Injection of a chemical into a varicose vein to cause inflammation and formation of fibrous tissue, which closes the vein
sedatives	Exert a calming or tranquilizing effect
skeletal muscle relaxants	Relieve muscle spasms and stiffness

(Continued)

Drug Classification	Description
spermicides	Chemically destroy sperm *Spermicidals consist of jellies, creams, and foams and do not require a prescription. They are commonly used within the woman's vagina for contraceptive purposes.*
statins	Lower cholesterol in the blood and reduce its production in the liver by blocking the enzyme that produces it
thrombolytics	Dissolve blood clots by destroying their fibrin strands *Thrombolytics are used to break apart, or lyse, thrombi.*
thyroid supplements	Replace or supplement thyroid hormones
topical anesthetics	Block sensation of pain by numbing the skin layers and mucous membranes *Topical anesthetics are applied directly in sprays, creams, gargles, suppositories, and other preparations. They are also used to numb the skin to make the injection of medication more comfortable.*
tranquilizers	Calm anxiousness or agitation without decreasing consciousness
uricosurics	Increase urinary excretion of uric acid, reducing the concentration of uric acid in the blood *Uricosurics are used in treatment of gout.*
uterine stimulants	Induce labor at term, control postpartum hemorrhage, and induce therapeutic abortion; also called *oxytocic agents* *Oxytocin is a pharmaceutically prepared chemical that is similar to the pituitary hormone oxytocin. Uterine stimulants are also used to treat infertility in females.*
vasoconstrictors	Narrow or constrict the diameter of blood vessels *Vasoconstrictors are used to decrease blood flow and increase blood pressure.*
vasodilators	Dilate the diameter of blood vessels *Vasodilators are used in treatment of angina pectoris and hypertension.*
vitamin B_{12}	Treats pernicious anemia *Vitamin B_{12} is delivered by nasal spray or intramuscular (IM) injection.*

Medical Specialties

Medical Specialty	Medical Specialist	Description of Medical Specialty
Allergy	Allergist	Diagnosis and treatment of allergic disorders caused by hypersensitivity to foods, pollens, dusts, and medicines
Anesthesiology	Anesthesiologist	Administration of agents capable of bringing about loss of sensation with or without loss of consciousness
Cardiology	Cardiologist	Diagnosis and treatment of heart and vascular disorders
General practice (GP)	General Practitioner (GP)	Coordination of total health care delivery to all members of the family, regardless of sex, including counseling; also known as *family medicine* *The GP encompasses several branches of medicine, including internal medicine, preventive medicine, pediatrics, surgery, obstetrics, and gynecology.*
Geriatrics	Geriatrician	Understanding of the physiological characteristics of aging and the diagnosis and treatment of diseases affecting elderly patients; also known as *gerontology*
Gynecology	Gynecologist	Diagnosis and treatment of diseases of the female reproductive organs
Hematology	Hematologist	Diagnosis and treatment of diseases of the blood and blood-forming tissues

(Continued)

Medical Specialty	Medical Specialist	Description of Medical Specialty
Immunology	Immunologist	Study of various elements of the immune system and their functions *Immunology includes treatment of immunodeficiency diseases such as AIDS; autoimmune diseases such as lupus erythematosus, allergies, and various cancer types related to the immune system.*
Internal medicine	Internist	Study of the physiological and pathological characteristics of internal organs and the diagnosis and treatment of these organs
Neonatology	Neonatologist	Care and treatment of neonates
Nephrology	Nephrologist	Diagnosis and management of kidney disease, kidney transplantation, and dialysis therapies
Neurosurgery	Neurosurgeon	Surgery of the brain, spinal cord, and peripheral nerves
Obstetrics	Obstetrician	Care of women during pregnancy, childbirth, and postnatal care
Oncology	Oncologist	Diagnosis, treatment, and prevention of cancer *Oncologists are internal medicine physicians who specialize in the treatment of solid tumors (such as carcinomas and sarcomas) and liquid tumors (including hematological malignancies such as leukemias).*
Ophthalmology	Ophthalmologist	Diagnosis and treatment of eye diseases, including prescribing corrective lenses
Optometry	Optometrist	Primary eye care, including testing the eyes for visual acuity, diagnosing and managing eye health, prescribing corrective lenses, and recommending eye exercises *An optometrist, licensed by the state, is not a medical doctor but is known as a Doctor of Optometry (OD).*
Orthopedics	Orthopedist	Prevention, diagnosis, care, and treatment of musculoskeletal disorders *Musculoskeletal disorders include injury to or disease of bones, joints, ligaments, muscles, and tendons.*
Otolaryngology	Otolaryngologist	Medical and surgical management of disorders of the ear, nose, and throat (ENT) and related structures of the head and neck

Medical Specialty	Medical Specialist	Description of Medical Specialty
Pathology	Pathologist	Study and cause of disease *A pathologist usually specializes in autopsy or in clinical or surgical pathology.*
Pediatrics	Pediatrician	Diagnosis and treatment of disease in infants, children, and adolescents
Physiatry	Physiatrist	Prevention, diagnosis, and treatment of disease or injury and the rehabilitation from resultant impairment and disability; also called *physical medicine* *Physiatrists are physicians who use physical agents such as light, heat, cold water, therapeutic exercise, mechanical apparatus and, sometimes, pharmaceutical agents.*
Plastic surgery	Plastic surgeon	Surgery to alter, replace, and restore a body structure due to a defect or for cosmetic reasons
Pulmonology	Pulmonologist	Diagnosis and treatment of diseases involving the lungs, its airways and blood vessels, and the chest wall (thoracic cage); also called *pulmonary medicine*
Psychiatry	Psychiatrist	Diagnosis, treatment, and prevention of disorders of the mind
Radiology	Radiologist	Diagnosis using x-ray and other diagnostic procedures, such as ultrasound (US), computed tomography (CT), and magnetic resonance imaging (MRI) *Radiology also employs various radiation techniques to treat disease through other subspecialties of radiology, such as interventional radiology and nuclear medicine.*
Rheumatology	Rheumatologist	Diagnosis and treatment of inflammatory and degenerative diseases of the joints
Surgery	Surgeon	Use of operative procedures to treat deformity, injury, and disease

(Continued)

Medical Specialty	Medical Specialist	Description of Medical Specialty
Thoracic surgery	Thoracic surgeon	Use of operative procedures to treat disease or injury of the thoracic area
Urology	Urologist	Diagnosis and treatment of the male urinary and reproductive systems and the female urinary system

Index of Diagnostic, Medical, and Surgical Procedures

This section provides a list of the diagnostic, medical, and surgical procedures covered in the textbook along with page numbers. Diagnostic procedures help the physician determine a patient's health status, evaluate the factors influencing that status, and determine a method of treatment. Medical and surgical procedures are performed to treat a specific disorder that is diagnosed by the physician.

Diagnostic Procedures

Medical and Surgical Procedures

Index of Oncological Terms

The following is a list of oncology disorders, diagnostic and surgical procedures and illustrations, as well as common abbreviations related to the medical specialty of oncology. For easy reference, page numbers for all of the terms below are included in the list.

Index

Note: An "f" following a page number indicates a figure; a "t" following a page number indicates a table.